Herbal Medicines in Pregnancy and Lactation

An Evidence-Based Approach

Edward Mills DPh MSc (Oxon)
Director, Division of Clinical Epidemiology
Canadian College of Naturopathic Medicine
North York, Ontario, Canada

Jean-Jacques Duguoa MSc (cand.) ND
Naturopathic Doctor
Toronto Western Hospital
Assistant Professor
Division of Clinical Epidemiology
Canadian College of Naturopathic Medicine
North York, Ontario, Canada

Dan Perri BScPharm MD MSc
Clinical Pharmacology Fellow
University of Toronto
Toronto, Ontario, Canada

Gideon Koren MD FACMT FRCP
Director of Motherisk
Professor of Medicine, Pediatrics and Pharmacology
University of Toronto
Toronto, Ontario, Canada

With a contribution from

Paul Richard Saunders PhD ND DHANP

informa
healthcare

New York London

First published in 2006 by the Taylor & Francis Group, LLC.

This edition published in 2010 by Informa Healthcare, Telephone House, 69-77 Paul Street, London EC2A 4LQ, UK.

Simultaneously published in the USA by Informa Healthcare, 52 Vanderbilt Avenue, 7th Floor, New York, NY 10017, USA.

Informa Healthcare is a trading division of Informa UK Ltd. Registered Office: 37–41 Mortimer Street, London W1T 3JH, UK. Registered in England and Wales number 1072954.

A CIP record for this book is available from the British Library.

Library of Congress Cataloging-in-Publication Data available on application

ISBN-13: 9780415373920

Orders may be sent to: Informa Healthcare, Sheepen Place, Colchester, Essex CO3 3LP, UK
Telephone: +44 (0)20 7017 5540
Email: CSDhealthcarebooks@informa.com
Website: http://informahealthcarebooks.com/

For corporate sales please contact: CorporateBooksIHC@informa.com
For foreign rights please contact: RightsIHC@informa.com
For reprint permissions please contact: PermissionsIHC@informa.com

CONTENTS

PREFACE

Exposures to over-the-counter products are frequent in pregnant women. Perhaps this is a paradoxical response to the decreased use of prescribed medications during pregnancy for fear of teratogenicity. For many women, natural health products such as herbal medicines or supplements may seem a reasonable alternative as the lay media often portrays natural medicines as safe. While the true incidence of natural product use in pregnancy is not known, some studies suggest that as high as sixty percent of pregnant women use natural therapies including herbal medicines either during pregnancy or while planning.[1] Pregnant women often consider the use of natural products such as peppermint tea or ginger to help with symptoms of pregnancy such as nausea and vomiting.[2] In one study of midwives practicing in North Carolina, half of the respondents admitted to recommending herbal medicines to their patients for pregnancy related conditions.[3] Further to this intended use, it must be remembered that nearly half of all pregnancies are unplanned and unexpected exposures to medicines and supplements in the first trimester are not rare.

Despite the prevalent use of natural health products by pregnant women, there is very little published evidence with regards to the safety and efficacy of natural health products during pregnancy and lactation. Many modern and classic texts warn against the use of natural product supplementation during pregnancy or lactation for up to one-third of the products listed in their monographs. However, most resources provide little information on the data used to evaluate reproductive toxicity apart from reports of historical use of herbs as abortifacients or uterine stimulants or animal data of genotoxicity or teratogenicity. Data on efficacy during pregnancy is similarly scarce from most texts.

To our knowledge, ours is the first text that aims to specifically address the lack of data of natural health product use in pregnancy and lactation. While it is not an exhaustive compendium of available supplements, it is a comprehensive listing of common herbs, vitamins and supplements used by pregnant women. Drawing on all available studies obtained through meta-analytic techniques, we have graded the quality of evidence on natural product safety during pregnancy and breastfeeding. Statements in traditional texts such as 'use of this herbal product should occur only after careful assessment of the benefits and risks' need clarification with up-to-date evidence from the medical literature. Busy healthcare providers need to have access to quick and reliable information they can use to help address patient concerns with regards to natural health product use in pregnancy or lactation. We hope that this text will be received as a valuable resource for all clinicians who treat pregnant patients. As natural health supplements continue to gain popularity, we anticipate that the utility for a text such as this will grow too.

Jean-Jacques Duguoa
Edward Mills
Dan Perri
Gideon Koren

References

1. Maats FH, Crowther CA. Patterns of vitamin, mineral, and herbal supplementation use prior to and during pregnancy. Aust NZ J Obstet Gynaecol 2002; 42:494–496.
2. Hollyer T, Boon H, Georgousis A, Smith M, Einarson A. The use of CAM by women suffering from nausea and vomiting during pregnancy. BMC Complementary and Alternative Medicine 2002; 2:5
3. Allaire AD, Moss M-K, Wells SR. Complementary and alternative medicine in pregnancy: a survey of North Carolina certified nurse-midmives. Obstet Gynecol 2000; 95:19–23.

Chapter 1

TRADITIONAL BOTANICAL MEDICINES

Paul Richard Saunders

Introduction

Pregnancy and subsequent lactation have been an essential part of human existence for millennia, but unfortunately the experience has not been easy for all women. Some of our earliest medicines were plants used to address the difficulties and complications of these biologic processes and to better prepare the expectant mother for pregnancy, delivery, and lactation. In many part of the world women still use herbal medicines even when attended by Western medicine.[1,2] This short review from an historical perspective will first examine some of the botanicals that have been used during pregnancy and delivery and then during lactation. Reference will also be made to some of the scientific literature on these botanical medicines.

Contraception and pregnancy

Although conception is a problem for some women, a more common problem is contraception. In rural Mindanao (the Philippines) women still drink kamias and other herbal preparations rather than use oral contraceptives.[2] Quisumbing's thorough study of Philippine medicinal plants identified over 60 plants used as abortifacients and over 130 plants used as emmenagogues.[3] Of interest is *Kibatalia blancoi* and *K. gitingesis* whose leaf and bark may have progesterone-like effects.[4,5] A 1995–1996 reproductive health survey of 6465 Paraguayan women of reproductive age found they were most familiar (88%) with yuyos, a variety of herbs usually drunk as a tea daily to prevent pregnancy.[6] Studies in India to find traditional, effective contraceptives have focused on *Hibiscus rosa-sinensis*, Rudrapushpaka, *Embelia ribes*, *Daucus carota*, *Butea monosperma*, *Sapindus trifoliatus*, *Mentha arvensis*, *Ferula jaeschkeana*, and several others because of their anti-implantation activity.[7] Herbs with potential as a male contraceptive are *Gossypium herbaceum* and *Tripterygium wilfordii*.[7]

In traditional Chinese medicine, a core of 10–20 herbs is used in pregnancy.[8] A review of traditional Chinese materia medica would, based on clinical tongue and pulse diagnosis, include plants used for liver cleansing, blood regulating, qi tonics, yin tonics and warming.[9] *Striga asiatica* is one herb being studied as a contraceptive.[10]

Moerman has published an exhaustive description of the plants used by native North Americans; abortifacients number over 100 and female gynecological aids nearly 350.[11] A large number of these plants came to the knowledge of European settlers by inquiry and observation with subsequent clinical use in patients. When the outcome was repeatedly successful this was recorded and the details of its use refined from repeated use by Eclectic physicians who differentiated between more effective and less well studied botanical medicines in *King's American Dispensatory*.[12]

Vitex agnus-castus has over a 2000-year history in female menstrual regulation including infertility. It has also been shown to have beneficial effects for lactation, making it in a sense a botanical alpha and omega of pregnancy and lactation.[13–15] Once the woman was pregnant *Rubus idaeus* leaf was used by the Cherokee for labor pains and by the Cree and Cherokee to slow uterine bleeding; benefits were attributed to its astringent and tannin properties.[16,17] It is a well-known partus preparator or parturient taken during pregnancy to tonify the uterus, maintain pregnancy and ease delivery.[18,19]

One complication of pregnancy is threatened miscarriage. A well-known herbal formula that prevents this is *Viburnum prunifolium*, *Leonurus cardiaca*, and *Mitchella repens*.[20] *Viburnum prunifolium* was used by the Delaware and Micmac to strengthen and tone the uterus during pregnancy, and by the Eclectics to calm uterine colic, for threatened miscarriage and painful uterine contractions.[21,22] *L. cardiaca* was regarded as a sedative for female nervousness and hysteria, and for general female complaints by the Cherokee, Delaware, Iroquois, Micmac, Mohegan, and Shinnecock as well as by the Eclectics.[23,24] *M. repens* was used by the Cherokee, Delaware, Iroquois and Menominee for a variety of complaints regarding the uterus.[25] The Eclectics considered it one of the most important herbs for successful pregnancy, to prevent miscarriage, throughout the pregnancy for complications, and in the last weeks to ease delivery.[26,27] This botanical formula was designed to address the uterine problems, anxiety, nervousness, and pain that could accompany a possible miscarriage.

As the pregnancy neared completion a partus preparator was often given to the expectant woman in the last 3–6 weeks to prepare the uterus for delivery and reduce the pain of delivery. Botanicals drawn upon to affect the uterine circulation and musculature included *M. repens*, *V. prunifolium*, *Caulophyllum thalictroides*, *Actea* (*Cimicifuga*) *racemosa*, *Aralia nudicaulis*, and for nervines included those such as *Leonurus cardiaca*, *Nepeta cataria*, and *Gelsemium sempervirens*.[26,28,29] The dose of *C. thalictroides* was minimal before and during labor to avoid fetal distress.[29,30] Its Native American use related to pregnancy and labor included the Cherokee, Menominee, Ojibwa, and Potawatomi.[31] *G. sempervirens* was used to calm the patient and help dilate the os in stalled labor.[32,33]

The preferred botanical to address post-labor pains was *G. sempervirens*.[32,33] Dose and timing were critical as administration too early or too frequent could slow the labor process and too much after labor could make the woman too drowsy to look after her newborn infant.[32]

Hemorrhage was the first severe complication after delivery as it could not only cause considerable blood loss and profound anemia, but also lead to death if unchecked. *Cinnamomum zeylanicum* was a preferred anti-hemorrhagic.[28,34,35] It also provided some anti-microbial protection from puerperal fever, a important complication arising from infection contracted during or after labor that took the life of many new mothers. *C. zeylanicum* is still used in traditional Chinese medicine for this type of fever.[36] Other anti-hemorrhagics included *Capsella bursa-pastoris* and *Geranium maculatum* whereas botanicals preferred for post-partum anti-fever were *Veratrum viride* and *Atropa belladonna*.[37]

In traditional Chinese medicine *Angelica sinensis* supplements blood, tones the uterus and is often used throughout the pregnancy. Its stimulating or inhibiting effect on the uterus is regulated by how long it is decocted in a larger formula.[38] In contrast, Western pharmacologists label it an abortifacient and strongly recommend against its use in pregnancy.[39] *Rehmannia glutinosa* is a nutritive tonic that nourishes yin and blood and can be of benefit in bleeding, *Paeonia lactiflora* can disperse blood thus controlling pain, and *Cyperus rotundus* can control bleeding as well as antepartum and post-partum headache pain.[40] Three additional traditional Chinese medicinal herbs of note are *Fritillaria cirrhosa* for regulating uterine contractions and blood loss after labor, *Poncirus trifoliata* to relieve pain and regulate uterine contractions, and *Codonopsis pilosula* to build qi, address weakness, fatigue, and loss of appetite – symptoms often present in the first trimester, near the end of pregnancy, or after delivery.[41]

An indirect use of traditional Chinese medicinal herbs is moxibustion (charcoal from *Artemisia argyi* and related species).[42] In a randomized human study it increased fetal activity during treatment and cephalic presentation after treatment and at delivery.[43] A study of recurrent spontaneous abortion using the traditional Chinese medicinal formula zhibai dihuang, with herbs to remove evil heat, dampness, replenish blood and activate circulation, altered anti-ABO group antibodies and yielded a high number of normal deliveries.[44]

Lactation

Mother's breast milk is still regarded as best and in some settings is the infant's only chance for survival. A study of new mothers attending breast-feeding clinics in Canada found up to 15% reported insufficient milk supply.[45] No doubt this has been a problem in some women, leading to efforts to identify herbal remedies across a diversity of cultures. Brückner has reviewed the herbal drugs most commonly used in Europe.[46] Bingel and Farnsworth have produced the most thorough review to date, identifying over 400 plants that have been used ethnomedically and recorded in the literature as galactagogues.[47] Not even 10% of the plants have been studied scientifically so their individual mechanism and effectiveness as galactagogues is generally unknown.

Breast pain, swelling, hardness, and even mastitis have been treated with *Phytolacca americana*, *Ricinus communis*, and *M. repens*, all of which can be applied topically before or between breast feeding. They must be cleansed from the breast prior to nursing.[48] A possible mechanism is their ability to facilitate flow from the gland through the nipple and to the infant.[47]

In Central America, Mayan and other native women use a variety of herbs to increase breast milk production. *Coffea arabica* and *Camellia sinensis* are two diuretics that contain caffeine, and caffeine and theophylline, respectively, and have been used – and shown experimentally – to promote lactation.[47] Caffeine in some infants can lead to insomnia and colic. *Euphorbia lancifolia* has been used by humans for centuries and may also increase milk production in cows.[49]

Emotions such as fear and anxiety may reduce the release of milk suggesting a role for herbs that reduce the psychological and physiological effects of emotions.[47] *Lactuca virosa* and *L. sativa* produce a dried sap used for sedation, whereas *L. biennis* has been used to ease breast pain and promote lactation.[50,51] *Anethum graveolens* is a sedative that has been used with some benefit.[47,52] Sedative plants often contain essential oils, compounds that dilate blood vessels, relax muscles, and enhance sleep. Noteworthy are *Origanum vulgare* employed in fomentations, *Lavandula officinal*, *L. angustifolia*, and *L. vera* that are added to baths or applied locally for pain, and *Mentha piperita*, *M. viridis*, and *Nepeta cataria* taken as an infusion.[53]

Beer, a well-known galactagogue, contains *Humulus lupulus*, noted for both its sedative action and estrogenic effect on breast tissue, and *Hordeum vulgare*, reputed to be galactogenic and to cause prolactin release.[47,54] *H. lupulus* can be applied to painful swellings such as of the breast, but is generally empirically contraindicated in depression.[55,56]

Other galactagogues of note include *Urtica dioica* and *U. urens* which can be applied topically or taken internally.[57] *Galega officinalis* has enjoyed more popularity in its native Europe than North America for it ability to stimulate milk production.[58,59] *Trigonella foenum-graecum* has historically been widely used in Europe and North Africa and some of the animal data are positive.[60,61] *Salvia officinalis* is used more as a lactation regulator, most often to reduce milk production and pain when the baby has been weaned.[62,63]

Ayurveda, the traditional medicine of India, has yielded such galactagogues as *Rauwolfia serpentina*, *R. oreogiton*, and *R. volkensii*, whose use is supported by endocrinology and findings from clinical trials that have focused on its alkaloid content. Reserpine, a dopamine-depleting agent can produce galactorrhea in women and decrease anxiety, and several other alkaloids have similar activity.[47] There is positive data for *Leptadenia reticulata* as well.[47] *Asparagus racemosus* was examined in a clinical trial where it was used in a herbal formula with six other herbs, but the results were not significant.[64] Current and future research could increase our knowledge about other herbs used traditionally in rural India.[65]

Traditional Chinese medicinal botanicals for enhancing milk production in humans include *Astragalus membranaceus*, *Taraxacum mongolicum*, *Tetrapanax papyrifera*, *Liquidambar taiwaniana*, and *Ligusticum chuaniong* (*L. striatum*) to name a few.[66] In general these are qi, yin, and/or blood tonics.

Summary

The use of medicinal plants to address infertility, maintain pregnancy, ease the birthing process, and aid in milk production or its cessation has been identified in many cultures, several of whom have complex medical systems.[1,2,4,6,9,11,65,67] Over 400 plants have been identified as ethnomedically affecting lactation.

Unfortunately, modern science has not maintained pace in the study of the mechanisms and relative benefit or potential harm of these plants. Women from many cultural backgrounds continue to use plants despite the presence of modern medications. More detailed study in this area could yield new information about mammalian reproductive endocrinology and physiology, plant pharmacognosy and constituent physiology, and identify the larger potential of at least some of these plants.

References

1. Mabina MH, Moodley J, Pitsoe SB. The use of traditional herbal medication during pregnancy. Trop Doct 1997; 27:84–86.
2. Quijano N Jr. Herbal contraceptives: exploring indigenous methods of family planning. Initiatives Popul 1986; 8:22, 31–35.
3. Quisumbing E. Medicinal plants of the Philippines. Caloocan City, Philippines: Katha Publishing, 1978:1079, 1110–1111.
4. Guerrero AM. Age-old methods of contraception. Initiatives Popul 1977; 3:20–25.
5. Quisumbing E. Medicinal plants of the Philippines. Caloocan City, Philippines: Katha Publishing, 1978:729.
6. Bull SS, Melian M. Contraception and culture: the use of yuyos in Paraguay. Health Care Women Int 1998; 19:49–60.
7. Chaudhery RR. The quest for a herbal contraceptive. Natl Med J India 1993; 6:199–201.
8. Wong HB. Effects of herbs and drugs during pregnancy and lactation. J Singapore Paediatr Soc 1979; 21:169–178.
9. Hsu HY. Oriental materia medica: a concise guide. Long Beach, CA: Oriental Healing Arts Institute, 1986:6–18.
10. Chaing HS, Merino-Chavez G, Yang LL, Wang FN, Hafez ES. Medicinal plants: conception/contraception. Adv Contracept Deliv Syst 1994; 10:355–363.
11. Moerman DE. Native American ethnobotany. Portland, OR: Timber Press, 1998:765, 799–801.
12. Felter HW, Lloyd JU. King's American Dispensatory, 18th ed, 1905. Reprinted, Sandy, OR: Eclectic Medical Publications, 1983:iii–iv.
13. McCutcheon AR, Chastebarry IN, Chandler F, eds. Herbs everyday reference for health professionals. Ottawa, ON: Canadian Pharmacists Association, Canadian Medical Association, 2000:76–68.
14. Witman G, Gerhard I, Runnebaum B. The efficacy of the herbal drug Mastodynon in femal infertility. Arch Gynecol Obstet 1993; 254:158–160.
15. Du Mee C. Vitex agnus castus. Aust J Herbal Med 1993; 5:63–65.
16. Moerman DE. Native American ethnobotany. Portland, OR: Timber Press, 1998:488–489.
17. Felter HW, Lloyd JU. King's American Dispensatory, 18th ed, 1905. Reprinted. Sandy, OR: Eclectic Medical Publications, 1983:1680–1683.
18. Scientific Committee. British herbal pharmacopoeia. Bournemouth, UK: British Herbal Medicine Association, 1995:182.
19. Mitchell WA Jr. Plant medicine in practice using the teachings of John Bastyr. St. Louis, MO: Elsevier Science, 2003:266.
20. Harper-Shove F. Prescriber and Clinical Repertory of Medicinal Herbs. Rustington, Sussex, UK: Health Science Press, 1938:99.

21. Moerman DE. Native American Ethnobotany. Portland, OR: Timber Press, 1998:595.
22. Felter HW, Lloyd JU. King's American Dispensatory, 18th ed, 1905. Reprinted. Sandy, OR: Eclectic Medical Publications, 1983:2059–2062.
23. Moerman DE. Native American Ethnobotany. Portland, OR: Timber Press, 1998:301.
24. Felter HW, Lloyd JU. King's American Dispensatory, 18th ed, 1905. Reprinted. Sandy, OR: Eclectic Medical Publications, 1983:1125–1126.
25. Moerman DE. Native American Ethnobotany. Portland, OR: Timber Press, 1998:345–346.
26. Mitchell WA Jr. Plant medicine in practice using the teachings of John Bastyr. St. Louis, MO: Elsevier Science, 2003:386.
27. Felter HW, Lloyd JU. King's American Dispensatory, 18th ed, 1905. Reprinted. Sandy, OR: Eclectic Medical Publications, 1983:1273–1274.
28. Harper-Shove F. Prescriber and clinical repertory of medicinal herbs. Rustington, Sussex, UK: Health Science Press, 1938:103–104.
29. Felter HW, Lloyd JU. King's American Dispensatory, 18th ed, 1905. Reprinted. Sandy, OR: Eclectic Medical Publications, 1983:468–472, 528–553, 916–923.
30. Wilson C. Useful Prescriptions. Cincinnati, OH: Lloyd Brothers Pharmacists, 1935: 102.
31. Moerman DE. Native American Ethnobotany. Portland, OR: Timber Press, 1998:144.
32. Felter HW, Lloyd JU. King's American Dispensatory, 18th ed, 1905. Reprinted. Sandy, OR: Eclectic Medical Publications, 1983:916–923.
33. Wilson C. Useful Prescriptions. Cincinnati, OH: Lloyd Brothers Pharmacists, 1935: 108.
34. Wilson C. Useful Prescriptions. Cincinnati, OH: Lloyd Brothers Pharmacists, 1935: 103.
35. Felter HW, Lloyd JU. King's American Dispensatory, 18th ed, 1905. Reprinted. Sandy, OR: Eclectic Medical Publications, 1983:557–560.
36. Hsu HY. Oriental materia medica a concise guide. Long Beach, CA: Oriental Healing Arts Institute, 1986:375–376.
37. Felter HW, Lloyd JU. King's American Dispensatory, 18th ed, 1905. Reprinted. Sandy, OR: Eclectic Medical Publications, 1983:431–434, 927–929, 331–340, 2050–2054.
38. Hsu HY. Oriental materia medica a concise guide. Long Beach, CA: Oriental Healing Arts Institute, 1986:540–542.
39. Barnes J, Anderson LA, Phillipson JD. Herbal medicines, 2nd ed. London, UK: Pharmaceutical Press, 2002:47–50.
40. Hsu HY. Oriental materia medica a concise guide. Long Beach, CA: Oriental Healing Arts Institute, 1986:148–149, 415–416, 546, 548–549.
41. Hsu HY. Oriental materia medica a concise guide. Long Beach, CA: Oriental Healing Arts Institute, 1986:407–409, 526–527, 679–680.
42. Bensky D, Gamble A. Chinese herbal medicine: materia medica, 2nd ed. Seattle, WA: Eastland Press, 1993:259–260.
43. Cardini F, Weixin H. Moxibustion for the correction of breech presentation: a randomized controlled trial. JAMA 1998; 280:1580–1584.
44. Li DJ, Li CJ, Zhu Y. Treatment of integrated traditional and western medicine in recurrent spontaneous abortion of immune abnormality type [English Abstract]. Zhongguo Zhong Xi YiJie He Za Zhi 1997; 17:390–392.

45. MacIntosh HC. What is the pharmacological basis for the action of herbs that promote lactation and how can they best be utilized Part I. Can J Herbalism 2003; XXIV:15–19, 36.
46. Brückner C. Anwendung and wert in europa gebräuchlicher lactationsördernder heilpflanzen (galactagoga) [English Abstract]. Pädiatr Grenzgeb 1989; 28:403–410.
47. Bingel AS, Farnsworth NR. Higher plants as potential sources of galactagogues. In: Wagner H, Farnsworth NR, eds. Economic and medicinal plant research volume 6. London, UK: Academic Press, 1994:1–54.
48. Felter HW, Lloyd JU. King's American Dispensatory, 18th ed, 1905. Reprinted. Sandy, OR: Eclectic Medical Publications, 1983:1471–1475, 1380–1383, 1273–1274.
49. Rosengarten F Jr. A neglected Mayan galactagogue – ixbut (Euphorbia lancifolia). J Ethnopharmacol 1982; 5:91–112.
50. Felter HW, Lloyd JU. King's American Dispensatory, 18th ed, 1905. Reprinted. Sandy, OR: Eclectic Medical Publications, 1983:1114–1117.
51. Moerman DE. Native American Ethnobotany. Portland, OR: Timber Press, 1998:294.
52. Felter HW, Lloyd JU. King's American Dispensatory, 18th ed, 1905. Reprinted. Sandy, OR: Eclectic Medical Publications, 1983:203.
53. Felter HW, Lloyd JU. King's American Dispensatory, 18th ed, 1905. Reprinted. Sandy, OR: Eclectic Medical Publications, 1983:1420, 1123–1124, 1254–1256, 1252.
54. Felter HW, Lloyd JU. King's American Dispensatory, 18th ed, 1905. Reprinted. Sandy, OR: Eclectic Medical Publications, 1983:996–1000.
55. Felter HW, Lloyd JU. King's American Dispensatory, 18th ed, 1905. Reprinted. Sandy, OR: Eclectic Medical Publications, 1983:998–1000.
56. Brinker F. Herb Contraindications and Drug Interactions. Sandy, OR: Eclectic Medical Publications, 2001:119.
57. Felter HW, Lloyd JU. King's American Dispensatory, 18th ed, 1905. Reprinted. Sandy, OR: Eclectic Medical Publications, 1983:2032–2034.
58. Felter HW, Lloyd JU. King's American Dispensatory, 18th ed, 1905. Reprinted. Sandy, OR: Eclectic Medical Publications, 1983:908.
59. Weiss RF. Herbal Medicine, 6th ed. Beaconsfield, UK: Beaconsfield Publishers, 1988:318.
60. Weiss RF. Herbal Medicine, 6th ed. Beaconsfield, UK: Beaconsfield Publishers, 1988:199, 336.
61. MacIntosh HC. What is the pharmacological basis for the action of herbs that promote lactation and how can they best be utilized part II. Can J Herbalism 2003; XXV:15–11, 38.
62. Felter HW, Lloyd JU. King's American Dispensatory, 18th ed, 1905. Reprinted. Sandy, OR: Eclectic Medical Publications, 1983:1705–1706.
63. Weiss RF. Herbal medicine, 6th ed. Beaconsfield, UK: Beaconsfield Publishers, 1988:228.
64. Sharma S, Ramji S, Kumari S, Bapna JS. Randomized controlled trial of Asparagus racemosus (Shatavari) as a lactogogue in lactational inadequacy. Indian Pediatr 1996; 33:675–677.
65. Anon. Learning from India's traditional birth attendants, the dais. Arrows Change. 199; 5:3.

66. Hsu HY. Oriental Materia Medica a Concise Guide. Long Beach, CA: Oriental Healing Arts Institute, 1986:521–523, 237–238, 311–312, 465, 446–447.
67. Raden-Sanusi HR, Werner R. The role of traditional healers in the provision of health care and family planning services: Malay traditional and indigenous medicine. Malays J Reprod Health 1985; 3(Suppl 1):S82–S89.

Chapter 2
PHARMACOGNOSY – THE SCIENCE OF NATURAL SOURCE MEDICINES

The study of medicinal plants and their properties is called **pharmacognosy**. This science has led to the development of many drugs in use today including aspirin (the basic salicylate structure was discovered from the white willow while aspirin was synthesized from meadowsweet), opioids (originally from opium poppies), the birth control pill (synthesized from steroid structures found in a wild Mexican yam), and chemotherapeutic agents like vincristine and vinblastine (from Madagascar periwinkle) or taxol (from the Pacific yew tree).

Today, herbal medicine is big business. However, there is much confusion about what herbal medicine is and is not. While pharmacognosy is a science that deals with the discovery of medicines from natural substances, it is certainly not the same as herbalism. According to the American Society of Pharmacognosy, its scope includes 'the study of the physical, chemical, biochemical and biological properties of drugs, drug substances, or potential drugs or drug substances of natural origin as well as the search for new drugs from natural sources. Research problems in pharmacognosy include studies in the areas of phytochemistry, microbial chemistry, biosynthesis, biotransformation, chemotaxonomy, and other biological and chemical sciences'. The term **herbalism** refers to a folk and traditional medicinal practice based on the use of plants and plant extracts. In essence, herbalism is the practice of herb-based care and pharmacognosy is the scientific study of herbs with medicinal purposes. Within the practice of herbalism there are a variety of different traditions including, for example, traditional Chinese medicine or the Indian ayurvedic medicine. Each of these has a unique paradigm on health, illness, and disease. Unlike pharmacognosists, herbalists are not particularly interested in specific active constituents found within a plant. Instead, they focus on the healing properties of the plant or part of plant (seed, root, leaf, etc.) and how it will benefit the body to heal itself. Although non-herbalists may also use herbal medicines in their clinical practice, they likely do so under a different health paradigm. Homeopaths also have a holistic approach to health, but their material medica uses a 'like cures like' philosophy of treating patients with ultra-dilute formulations unlikely to contain significant (if any) 'active' ingredient. **Homeopathy**, then, is unlike herbal medicine, herbalism, or pharmacognosy. It has not been included in this text.

The current trend in natural product use follows many different health paradigms – some are popular because of their use in traditional Chinese medicine or Ayurveda, some from the widespread use of herbal medicine in Europe, and some due to increasing published studies on natural medicines, somewhat representative of the renewed interest in pharmacognosy. So, irrespective of the particular health paradigm from which the natural health products summarized in this text are derived, we will adopt the pharmacology perspective (or perhaps in this case, pharmacognosy would be the more accurate term). As such, individual constituents (chemical entities) of each natural product are discussed with regard to their pharmacologic or toxicologic properties. Since this likely represents a new vocabulary for most healthcare professionals, some common classes of herbal constituents are described below.

Glossary of terms used in natural product pharmacology (pharmacognosy)

A true understanding of the nature of plant constituents demands a solid foundation in organic chemistry since many constituent names are based on the compound's chemical structure. An explanation of the structure–function relationship of plant constituents is beyond the scope of this text. Whenever possible, chemical constituents will be described here by their pharmacologic function or unique physicochemical properties rather than their structural forms. However, more often than not, the constituents derived from plants are grouped according to their structural similarity rather than functional effect. In these cases, the chemistry is simplified such that undergraduate level organic chemistry knowledge will suffice. Further details can be found in the texts recommended at the end of this chapter.

Alkaloids are chemicals formed from amino acids. True alkaloids contain a heterocyclic ring structure containing nitrogen while proto alkaloids do not have the nitrogen in the ring. Pseudo-alkaloids are related compounds that contain a heterocyclic ring structure containing nitrogen but are not derived from amino acids. Alkaloids are highly reactive substances with biologic activity in low doses. In plants, most alkaloids (which are bases) form salts with acids. Alkaloids may be monocyclic, bicylic, or polycylic. Alkaloids may occur as pyridine-piperidines, tropanes, quinolines, isoquinolines, indoles, imidazoles, steroidals, purine bases, and alkaloidal amines. Drug examples of alkaloids include atropine, ipecac, nicotine, colchicine, caffeine, theophylline, quinine, vinblastine, tubocurarine, reserpine, yohimbine, morphine, and the ergot alkaloids. They are usually bitter-tasting white solids (although nicotine is a brown liquid). Apart from their similar structural roots, alkaloids are not related and thus do not necessarily share any pharmacologic properties.

Anthocyanins are plant pigments that strongly absorb in the ultraviolet (UV) spectrum and thus have a role in attracting insects (by carnivorous plants or for pollination purposes) as well as UV protection. Plants containing anthocyanins can be of a variety of colors. They are usually red, purple, or blue but depending on their oxidation state may even be yellow or colorless. Over 300 different anthocyanins have been identified in plants. They are one class of flavonoid compounds that are very popular today due to their possible health benefits as antioxidants. The most popular supplements are grape seed extract, pine bark extract, and green tea. Anthocyanin-containing plants have also been used historically as anti-inflammatories and for enhancing vision. Cranberries, bilberries, apples, eggplant, and radish all contain anthocyanins. Anthocyanins also contribute to the color changes of leaves in autumn.

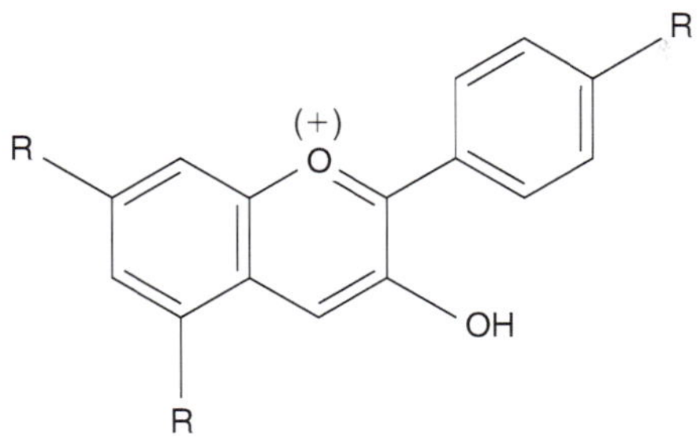

Figure 2.1 Basic structure of anthocyanins.

Anthraquinones have a three-ring structure and have been used for centuries as purgatives and dyes. They are usually found in plants in a glycoside form (i.e. attached to sugar molecules). Anthraquinone laxatives irritate the bowel wall, provoking increased muscle contractions and peristaltic movements. Examples include senna, cascara sagrada, rhubarb, yellow dock, and aloe. Anthraquinones may also have antiviral, antibacterial, and cytotoxic properties.

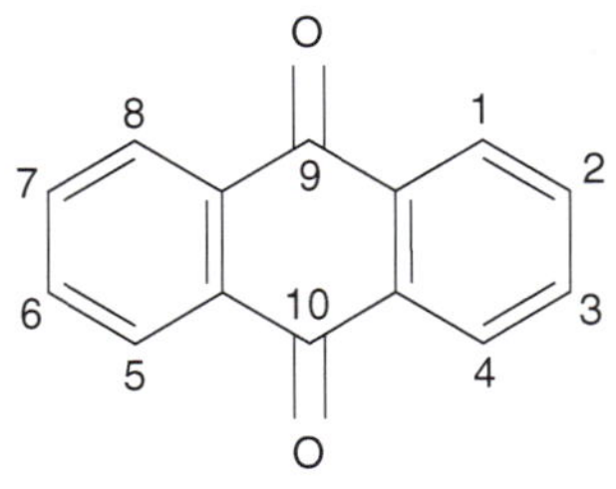

Figure 2.2 Basic structure of anthraquinones.

Coumarins are derived from cinnamic acid and are usually found in grasses and the pea family (such as clover). Coumarins are responsible for the scent of fresh cut grass. Dicumarol, the fermentation product of coumarin that is thought to inhibit vitamin K effects on coagulation biosynthesis due to its similarity in structure to vitamin K, is the anticoagulant from which warfarin was synthesized. Many coumarins, if injected, are anticoagulants but most plant coumarins are neutralized in the digestive tract and so have very little anticoagulant effects when ingested. Derivatives of coumarins have antifungal properties (like umbelliferone from the parsley family) and vascular tone effects (like esculin from horse chestnut).

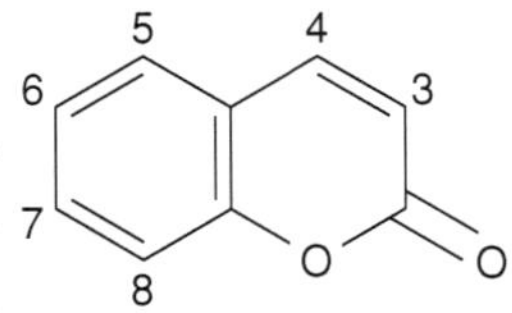

Figure 2.3 Basic structure of coumarins.

Flavonoids are commonly found as pigments in flowering plants. Over 2000 different flavonoid compounds have been found in plants in either the free state or as glycosides. They are polyphenolic compounds with a base structure that consists of two aromatic rings joined with a three-carbon chain – the so-called 'C6-C3-C6' carbon skeleton. The three-carbon chain may be part of a more complex structure including ringed moieties. The nature of the functional groups at this central complex determines the subclass of flavonoids. Some examples include flavones (such as apigenin found in celery and other herbaceous plants of the *Labiatae*, *Umbelliferae*, and *Compositae* families), flavonols (found in woody flowering plants like quercitol or kaempferol from *Sambucus nigra*), flavonones, and anthocyanins. Flavonoids found in colorful fruits and vegetables have powerful antioxidant properties. Flavonoids are the reason why green tea, grape seed extract and pine bark extract have been so popular over the past few years.

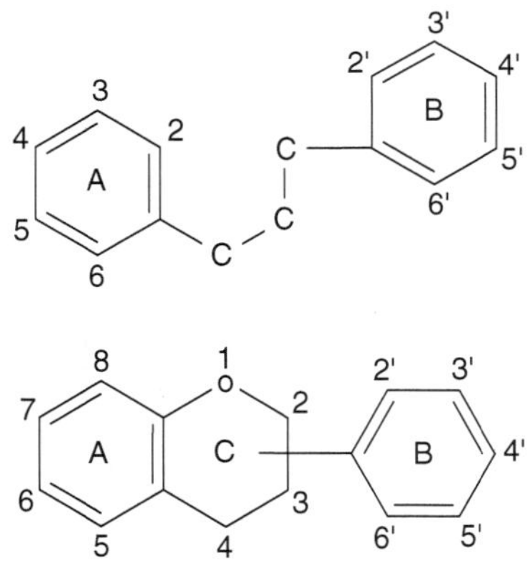

Figure 2.4 Two variants of the basic structure of flavanoids.

Isoflavonoids are similar in structure to flavonoids but have one of their benzene rings at a slightly different position. Unlike most flavonoids, isoflavonoids are colorless and are limited to legume plants. Soy isoflavones are touted as agents that may lower low-density lipoprotein (LDL) cholesterol and triglycerides as well as helping with menopausal symptoms and complications.

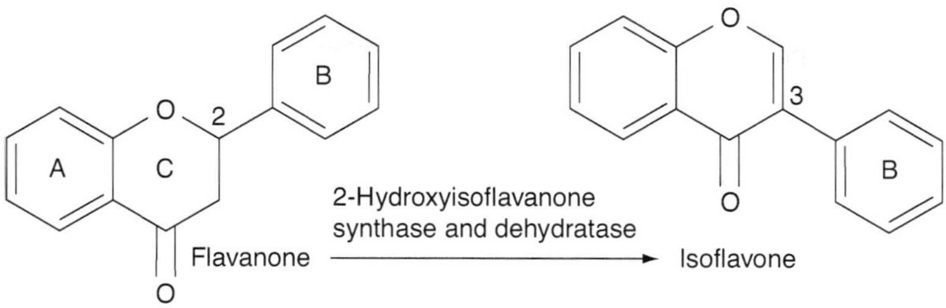

Figure 2.5 The conversion of flavonone to isoflavone.

Glucosinolates is a term often used to refer to a group of bound toxins such as the cyanogenic and isothiocyanate glycosides. Some glycosides produce hydrocyanic acid when hydrolyzed. These are referred to as **cyanogenic glycosides**. Amygdalin, found in apricot pits and bitter almonds, or prunasin, found in wild cherry bark, for example, are cyanogenic glycosides. The hydrolysis of the glycoside sinigrin from plants in the mustard family leads to allyl isothiocyanate – mustard oil. Plants from the mustard family as well as the cyanogenic glycosides have been used due to their anticarcinogenic properties. Laetrile (amygdalin) was a very popular cancer remedy in the 1980s despite clinical evidence of a lack of effect. Unfortunately, after pure amygdalin was banned, patients tried ingesting large amounts of apricot kernels, which led to several deaths because apricot kernels also contain an enzyme that hydrolyzes amygdalin and releases cyanide. Subsequent research showed that amygdalin alone can lead to cyanide poisoning.

Glycosides are compounds that contain a carbohydrate (glycone) and non-carbohydrate (aglycone) moiety joined by an acetal group. Although their chemical names can be quite complex, they can be recognized from their trivial names which are formed from the source plant name and the suffix '-in' such as salicin which is found in *Salix* (willow). Salicin is an **alcohol glycoside** found in willow bark that yields salicyl alcohol when hydrolyzed. Salicin has anti-inflammatory properties probably due to its oxidation into salicylic acid. It is shown here.

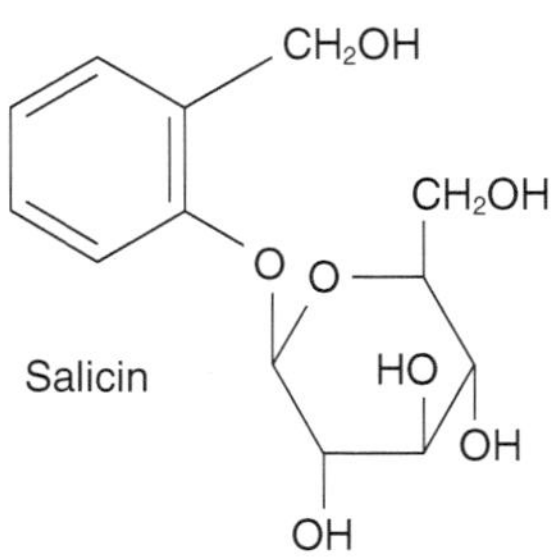

Figure 2.6 Salicin, an example of an alcohol glycoside.

Classification of glycosides is difficult since it can be done either by the sugar or the non-sugar group or by pharmaceutic viewpoint. Glycosides are ubiquitous within plants and their aglycone groups include, among others, tannins, aldehydes, alcohols, saponins, anthraquinones, lactones, flavanols, phenols, and isocyanates. The anthraquinones described earlier are found in plants as glycosides. Glucosinolates, a form of glycoside toxin, are described above. Glucovanillin is an **aldehyde glycoside** that is hydrolyzed to vanillin (an aldehyde) – the principal flavoring constituent of vanilla. Uva ursi, or bearberry, has a long tradition in folk medicine as a urinary antiseptic. Arbutin is a **phenol glycoside** found in bearberry (a small evergreen shrub) that can be hydrolyzed to the phenol hydroquinone – the agent that made arbutin a popular choice for urinary tract infections prior to sulfa antibiotics. Today hydroquinone is commonly used topically as a skin bleacher. The combination of sapogenin and a sugar yields a **saponin glycoside** which is described below as saponin. Sapogenins have steroid or triterpenoid aglycone structures. Cardiac glycosides, like digitoxin, are an example of a sapogenin with a steroid aglycone. These are discussed in greater detail under saponins.

Lignans are plant products formed by the coupling of two para-propylphenol (phenylpropanoid) moieties at their β carbon atoms. The three structures below represent different lignan skeletal types.

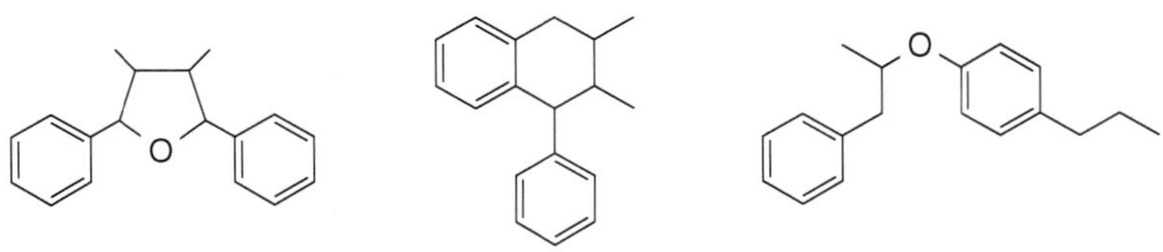

(1) (2) (3)

Figure 2.7 Three different skeletal structures of lignans.

If the two C_6C_3 units (4) are linked by a β,β′-bond the parent structure lignane (5) is used as the basis for naming the lignan.

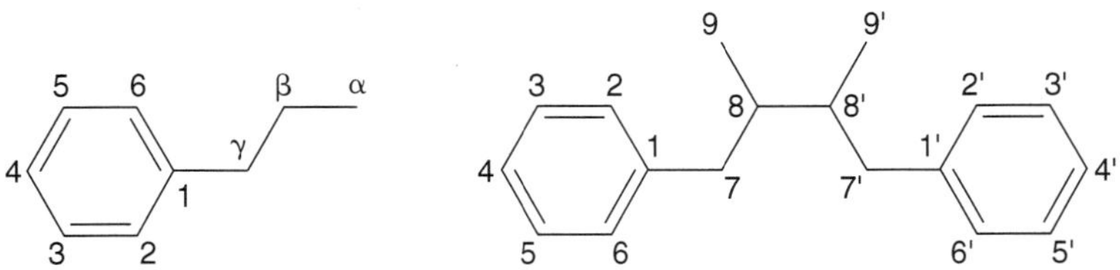

(4) (5)

Figure 2.8 β-β′-bond linkage of two C_6C_3 units to form a lignan (lignane).

If the two C_6C_3 units (**4**) are linked by a bond other than a β,β′-bond the parent structure, neolignane, is used as the basis for naming the neolignan such as 3,3′-neolignane shown below.

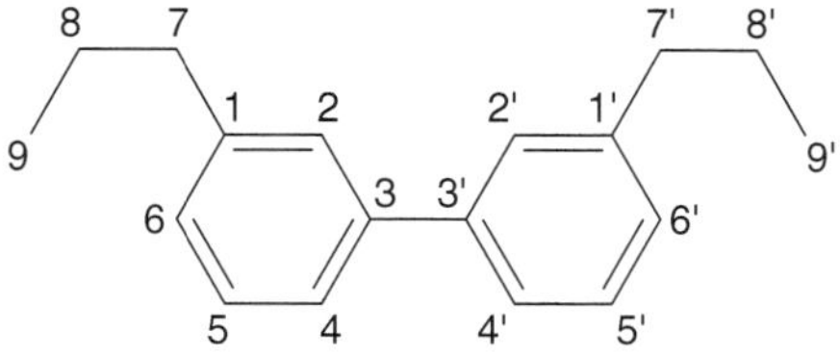

Figure 2.9 Non- β-β′-bond linkage of two C_6C_3 units to form a neolignan (3,3'-neolignane).

Lignans and neolignans play a role in plant defense as they have antimicrobial, antifungal, and insect repellant properties. Podophyllum is the dried rhizome and roots of *Podophyllum peltatum* (also known as mayapple or American mandrake). A resin from podophyllin (called podophyllotoxin) is a lignan that is used topically in the treatment of warts due to its antimitotic properties. The chemotherapeutic drug etoposide is a semisynthetic podophyllotoxin derivative. Podophyllotoxin is also a potent purgative. Other lignans, such as secoisolariciresinol, are considered to be phytoestrogens. Flaxseed has become very popular as a natural product therapy in women's health due to its very high lignan content. Other benefits of flaxseed, such as its potential role in lowering LDL cholesterol, are also attributed to its lignan content. Much of the natural product lay literature incorrectly states that lignans are synonymous with phytoestrogens. The chemical structures, and thus function, of lignans are quite variable. As discussed here, podophyllotoxin, a prototypic lignan, is used for papillomas and not as a phytoestrogen. It is shown here.

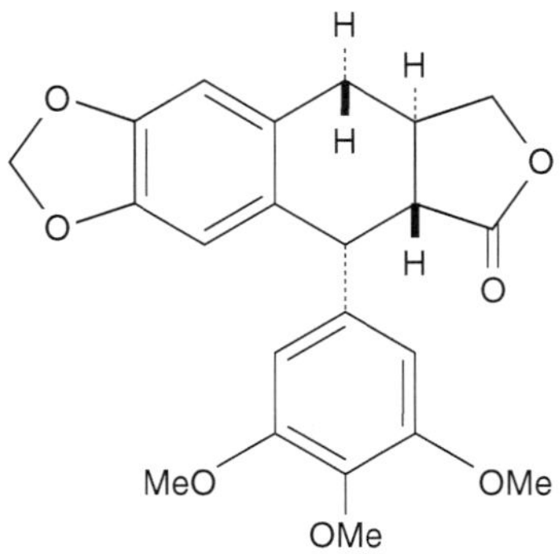

Figure 2.10 Podophyllotoxin, an example of a lignan.

Saponins are compounds that form colloidal solutions in water and foam on shaking. The name comes from the soapwort plant (*Saponaria*) the root of which was used as a soap. They consist of a polycyclic aglycone derived from squalene that is either a choline steroid or a cyclic triterpenoid (see terpenoids for description) attached via C3 and an ether bond to a sugar side chain, thus making them glycosides. Certain saponins called 'sapotoxins' are used as fish poisons. They have even been used in poison arrow tips. When ingested, saponins are usually safe in humans; however, when injected, their detergent effect on the lipid cell membrane leads to hemolysis. A large variety of plants contain saponins. The physiologic effects of saponins depend on the particular aglycone. Saponins from wild yam or fenugreek are precursors to estrogens or progestogens. They also exert lipid-lowering effects. The **cardiac glycosides**, like digitoxigenin from the foxglove plant, have a steroid aglycone group. These agents enhance cardiac contractility by increasing intracellular myocyte calcium concentration through effects on the Na^+/K^+ ATPase pump. Many plants have cardiac glycosides including lily-of-the-valley, Christmas rose, oleander, squill, and ouabain. Glycyrrhizin is a saponin from licorice that has been used as an expectorant and sweetener. When it is hydrolyzed in the body it forms glycyrrhetinic acid which inhibits enzymes that metabolize prostaglandins E2 and F2α. Physiologically, this leads to a reduction in gastric acid secretion and stimulation of uterine smooth muscle. A metabolite of glycyrrhetinic acid can inhibit 11-β-hydroxysteroid dehydrogenase which converts active cortisol to inactive cortisone in the kidneys. The net effect is sodium and water retention, hypokalemia, and hypertension. Ginseng contains a mixture of triterpenoid saponins, several of which are steroidal triterpenes called ginsenosides. These are thought to be responsible for ginseng's biologic properties. The skeleton structure for the triterpenoid saponins of ginseng (ginsenosides) is shown below.

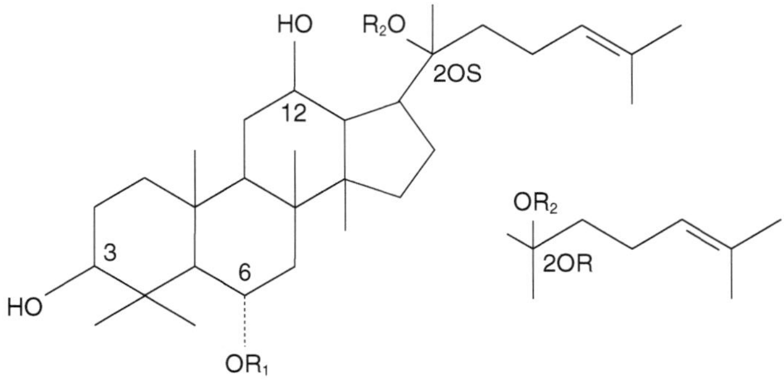

Figure 2.11 Typical skeletal structure of triterpenoid saponins found in ginseng (ginsenosides).

Tannins are plant polyphenols that contain hydroxyl or carboxyl groups that can form strong complexes with proteins. The ability of tannins to precipitate proteins enables the conversion of animal hides to leather. Tannins are also responsible for the 'puckering' taste of red wine or unripe fruit. Tannins are broadly categorized into two forms – hydrolyzable and non-hydrolyzable.

Hydrolyzable tannins have a polyol (like D-glucose) central core and hydroxyl groups that are esterified with phenolic compounds. Hydrolyzable tannins are usually present in low amounts in plants. Tannins can combine with proteins and make them resistant to proteolytic enzymes. When used in living tissues this action is referred to as an 'astringent' effect. Astringents have historically been applied topically to burns and wounds or taken internally for gastrointestinal tract disorders like ulcers or gastritis. When superficial proteins in exposed tissues are precipitated, a protective and mildly antiseptic coat is thought to form that enables regeneration of tissue to occur below. The astringent effects of tannins from witch hazel leaves or nutgall have been known for centuries. A typical polymer of gallic acid is shown below. Tannic acid is a polymer of about eight monomers of gallic acid and glucose.

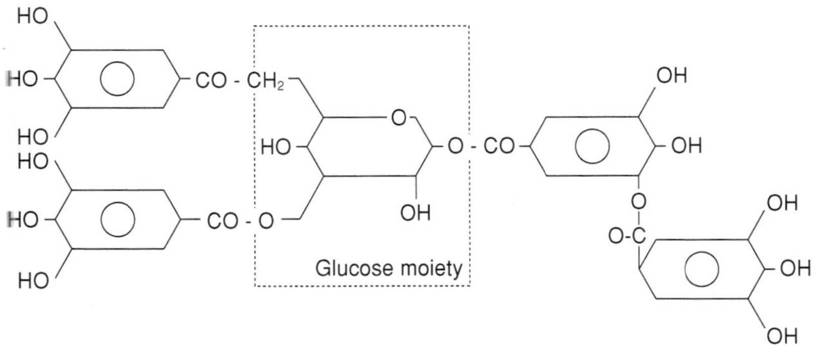

Figure 2.12 Structure of a hydrolyzable tannin formed as a polymer of gallic acid with a polyol (glucose moiety) at the core.

Non-hydrolyzable tannins (also called condensed tannins based on their small molecular size) are composed of flavonoid units linked by carbon-to-carbon bonds that cannot be cleaved by hydrolysis. When non-hydrolyzable tannins are heated in acidic solutions they form anthocyanidin pigments (described earlier) leading to their other synonym, proanthocyanidins. Proanthocyanidins (also referred to as pycnogenols) lead to anthocyanidins that are effective antioxidants and free radical scavengers. As discussed earlier, they are found in pine bark, grape seed, and green tea. A trimer of catechin is shown here.

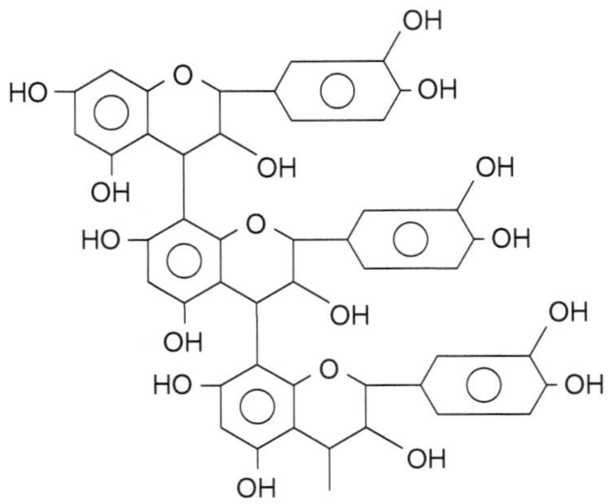

Figure 2.13 Structure of a non-hydrolyzable tannin formed as a trimer of catechin without a polyol at its core.

Terpenes and terpenoids are synthesized from a 5-carbon isoprene molecule (C_5H_8). Terpenes are hydrocarbons and terpenoids are oxygen-containing hydrocarbons. Since all these molecules are made from isoprene, they can also be called isoprenoids. Two isoprene units form a 10-carbon molecule called a monoterpene. Terpenoids can be classified based on the number of isoprene units (hence carbons) that make up their skeleton structure. These are summarized in the table below:

Table 2.1 Nomenclature of terpenoids

Terpenoid	*Isoprenes*	*Formula*	*Example*
Monoterpenoids	2	$C_{10}H_{16}$	Cineole (found in eucalyptus)
Sesquiterpenoids	3	$C_{15}H_{24}$	Valerenic acid (found in valerian)
Diterpenoids	4	$C_{20}H_{32}$	Taxol (from Pacific yew)
Triterpenoids	6	$C_{30}H_{48}$	Glycyrrhetic acid (from licorice)
Tetraterpenoids	8	$C_{40}H_{60}$	Lycopene (carotenoids)

A subgroup of structurally related sesquiterpenes are limited to only few families of plants such as *Asteraceae*. These are called **sesquiterpene lactones** and usually are responsible for the bitter taste and toxicity of many plants in which they are found. Artemisinin, a sesquiterpene lactone from *Artemisia annua* has a long history of use for its antimalarial properties. Parthenolide is a sesquiterpene lactone found in feverfew which has been shown to reduce the frequency and severity of migraine. Many triterpenoids exist as pentacyclic structures resembling steroid skeletons. Others have a tetracyclic structure. Since most are alcohols they can combine with sugars to form glycosides. Pentacyclic triterpenoids are often saponins. Carotenoids are found in brightly colored fruits and vegetables. Lycopene and other carotenoids are powerful antioxidants.

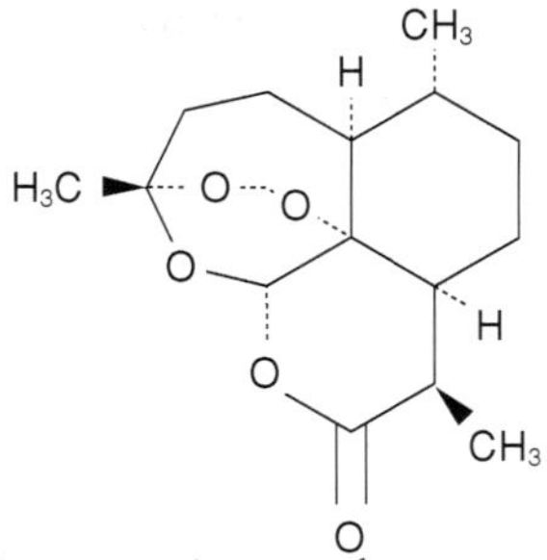

Figure 2.14 Artemisinin, a sesquiterpene lactone with antimalarial properties.

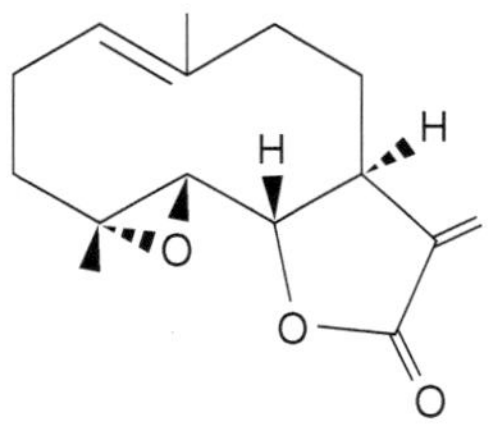

Figure 2.15 Parthenolide, a sesquiterpene lactone found in feverfew.

Volatile oils are the fragrant or aromatic plant compounds that evaporate when exposed to air at normal temperatures. They are also called essential oils as these oils impart the odoriferous character or 'essence' of the plant. Spices are made from plant parts that contain volatile oils. Volatile oils are also used in aromatherapy, as flavoring agents, and in the perfume industry. Volatile oils may also have medical properties such as the antiseptic or expectorant properties of eucalyptus oil or disinfectant properties such as pine oil. Structurally, volatile oils are either terpenoid derivatives (like those volatile oils characteristic of menthol, camphor, lemon and pine) or phenylpropanoids (like those in cinnamon, cloves, and wintergreen).

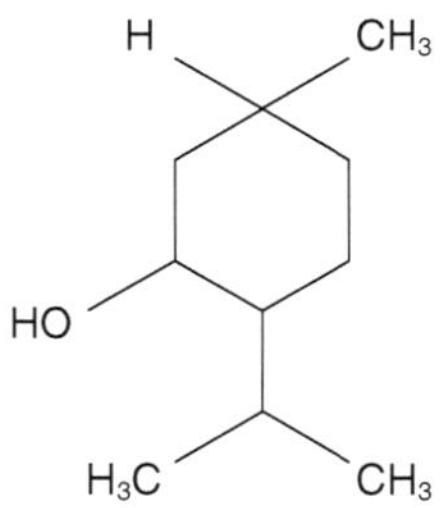

Figure 2.16 Menthol, a volatile oil and terpenoid derivative.

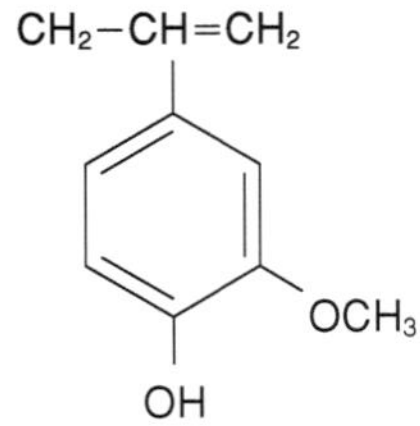

Figure 2.17 Eugenol (from cloves)

Suggested reading

Bisset NG, Wichtl M, eds. Herbal Drugs and Phytopharmaceuticals. Boca Raton: CRC Press, 1994.

Bruneton J. Pharmacognosy: Phytochemistry Medicinal Plants, 2nd ed. Hampshire, UK: Intercept, 1999.

Dewick PM. Medicinal Natural Products: A Biosynthetic Approach. Chichester: John Wiley and Sons, 1997.

Evans WC. Trease and Evans Pharmacognosy, 14th ed. London: WB Saunders Company Ltd, 1996.

Heinrich M, Barnes J, Gibbons S, Williamson EM. Fundamentals of Pharmacognosy and Phytotherapy. Edinburgh: Churchill Livingstone, 2004.

Huang KC. The Pharmacology of Chinese herbs, 2nd ed. Boca Raton: CRC Press, 1999.

Robbers JE, Speedie MK, Tyler VE. Pharmacognosy and Pharmacobiotechnology. Baltimore: Williams and Wilkins, 1996.

Chapter 3
METHODOLOGY

In keeping with the principles of evidence-based practice, we have endeavored to identify all the relevant literature on the specific health products examined. Our search strategy employed systematic searching of the following databases:

- AltHealthWatch
- AMED
- CinAhl
- Cochrane Database of Systematic Reviews
- Cochrane CENTRAL Controlled Trials Database
- E-Psyche
- DARE
- MedLine

The MeSH terms used for searching included 'pregnancy', 'lactation', and 'breastfeeding'. For individual health products, we searched using both the common and Latin names, and where appropriate, we searched using known synonyms. In the case of a well-known active ingredient or constituent, this term was also used in the search for its safety during pregnancy and lactation. The principal databases used were:

- Pubmed
- Cochrane Trial Registry (CENTRAL) and Cochrane Review database
- AMED
- CINAHL
- E-Psyche

To ensure that reports, trials, and other forms of evidence were not overlooked owing to the variety of common names for each individual herb, e.g. *Panax ginseng* is also known as ren shen in traditional Chinese medicine, the following additional databases were consulted:

- www.naturalstandard.com
- www.naturaldatabase.com
- The Complete German Commission E Monographs by the American Botanical Council

Each relevant journal article was collected and referenced in our database. The nature of the findings and the grade of evidence were then assessed and compiled in our final report.

The grade of evidence for indications was evaluated as follows:

Grade	*Level of evidence*
A	Very strong scientific evidence Statistically significant evidence of benefit from one or more systematic reviews or meta-analyses
B1	Strong scientific evidence Statistically significant evidence of benefit from one or more properly conducted randomized controlled trials (RCTs).
B2	Good scientific evidence Statistically significant evidence of benefit from one or more RCTs. The RCTs, however, are either of small sample size or have discrepancies in their methodologies
C	Fair scientific evidence Statistically significant evidence of benefit from one or more cohort studies or outcome studies
D	Weak scientific evidence Evidence from case series
E	Theoretical and/or clinical evidence Evidence from case reports or expert opinion or laboratory studies
F	Historical or traditional evidence Historical or traditional evidence of use by medical professionals, herbologists, scientists or aboriginal groups

The level of evidence for harm was evaluated as follows:

Level	*Evidence*
1a	Very strong scientific evidence Statistically significant evidence from one or more systematic reviews or RCTs
1b	Strong scientific evidence Statistically significant evidence from one or more cohort studies or control studies
1c	Good scientific evidence Evidence from one or more case series
2	Fair scientific evidence Evidence based on case reports
3	In vitro scientific evidence Evidence based on scientific studies conducted on animals, insects or microorganisms, or laboratory studies on human cells
4	Theoretical evidence Evidence based on scientific theory or expert opinion
5	Unknown No available information

Chapter 4
HERBAL MEDICINES

Herbal medicines are increasingly popular among the general public, particularly women of childbearing age. These medicines are not only viewed as having clinical benefits but are also generally believed to be safe. In some cases, a systematic review of the evidence-based medicine literature shows that this is not the case.

In pregnancy, soon-to-be mothers are concerned about all medications that may affect their health, the health of their fetus, and the pregnancy outcome. When it comes to the types of evidence for herbal medicines during pregnancy and lactation, not all evidence is created equally. The type of evidence for the safety of herbal medicines during pregnancy and lactation ranges from theoretical to animal studies, to case reports, to cohort studies and finally to randomized controlled trials.

This chapter aims to provide healthcare practitioners and mothers-to-be with the best available evidence-based safety information on the products they may choose to use or not to use during pregnancy and lactation. We selected 60 herbal medicines in total. In choosing these herbs, we set forth a number of selection criteria. These are outlined below.

Herbs that are frequently used during pregnancy, e.g. black and blue cohosh, red raspberry, evening primrose oil
Herbs that are used to treat pregnancy-related complaints, e.g. ginger
Herbs that are known abortifacients, e.g. pennyroyal, parsley
Herbs that have narrow therapeutic indices and are toxic, e.g. digitalis, deadly nightshade, ephedra
Herbs that are used more often by women than men, e.g. red clover, don quai
Herbs that are known to have hormonal effects, e.g. chastetree
The most frequently used herbs, e.g. St. John's wort (depression), garlic (hyperlipidemia), ginkgo (memory), Echinacea (immune system)

Systematic reviews on all 60 herbal medicines are presented as follows:

Common name
The name by which the herb is commonly referred to, e.g. garlic.

Latin name
The Latin name (genus, species) of the herb, e.g. *Allium sativum*. In some cases, more than one species of the herb has the same therapeutic effect, e.g. *Panax* spp.

Synonyms
Other names by which the herb may be known.

Indications
The main therapeutic indications for the herb. According to evidence-based medicine principles, the indications for the herb are evaluated based on grades/levels of evidence (see Chapter 3).

Pregnancy
The safety of the herb during pregnancy. According to evidence-based medicine principles, the safety of the herb during pregnancy is evaluated based on grades/levels of evidence (see Chapter 3).

Lactation
The safety of the herb during lactation. According to evidence-based medicine principles, the safety of the herb during lactation is evaluated based on grades/levels of evidence (see Chapter 3).

Contraindications
Conditions and diseases in which the herb should not be taken.

Caution
Conditions or diseases in which the herb should be used with caution.

Constituents
The main pharmacological constituents in the herb.

Toxicity
The toxicity of the herb (lethal dose (LD_{50}) where available).

Pharmacology
General pharmacological properties of the herb.

Drug interactions
Drugs that may interact with the herb.

Parts used
The part that provides the therapeutic benefits of the herb, e.g. root, leaf, stem.

ALFALFA
Medicago sativa

Synonyms/common names/related compounds[1]
Feuille de luzerne, lucerne, medicago, phytoestrogen, purple medick

Indications

Menopausal symptoms (with sage):[2]	Evidence grade B2
Elevated cholesterol:[3–5]	Evidence grade D
Atherosclerosis:[6,7]	Evidence grade E
Diabetes:[8,9]	Evidence grade E

Pregnancy

Estrogenic activity:[10–13]	Evidence level 3

A study on the effects of dietary genistein exposure during development found that dietary genistein produced effects in multiple estrogen-sensitive tissues in both male and female rats.[10] Another study reported estrogenic activity of genistein and daidzein in human cells in vitro and in rats.[11] The phytoestrogen coumestrol, contained in alfalfa, was reported to be 35 times more potent than the phytoestrogens genistein, biochanin A, formononetin and daidzein.[12] A review article on the potential value of plants as sources of anti-fertility agents reported that alfalfa has estrogenic activity.[13]

Isolated compounds have uterine-stimulating activity:[14]	Evidence level 4

A review article on the potential value of plants as sources of anti-fertility agents reported that alfalfa was a uterine stimulant and that its constituent stachydrine was a uterine stimulant.[14]

Emmenagogue:[15]	Evidence level 4

A herbal medicine compendium reported that alfalfa is an emmenagogue.[15] There are no reports in the scientific literature of alfalfa being an emmenagogue.

Anti-gonadotrophic activity:[14]	Evidence level 4

A review article on the potential value of plants as sources of anti-fertility agents reported that alfalfa had anti-gonadotrophic activity in rats where the acid extract interfered with the growth of the seminal vesicles and potentiated the action of estrogens.[14]

Consumed as food

Minimal risk:[15–18]	Evidence level 3

In a study on the effects of alfalfa feeding on pregnancy and lactation in beef heifers, no adverse effects were reported when alfalfa was consumed in food amounts.[16] A herbal medicine compendium reported that when consumed as food, alfalfa is believed to be of minimal risk.[15]

Lactation

Estrogenic activity:[10–12]	Evidence level 3

A study on the effects of dietary genistein exposure during development found that dietary genistein produced effects in multiple estrogen-sensitive tissues in both male and female rats.[10] Another study reported estrogenic activity of genistein and diadzein in human cells in vitro and in rats.[11] The phytoestrogen coumestrol, contained in alfalfa, was reported to be 35 times more potent than the phytoestrogens genistein, biochanin A, formononetin and daidzein.[12]

Lactogenic:[14]	Evidence level 4

A review article on the potential value of plants as sources of anti-fertility agents reported that alfalfa seeds may be lactogenic.[14]

Consumed as food

Minimal risk:[15–17]	Evidence level 3

In a study on the effects of alfalfa feeding on pregnancy and lactation in beef heifers, no adverse effects were reported with alfalfa consumed in food amounts.[16] A herbal medicine compendium reported that when consumed as food, alfalfa is believed to be of minimal risk.[15]

Contraindications
Systemic lupus erythematosus[19,20]

Caution
- Hormone sensitive conditions such as breast, uterine, or ovarian cancer, endometriosis and fibroids[12,21]
- Diabetes [15]

Constituents
- Saponins[15,22]
- Flavonoids[23]
- Phytoestrogens:[1,12,24] coumestrol, genistein, biochanin A, and daidzein
- Vitamins A, C, E, and K[15]

- Manganese[15,25]
- Stachydrine[14]

Toxicity

In a 6-week study, no signs of toxicity were reported in six humans consuming 160 g a day of alfalfa for 3 weeks followed by 80 g of alfalfa a day for 3 weeks.[5]

Pharmacology

- The phytoestrogens coumetrol, genistein, biochanin A and daidzein have been shown to have estrogenic properties.[10–12,24]
- The saponin constituents in alfalfa leaves were shown to decrease total cholesterol levels without affecting high-density lipoprotein levels.[15]
- Alfalfa constituents may decrease cholesterol absorption and increase fecal excretion of neutral steroids and bile acids.[15,26]
- Alfalfa contains manganese which might be responsible for its hypoglycemic effects.[15]
- Alfalfa contains medicagol, which appears to have anti-fungal properties.[1]

Drug interactions[1]

Anti-coagulants[15]
Photosensitizing drugs[27]
Oral contraceptives[1,15]
Hormone therapy[15]
Warfarin (Coumadin)[15]

Parts used

Above ground parts[28]

References

1. Jellin JM, Batz F, Hitchens K. Natural Medicines Comprehensive Database, 3rd ed. Stockton, CA: Therapeutic Research Faculty, 2002:1530.
2. De Leo V, Lanzetta D, Cazzavacca R, Morgante G. [Treatment of neurovegetative menopausal symptoms with a phytotherapeutic agent]. Minerva Ginecol 1998; 50:207–211.
3. Malinow MR, Connor WE, McLaughlin P et al. Cholesterol and bile acid balance in Macaca fascicularis. Effects of alfalfa saponins. J Clin Invest 1981; 67:156–162.
4. Molgaard J, von Schenck H, Olsson AG. Alfalfa seeds lower low density lipoprotein cholesterol and apolipoprotein B concentrations in patients with type II hyperlipoproteinemia. Atherosclerosis 1987; 65:173–179.
5. Malinow MR, McLaughlin P, Stafford C. Alfalfa seeds: effects on cholesterol metabolism. Experientia 1980; 36:562–564.
6. Malinow MR. Experimental models of atherosclerosis regression. Atherosclerosis 1983; 48:105–118.
7. Malinow MR, McLaughlin P, Naito HK, Lewis LA, McNulty WP. Effect of alfalfa meal on shrinkage (regression) of atherosclerotic plaques during cholesterol feeding in monkeys. Atherosclerosis 1978; 30:27–43.

8. Swanston-Flatt SK, Day C, Bailey CJ, Flatt PR. Traditional plant treatments for diabetes. Studies in normal and streptozotocin diabetic mice. Diabetologia 1990; 33:462–464.
9. Gray AM, Flatt PR. Pancreatic and extra-pancreatic effects of the traditional anti-diabetic plant, Medicago sativa (lucerne). Br J Nutr 1997; 78:325–334.
10. Delclos KB, Bucci TJ, Lomax LG et al. Effects of dietary genistein exposure during development on male and female CD (Sprague-Dawley) rats. Reprod Toxicol 2001; 15:647–663.
11. Casanova M, You L, Gaido KW et al. Developmental effects of dietary phyto-estrogens in Sprague-Dawley rats and interactions of genistein and daidzein with rat estrogen receptors alpha and beta in vitro. Toxicol Sci 1999; 51:236–244.
12. Elakovich SD, Hampton JM. Analysis of coumestrol, a phytoestrogen, in alfalfa tablets sold for human consumption. J Agric Food Chem 1984; 32:173–175.
13. Farnsworth NR, Bingel AS, Cordell GA, Crane FA, Fong HH. Potential value of plants as sources of new anti-fertility agents II. Pharm Sci 1975; 64:717–753.
14. Farnsworth NR, Bingel AS, Cordell GA, Crane FA, Fong HH. Potential value of plants as sources of new anti-fertility agents I. J Pharm Sci 1975; 64:535–598.
15. Newall CA, Anderson LA, Phillipson JD. Herbal Medicines: A Guide for Health-care Professionals. London, UK: Pharmaceutical Press, 1996:296.
16. Vanzant ES, Cochran RC, Johnson DE. Pregnancy and lactation in beef heifers grazing tallgrass prairie in the winter: influence on intake, forage utilization, and grazing behavior. J Anim Sci 1991; 69:3027–3038.
17. Coffey KP, Paterson JA, Saul CS et al. The influence of pregnancy and source of supplemental protein on intake, digestive kinetics and amino acid absorption by ewes. J Anim Sci 1989; 67:1805–1814.
18. Guay KA, Brady HA, Allen VG et al. Matua bromegrass hay for mares in gestation and lactation. J Anim Sci 2002; 80:2960–2966.
19. Malinow MR, Bardana EJ Jr, Pirofsky B, Craig S, McLaughlin P. Systemic lupus erythmatosus-like syndrome in monkeys fed alfalfa sprouts: role of a nonprotein amino acid. Science 1982; 216:415.
20. Roberts JL, Hayashi JA. Exacerbation of SLE associated with alfalfa ingestion. N Engl J Med 1983; 308:1361.
21. Kurzer MS, Xu X. Dietary phytoestrogens. Annu Rev Nutr 1997; 17:353–381.
22. Malinow MR, McLaughlin P, Stafford C et al. Comparative effects of alfalfa saponins and alfalfa fiber on cholesterol absorption in rats. Am J Clin Nutr 1979; 32:1810–1812.
23. Stochmal A, Piacente S, Pizza C et al. Alfalfa (Medicago sativa L.) flavonoids. 1. Apigenin and luteolin glycosides from aerial parts. J Agric Food Chem 2001; 49:753–758.
24. Leung AY, Foster S. Encyclopedia of Common Natural Ingredients Used in Food, Drugs and Cosmetics. New York, NY: John Wiley & Sons, 1996:649.
25. Rubenstein AH, Levin NW, Elliott GA. Manganese-induced hypoglycemia. Lancet 1962:1348–1351.
26. The Review of Natural Products by Facts and Comparisons. St. Louis, MO: Wolters Kluwer Co., 1999.
27. Brown R. Potential interactions of herbal medicines with anti-psychotics, anti-depressants and hypnotics. Eur J Herbal Med 1997; 3:25–28.
28. Brinker F. Herb Contraindications and Drug Interactions. Sandy, OR: Eclectic Medical Publications, 2001:432.

ALOE
Aloe spp.

Synonyms/common names/related substances[1]

A. vera (A. barbadensis), A. ferox, A. africana, A. arborescens natalenis, A. capensis, A. leaf gel, *A. perfoliata, A. perryi, A. spicata*, salvia, cape aloes, Barbados aloe, Curacao aloe, hepatic aloes, aloe dried juice from leaf, aloe juice, burn plant, elephant's gall, hsiang-dan, lily of the desert, lu-hui, miracle plant, plant of immortality

Indications

Oral

Chronic constipation:[2–6]	Evidence grade B1
Solid tumors (with melatonin):[7]	Evidence grade C
Elevated cholesterol and triglycerides, hyperglycemia and low high-density lipoprotein cholesterol (with husk of Isabgol):[8]	Evidence grade C
Chronic venous leg ulcers:[9]	Evidence grade C
Fibromyalgia, chronic fatigue syndrome:[10]	Evidence grade C
Diabetes type 2:[11–13]	Evidence grade E
Bronchial asthma (aloe vera gel):[14]	Evidence grade E

Topical

Psoriasis vulgaris:[15]	Evidence grade B1
Herpes simplex type II:[16,17]	Evidence grade B1
Seborrheic dermatitis:[18]	Evidence grade B1
Radiation induced dermatitis:[19]	Evidence grade B2
Occupational dry skin, irritant contact dermatitis:[20]	Evidence grade B2
Burn wounds:[21]	Evidence grade C
Alveolar osteitis:[22]	Evidence grade C

Chronic venous leg ulcers:[9]	Evidence grade C
Anti-arthritic, anti-inflammatory (*A. africana*):[23]	Evidence grade E
Anti-inflammatory (*A. vera*):[24]	Evidence grade E
Wounds (*A. vera*):[24,25]	Evidence grade E

Pregnancy

Oral

Potentially nephrotoxic:[26]	Evidence level 2
Potential hepatic dysfunction:[26]	Evidence level 2

A case of acute oliguric renal failure and liver dysfunction was reported in the literature following traditional therapeutic use of cape aloes.[26]

Potential abortifacient:[27]	Evidence level 4
Emmenagogue:[27]	Evidence level 4

A review article on the potential value of plants as sources of anti-fertility agents reported that aloe species are potential abortifacients and emmenagogues.[27]

Potentially genotoxic:[3,28,29]	Evidence level 3
Potentially mutagenic:[3,28,29]	Evidence level 3
Potentially carcinogenic:[3,28,29]	Evidence level 3

Aloe-emodin, a 1,8-dihydroxyanthraquinone found in aloe, is potentially carcinogenic, mutagenic and genotoxic in mice.[3,28,29]

Topical

Aloe vera gel – minimal risk:[3,30]	Evidence level 4

A herbal medicine compendium reported that the external use of aloe vera gel is not a concern during pregnancy. The external use of aloe was not reported in the scientific literature as contraindicated or safe during pregnancy or lactation.

Lactation

Oral

Potentially genotoxic:[3,28,29]	Evidence level 3

Potentially mutagenic:[3,28,29]	Evidence level 3

Potentially carcinogenic:[3,28,29]	Evidence level 3

Although it is unclear if aloe components cross into breast milk, these components are potentially genotoxic/mutagenic and carcinogenic to the nursing infant.[3,28,29]

Avoid during lactation:[3,31]	Evidence level 4

A herbal safety and drug interaction compendium and a herbal medicine compendium reported that aloe species should be avoided during lactation.[3,31]

Potential laxative:[3,28]	Evidence level 4

A herbal safety and drug interaction compendium and a herbal medicine compendium reported that aloe species may cause diarrhea in the infant due to aloe's laxative effect.[3,28]

Topical

Use with caution:	Evidence level 4

Infants nursing from a breast to which aloe has been topically applied may be susceptible to the same risks as if aloe components where ingested.

Contraindications[2,3,26,30,32]

Menstruation (especially menorrhagia and metrorrhagia)
Actively inflamed hemorrhoids
Intestinal obstruction
Acutely inflamed intestinal diseases (e.g. Crohn disease, ulcerative colitis, appendicitis)
Abdominal pain of unknown origin
Kidney dysfunction
Children under 12 years of age

Caution

If used for more than 8–10 days
Postsurgical wounds[33]

Constituents

- Anthroquinone glycosides:[3,30] aloin A, aloin B, aloinoside A, aloinoside B, 7-hydroxyaloins, emodin
- Anthraquinone:[34] aloe-emodin (1,8-dihydroxyanthraquinone)
- Aloresin A[30]

Toxicology

- Aloe-emodin is potentially carcinogenic and genotoxic.[29,35]
- Acemannan exhibited significant cytotoxicity to human gingival fibroblasts; however, in animals, oral administration of acemannan was found to be safe.[36–38]

Pharmacology

- The anthraquinones (dried latex) in aloe exert a laxative and purgative effect whereas aloe gel does not.[3]
- Aloe and aloe gum may have a hypoglycemic effect.[11–13]
- With husk of Isabgol, aloe significantly reduced total cholesterol, triglycerides, fasting and postprandial blood sugar levels in diabetic patients, and total lipids and increased high-density lipoprotein cholesterol.[8]
- Aloe vera gel has been shown to delay wound healing in women following cesarean delivery or laparotomy.[33]
- Topical application – *A. africana* was found to have anti-arthritic and anti-inflammatory effects.[23]
- Aloe vera gel was found to enhance phagocytosis in human bronchial asthma.[14]
- Aloe vera gel was found to reduce pruritus by inhibiting thromboxane formation in vivo, inactivating bradykinin in vitro, and inhibiting histamine.[39]
- Aloe vera gel may have anti-bacterial and anti-fungal effects.[39]
- The addition of aloe vera gel to a mild soap had a protective effect on the skin of patients undergoing radiation therapy.[19]

Drug interactions

Anti-glycemic drugs[11–13]
Cardiac glycosides[3]
Diuretics[2]
Oral drugs[31]

Parts used[3,30]

Dried latex and gel from leaves

References

1. Jellin JM, Batz F, Hitchens K. Natural Medicines Comprehensive Database, 3rd ed. Stockton, CA: Therapeutic Research Faculty, 2002:1530.
2. Blumenthal M, Busse WR, Goldberg A et al. The Complete German Commission E Monographs: Therapeutic Guide to Herbal Medicines. Boston, MA: American Botanical Council, 1998.
3. Newall CA, Anderson LA, Phillipson JD. Herbal Medicines: A Guide for Health-care Professionals. London, UK: Pharmaceutical Press, 1996:296.
4. Wichtl M, Czygan FC, Frohne D et al. Herbal Drugs and Phytopharmaceuticals. Stuttgart, DE: Medpharm-CRC, Press, 1994:566.
5. Odes HS, Madar Z. A double-blind trial of a celandin, aloevera and psyllium laxative preparation in adult patients with constipation. Digestion 1991; 49:65–71.

6. Chapman DD, Pittelli JJ. Double-blind comparison of alophen with its components for cathartic effects. Curr Ther Res Clin Exp 1974; 16:817–820.
7. Lissoni P, Giani L, Zerbini S, Trabattoni P, Rovelli F. Biotherapy with the pineal immunomodulating hormone melatonin versus melatonin plus aloe vera in untreatable advanced solid neoplasms. Nat Immun 1998; 16:27–33.
8. Agarwal OP. Prevention of atheromatous heart disease. Angiology 1985; 36:485–492.
9. Atherton P. Aloe vera: magic or medicine? Nurs Stand 1998; 12:49–52, 54.
10. Dykman KD, Tone C, Ford C, Dykman RA. The effects of nutritional supplements on the symptoms of fibromyalgia and chronic fatigue syndrome. Integr Physiol Behav Sci 1998; 33:61–71.
11. Al-Awadi FM, Gumaa KA. Studies on the activity of individual plants of an antidiabetic plant mixture. Acta Diabetol Lat 1987; 24:37–41.
12. Al-Awadi FM, Khattar MA, Gumaa KA. On the mechanism of the hypoglycaemic effect of a plant extract. Diabetologia 1985; 28:432–434.
13. Ghannam N, Kingston M, Al-Meshaal IA et al. The anti-diabetic activity of aloes: preliminary clinical and experimental observations. Horm Res 1986; 24:288–294.
14. Shida T, Yagi A, Nishimura H, Nishioka I. Effect of Aloe extract on peripheral phagocytosis in adult bronchial asthma. Planta Med 1985:273–275.
15. Syed TA, Ahmad SA, Holt AH et al. Management of psoriasis with Aloe vera extract in a hydrophilic cream: a placebo-controlled, double-blind study. Trop Med Int Health 1996; 1:505–509.
16. Syed TA, Afzal M, Ashfaq AS. Management of genital herpes in men with 0.5% Aloe vera extract in a hydrophilic cream. A placebo-controlled double-blind study. J Derm Treatment 1997; 8:99–102.
17. Syed TA, Cheema KM, Ahmad SA. Aloe vera extract 0.5% in hydrophilic cream versus aloe vera gel for the measurement of genital herpes in males. A placebo-controlled, double-blind, comparative study. J Eur Acad Dermatol Venerol 1996; 7:294–295.
18. Vardy AD, Cohen AD, Tchetov T. A double-blind, placebo-controlled trial of Aloe vera (A. barbadensis) emulsion in the treatment of seborrheic dermatitis. J Derm Treatment 1999; 10:7–11.
19. Olsen DL, Raub WJ, Bradley C et al. The effect of aloe vera gel/mild soap versus mild soap alone in preventing skin reactions in patients undergoing radiation therapy. Oncol Nurs Forum 2001; 28:543–547.
20. West DP, Zhu YF. Evaluation of aloe vera gel gloves in the treatment of dry skin associated with occupational exposure. Am J Infect Control 2003; 31:40–42.
21. Visuthikosol V, Chowchuen B, Sukwanarat Y, Sriurairatana S, Boonpucknavig V. Effect of aloe vera gel to healing of burn wound a clinical and histologic study. J Med Assoc Thai 1995; 78:403–409.
22. Poor MR, Hall JE, Poor AS. Reduction in the incidence of alveolar osteitis in patients treated with the SaliCept patch, containing Acemannan hydrogel. J Oral Maxillofac Surg 2002; 60:374–379.
23. Davis RH, Shapiro E, Agnew PS. Topical effect of aloe with ribonucleic acid and vitamin C on adjuvant arthritis. J Am Podiatr Med Assoc 1985; 75:229–237.
24. Davis RH, Donato JJ, Hartman GM, Haas RC. Anti-inflammatory and wound healing activity of a growth substance in Aloe vera. J Am Podiatr Med Assoc 1994; 84:77–81.
25. Fulton JEJ. The stimulation of postdermabrasion wound healing with stabilized aloe vera gel-polyethylene oxide dressing. J Dermatol Surg Oncol 1990; 16:460–467.

26. Luyckx VA, Ballanti-ne R, Claeys M et al. Herbal remedy-associated acute renal failure secondary to Cape aloes. Am J Kidney Dis 2002; 39:E13.
27. Farnsworth NR, Bingel AS, Cordell GA, Crane FA, Fong HH. Potential value of plants as sources of new anti-fertility agents I. J Pharm Sci 1975; 64:535–598.
28. Brinker F. Herb Contraindications and Drug Interactions. Sandy, OR: Eclectic Medical Publications, 2001:432.
29. Muller SO, Eckert I, Lutz WK, Stopper H. Genotoxicity of the laxative drug components emodin, aloe-emodin and danthron in mammalian cells: topoisomerase II mediated? Mutat Res 1996; 371:165–173.
30. Brinker F. The Toxicology of Botanical Medicines. Sandy, Oregon: Eclectic Medical Publications, 2000:296.
31. Brinker F. Herb Contraindications and Drug Interactions. Sandy, OR: Eclectic Institute Inc., 1997:146.
32. McGuffin M, Hobbs C, Upton R, Goldberg A. American Herbal Products Association's Botanical Safety Handbook. Boca Raton, FL: CRC Press, 1997:231.
33. Schmidt JM, Greenspoon JS. Aloe vera dermal wound gel is associated with a delay in wound healing. Obstet Gynecol 1991; 78:115–117.
34. Muller-Jakic B, Breu W, Probstle A et al. In vitro inhibition of cyclooxygenase and 5-lipoxygenase by alkamides from Echinacea and Achillea species. Planta Med 1994; 60:37–40.
35. Westendorf J, Marquardt H, Poginsky B et al. Genotoxicity of naturally occurring hydroxyanthraquinones. Mutat Res 1990; 240:1–12.
36. Fogleman RW, Shellenberger TE, Balmer MF, Carpenter RH, McAnalley BH. Subchronic oral administration of acemannan in the rat and dog. Vet Hum Toxicol 1992; 34:144–147.
37. Fogleman RW, Chapdelaine JM, Carpenter RH, McAnalley BH. Toxicologic evaluation of injectable acemannan in the mouse, rat and dog. Vet Hum Toxicol 1992; 34:201–205.
38. Tello CG, Ford P, Iacopino AM. In vitro evaluation of complex carbohydrate denture adhesive formulations. Quintessence Int 1998; 29:585–593.
39. Klein AD, Penneys NS. Aloe vera. J Am Acad Dermatol 1988; 18:714–720.

ASHWAGANDHA
Withania somnifera

Synonyms/common names/related compounds[1]

Ajagandha, amangura, amukkirag, asan, asgand, asgandh, asgandha, ashagandha, ashvagandha, ashwaganda, asoda, asundha, asvagandha, aswagandha, avarada, ayurvedic ginseng, clustered wintercherry, ghoda asoda, Indian ginseng, kanaje hindi, kuthmithi, samm al ferakh, turangi-ghanda, winter cherry, withania

Indications

Osteoarthritis (with *Boswellia*, turmeric, and zinc):[2]	Evidence grade B2
Diabetes type 2:[3]	Evidence grade C
Hypercholesterolemia:[3]	Evidence grade C
Stress:[4]	Evidence grade E
Cancer:[5]	Evidence grade E

Pregnancy

Reduces fertility:[6]	Evidence level 3

A review article on the potential value of plants as sources of anti-fertility agents reported that ashwagandha caused a reduction in fertility in rats.[6]

Abortifacient:[7,8]	Evidence level 4
Uterine stimulant constituent:[6]	Evidence level 4

A review article on the potential value of plants as sources of anti-fertility agents reported that ashwagandha was a potential abortifacient and that its constituent, nicotine, was a uterine stimulant.[6]

Lactation

Unknown:	Evidence level 5

There are no reports in the scientific literature of ashwagandha being either safe or contraindicated during lactation.

Constituents

Alkaloids:[9,10] isopelletierine, anaferine
Steroidal lactones:[9–11] withanolides, aithaferins
Saponins[9,10]

Toxicity

- LD_{50} (intraperitoneal):[12] 432–465 mg/kg
- Doses of 1000 mg/kg produced fatalities in mice.[13]
- Doses of 500–750 mg/kg given to total cumulative doses of 7.5–10 g were apparently safe.[13]

Pharmacology[1]

- Ashwagandha was reported to have analgesic, anti-pyretic, anxiolytic, immunomodulatory, sedative, hypotensive, anti-inflammatory, and antioxidant effects.[1,9,10,14–16]
- During stress, ashwagandha suppresses the increases of plasma corticosterone, blood urea nitrogen, blood lactic acid, and the increase of dopamine receptors in the corpus striatum of the brain.[9,14]
- Ashwagandha may have anxiolytic effects by acting as a γ-aminobutyric acid (GABA) mimetic agent and anti-convulsant activity by binding to GABA receptors.[14]
- Ashwagandha stimulates respiratory function, smooth muscle relaxation, and thyroid hormone synthesis and secretion.[14]
- The ashwagandha constituent withanolides cause mobilization of macrophages, phagocytosis, and lysosomal enzymes.[9]
- Ashwagandha reduces cyclophosphamide-induced immunosuppression and leukopenia and increases bone marrow cell and white blood cell count in radiation-treated animals.[15,17]
- Ashwagandha has diuretic effects.[3]

Drug interactions

Benzodiazepines[14]
Central nervous system depressants[14]
Immunosuppressant drugs[15,17]
Thyroid hormone[14]

Parts used[1]

Root and berry

References

1. Jellin JM, Batz F, Hitchens K. Natural Medicines Comprehensive Database, 3rd ed. Stockton, CA: Therapeutic Research Faculty, 2002:1530.
2. Kulkarni RR, Patki PS, Jog V, Gandage SG, Patwardhan B. Treatment of osteoarthritis with a herbomineral formulation: a double-blind, placebo-controlled, cross-over study. J Ethnopharmacol 1991; 33:91–95.

3. Andallu B, Radhika B. Hypoglycemic, diuretic and hypocholesterolemic effect of winter cherry (Withania somnifera, Dunal) root. Indian J Exp Biol 2000; 38:607–609.
4. Rege NN, Thatte UM, Dahanukar S. Adaptogenic properties of six rasayana herbs used in Ayurvedic medicine. Phytother Res 1999; 13:275–291.
5. Devi PU. Withania somnifera Dunal (Ashwagandha): potential plant source of a promising drug for cancer chemotherapy and radiosensitization. Indian J Exp Biol 1996; 34:927–932.
6. Farnsworth NR, Bingel AS, Cordell G, Crane FA, Fong HH. Potential value of plants as sources of new anti-fertility agents I. J Pharm Sci 1975; 64:535–598.
7. Brinker F. Herb Contraindications and Drug Interactions., 3rd ed. Sandy, OR: Eclectic Medical Publications, 2001:432.
8. McGuffin M, Hobbs C, Upton R, Goldberg A. American Herbal Products Association's Botanical Safety Handbook. Boca Raton, FL: CRC Press, 1997:231.
9. Mishra LC, Singh BB, Dagenais S. Scientific basis for the therapeutic use of Withania somnifera (åshwagandha): a review. Altern Med Rev 2000; 5:334–346.
10. Bhattacharya SK, Satyan KS, Ghosal S. Anti-oxidant activity of glycowithanolides from Withania somnifera. Indian J Exp Biol 1997; 35:236–239.
11. Abou-Douh AM. New withanolides and other constituents from the fruit of Withania somnifera. Arch Pharm (Weinheim) 2002; 335:267–276.
12. Malhotra CL, Mehta VL, Das PK et al. Studies on Withania-ashwagandha, Kaul. V. The effect of total alkaloids (ashwagandholine) on the central nervous system. Indian J Physiol Pharmacol 1965; 9:127–136.
13. Devi PU, Sharada AC, Solomon FE et al. In vivo growth inhibitory effect of Withania somnifera (Ashwagandha) on a transplantable mouse tumor, Sarcoma 180. Indian J Exp Biol 1992; 30:169–172.
14. Upton R. Ashwagandha Root (Withania somnifera): Analytical, quality control, and therapuetic monograph. Santa Cruz, CA: American Herbal Pharmacopoeia, 2000:1–25.
15. Davis L, Kuttan G. Effect of Withania somnifera on cyclophosphamide-induced urotoxicity. Cancer Lett 2000; 148:9–17.
16. Archana R, Namasivayam A. Anti-stressor effect of Withania somnifera. J Ethnopharmacol 1999; 64:91–93.
17. Davis L, Kuttan G. Suppressive effect of cyclophosphamide-induced toxicity by Withania somnifera extract in mice. J Ethnopharmacol 1998; 62:209–214.

ASTRAGALUS
Astragalus membranaceus

Synonyms/common names/related substances[1]

Astragali, beg kei, bei qi, buck qi, huang qi, huang qi, hwanggi, membranous milk vetch, milk vetch, Mongolian milk, ogi

Indications

Chronic hepatitis (within a Chinese herbal preparation):[2]	Evidence grade B2
Human immunodeficiency virus infection (within a Chinese herbal preparation)[3,4]	Evidence grade B2
Chronic nephritis:[5]	Evidence grade B2
Minimal brain dysfunction:[6]	Evidence grade B2
Immune stimulation:[7,8]	Evidence grade C
Leucopenia:[8]	Evidence grade C
Chemotherapy side effects:[9]	Evidence grade C
Post acute myocardial infarction:[10]	Evidence grade C
Acute viral myocarditis (with drugs and other supplements):[11,12]	Evidence grade C
Congestive heart failure:[13]	Evidence grade C
Chronic renal failure:[14]	Evidence grade C
Liver protection:[15,16]	Evidence grade E
Cancer:[4]	Evidence grade E
Herpes simplex I:[6]	Evidence grade E

Pregnancy

Unknown:	Evidence level 5

There is no report in the scientific literature of astragalus being either safe or contraindicated during pregnancy.

Other Astragalus *species*

Unsafe during pregnancy:[17,18] Evidence level 3

Estrogenic:[19] Evidence level 4

Other *Astragalus* spp., such as *A. lentiginosis* or *A. mollissimus* (locoweed), have been reported to have harmful effects during animal pregnancies.[17] Ingestion of locoweed (*Astragalus* spp.) by pregnant livestock may result in fetal malformations, delayed placentation, reduced placental and uterine vascular development, hydrops amnii, hydrops allantois, abnormal cotyledonary development, interruption of fetal fluid balance, and abortion.[18] During pregnancy, the toxic agent in locoweed (swainsonine) is believed to pass through the placental barrier to the fetus.[18] A review article on the potential value of plants as sources of anti-fertility agents reported that *A. hypogaea*, *A. lentiginosis*, *A. miser*, and *A. sinicus* have estrogenic activity.[19] *A. membranaceus* is not reported in the scientific literature as containing the toxic agent swainsonine.

Lactation

Unknown: Evidence level 5

There is no report in the scientific literature of astragalus being either safe or contraindicated during lactation.

Other Astragalus *species*

Unsafe during lactation:[18] Evidence level 3

During lactation, the toxic agent in locoweed (swainsonine) is believed to pass through the milk to the neonate.[18] *A. membranaceus* is not reported in the scientific literature as containing the toxic agent swainsonine.

Constituents[20,21]

Saponins: astragaloside
Flavonoids
Polysaccharides
Coumarins
Trace minerals
Amino acids

Toxicity

- LD_{50} in mice (intraperitoneal): 39.8 g/kg.[22]
- Doses greater than 28 g/day may cause immunosuppression.[21]
- Aqueous extracts of 1.25 mg/mL modestly increased the incidence (16%) of aberrant cells in vitro.[23]

Pharmacology

- Astragalus is an antioxidant where it inhibits free radical production, increases superoxide dismutase, and decreases lipid peroxidation.[21]
- Astragalus acts as an immune stimulant by increasing the effects of interferon, by increasing antibody levels of IgA and IgG in nasal secretions, by improving the response of mononuclear cells and by stimulating lymphocyte production.[7,21]
- Astragalus may restore or improve immune function in cases of immune deficiency.[7,24]
- Lower doses appear to stimulate the immune system, while doses in excess of 28 g/day may suppress immunity.[21]
- Astragalus may increase proliferation and differentiation of bone marrow stem cells and progenitor cells when administered intravenously.[21]
- Astragalus decreases liver enzymes serum glutamate pyruvate transaminase and alanine aminotransferase.[2,15,21]
- Astragalus causes vasodilation and increases cardiac output.[21]
- Astragalus has anti-bacterial activity.[21]

Drug interactions

Cyclophosphamide[21,24]
Immunosuppressants[21]

Parts used

Root[1]

References

1. Jellin JM, Batz F, Hitchens K. Natural Medicines Comprehensive Database, 3rd ed. Stockton, CA: Therapeutic Research Faculty, 2002:1530.
2. Batey RG, Bensoussan A, Fan YY, Bollipo S, Hossain MA. Preliminary report of a randomized, double-blind placebo-controlled trial of a Chinese herbal medicine preparation CH-100 in the treatment of chronic hepatitis C. J Gastroenterol Hepatol 1998; 13:244–247.
3. Burack JH, Cohen MR, Hahn J, Abrams DI. Pilot randomized controlled trial of Chinese herbal treatment for HIV-associated symptoms. J Acquir Immune Defic Syndr Hum Retrovirol 1996; 12:386–393.
4. Chu DT, Lin JR, Wong W. [The in vitro potentiation of LAK cell cytotoxicity in cancer and aids patients induced by F3–a fractionated extract of Astragalus membranaceus]. Zhonghua Zhong Liu Za Zhi 1994; 16:167–171.
5. Su ZZ, He YY, Chen G. [Clinical and experimental study on effects of man-shen-ling oral liquid in the treatment of 100 cases of chronic nephritis]. Zhongguo Zhong Xi Yi Jie He Za Zhi 1993; 13:269–272, 259–620.
6. Zhang H, Huang J. [Preliminary study of traditional Chinese medicine treatment of minimal brain dysfunction: analysis of 100 cases]. Zhong Xi Yi Jie He Za Zhi 1990; 10:278–279, 260.

7. Sun Y, Hersh EM, Talpaz M et al. Immune restoration and/or augmentation of local graft versus host reaction by traditional Chinese medicinal herbs. Cancer 1983; 52:70–73.
8. Weng XS. [Treatment of leucopenia with pure Astragalus preparation – an analysis of 115 leucopenic cases]. Zhongguo Zhong Xi Yi Jie He Za Zhi 1995; 15:462–464.
9. Li NQ. [Clinical and experimental study on shen-qi injection with chemotherapy in the treatment of malignant tumor of digestive tract]. Zhongguo Zhong Xi Yi Jie He Za Zhi 1992; 12:588–592, 579.
10. Chen LX, Liao JZ, Guo W. [Effects of Astragalus membranaceus on left ventricular function and oxygen free radical in acute myocardial infarction patients and mechanism of its cardiotonic action]. Zhongguo Zhong Xi Yi Jie He Za Zhi 1995; 15:141–143.
11. Gu W, Yang YZ, He M. [A study on combination therapy of Western and traditional Chinese medicine of acute viral myocarditis]. Zhongguo Zhong Xi Yi Jie He Za Zhi 1996; 16:713–716.
12. Yan HJ. [Clinical and experimental study of the effect of kang er xin-I on viral myocarditis]. Zhong Xi Yi Jie He Za Zhi 1991; 11:468–470, 452.
13. Luo HM, Dai RH, Li Y. [Nuclear cardiology study on effective ingredients of Astragalus membranaceus in treating heart failure]. Zhongguo Zhong Xi Yi Jie He Za Zhi 1995; 15:707–709.
14. Sheng ZL, Li NY, Ge X. [Clinical study of baoyuan dahuang decoction in the treatment of chronic renal failure]. Zhongguo Zhong Xi Yi Jie He Za Zhi 1994; 14:268–270, 259.
15. Fu QL. [Experimental study on yiqi-huoxue therapy of liver fibrosis]. Zhongguo Zhong Xi Yi Jie He Za Zhi 1992; 12:228–229, 198.
16. Zhang BZ, Ding F, Tan L. [Clinical and experimental study on yi-gan-ning granule in treating chronic hepatitis B]. Zhongguo Zhong Xi Yi Jie He Za Zhi 1993; 13:597–599, 580.
17. Panter KE, James LF, Stegelmeier BL, Ralphs MH, Pfister JA. Locoweeds: effects on reproduction in livestock. J Nat Toxins 1999; 8:53–62.
18. Bunch TD, Panter KE, James L. Ultrasound studies of the effects of certain poisonous plants on uterine function and fetal development in livestock. J Anim Sci 1992; 70:1639–1643.
19. Farnsworth NR, Bingel AS, Cordell GA, Crane FA, Fong HH. Potential value of plants as sources of new anti-fertility agents II. J Pharm Sci 1975; 64:717–753.
20. Leung AY, Foster S. Encyclopedia of Common Natural Ingredients Used in Food, Drugs and Cosmetics, 2nd ed. New York, NY: John Wiley & Sons, 1996:649.
21. Upton R. Astragalus Root: Analytical, quality control, and therapeutic monograph. Santa Cruz, CA: American Herbal Pharmacopoeia, 1999:1–25.
22. Cheng H, But P. Pharmacology and applications of Chinese materia medica. Vol. 2. Singapore: World Scientific, 1987:1041–1046.
23. Tadaki S, Yamada S, Miyazawa N et al. [Clastogenicity of Eucommiae and Astragali Radix]. Jap J Toxicol Environ Health 1995; 41:463–469.
24. Chu DT, Wong WL, Mavligit GM. Immunotherapy with Chinese medicinal herbs. II. Reversal of cyclophosphamide-induced immune suppression by administration of fractionated Astragalus membranaceus in vivo. J Clin Lab Immunol 1988; 25:125–129.

BARBERRY
Berberis vulgaris

Synonyms/common names/related substances[1]

European barberry, pepperidge, sow berry, jaundice berry, berberry, berbis, common barberry, epine-vinette, espino cambrón, pipperidge, piprage, sauerdorn, vinettier, agracejo, *Berberidis cortex*, *B. fructus*, *B. radicis cortex*, *B. radix*, berberitze

Indications

Berberine

Chloroquine-resistant malaria (with pyrimethamine):[2]	Evidence grade B1
Infectious diarrhea:[3,4]	Evidence grade B1
Trachoma (*Chlamydia trachomatis* eye infection):[5,6]	Evidence grade B2
Congestive heart failure:[7]	Evidence grade C
Upper respiratory tract infections:[8,9]	Evidence grade E
Anti-*Helicobacter pylori*:[10]	Evidence grade E
Cancer prevention:[11–13]	Evidence grade E

Pregnancy

May cause newborn jaundice (kernicterus):[14]	Evidence level 3

In rats, berberine displaces bilirubin bound to albumin.[14] Berberine (10–20 μg/g) was administered intraperitoneally to adult rats on a daily basis for 1 week.[14] After 1 week, a significant decrease in mean bilirubin serum protein binding was observed, due to an in vivo displacement effect by berberine.[14] Persistent elevation in serum concentrations of unbound and total bilirubin was also observed.[14]

Uterine stimulant:[15,16]	Evidence level 4

A review article on the potential value of plants as sources of anti-fertility agents reported that barberry was a uterine stimulant.[16] The alkaloids palmatine, berberine, jatrorrhizine and columbamine, contained in barberry, are believed to act as uterine stimulants.[15,17]

Lactation

May cause or aggravate newborn jaundice (kernicterus):[14]	Evidence level 3

In rats, berberine displaces bilirubin bound to albumin.[14] Berberine (10–20 μg/g) was administered intraperitoneally to adult rats on a daily basis for 1 week.[14] After 1 week, a significant decrease in mean bilirubin serum protein binding was observed, due to an in vivo displacement effect by berberine.[14] Persistent elevation in serum concentrations of unbound and total bilirubin was also observed.[14]

Contraindication

Newborn jaundice (kernicterus)[14]

Toxic constituents

- Isoquinoline alkaloids:[17] oxyacanthine, berbamine, berberine, palmatine, jatorrhizine, columbamine
- Tannins[17]

Toxicology

LD_{50} of berberine in humans:[15] 27.5 mg/kg

Pharmacology

- Berberine was found to displace bilirubin bound to albumin in vitro.[14] Berberine was found to be about 10 times superior to phenylbutazone, a known potent displacer of bilirubin, and about 100 times superior to papaverine, a berberine-type alkaloid.[14]
- The constituents berberine and oxyacanthine have been shown to have anti-bacterial activity.[8,9,18,19]
- Berberine has been shown to have amebicidal, anti-parasitic (trypanocidal) and anti-fungal activity.[18,20–22]
- Berberine and β-hydrastine were shown to have anti-*Helicobacter pylori* activity in vitro.[10]
- In low doses, berberine may act as a cardiac and respiratory stimulant, whereas in high doses it may act as a cardiac and respiratory depressant.[15,18,23]
- Berberine was shown to have anti-platelet activity.[24]
- Barberine, oxyacanthine, and barbamine were shown to have anti-inflammatory effects.[25–28]
- Barberine was found to have an anti-diarrheal effects.[30]
- Barberine was found to inhibit parathyroid hormone-stimulated bone resorption, inhibit osteoclastic bone resorption and prevent a decrease in bone mineral density of the lumbar vertebra.[32]

Drug interactions

Anti-coagulant drugs[24]
Highly protein-bound drugs[14]

Parts used[17]

Root

References

1. Jellin JM, Batz F, Hitchens K. Natural Medicines Comprehensive Database, 3rd ed. Stockton, CA: Therapeutic Research Faculty, 2002:1530.
2. Sheng WD, Jiddawi MS, Hong XQ, Abdulla SM. Treatment of chloroquine-resistant malaria using pyrimethamine in combination with berberine, tetracycline or cotrimoxazole. East Afr Med J 1997; 74:283–284.
3. Rabbani GH, Butler T, Knight J, Sanyal SC, Alam K. Randomized controlled trial of berberine sulfate therapy for diarrhea due to enterotoxigenic Escherichia coli and Vibrio cholerae. J Infect Dis 1987; 155:979–984.
4. Swabb EA, Tai YH, Jordan L. Reversal of cholera toxin-induced secretion in rat ileum by luminal berberine. Am J Physiol 1981; 241:G248–252.
5. Khosla PK, Neeraj VI, Gupta SK, Satpathy G. Berberine, a potential drug for trachoma. Rev Int Trach Pathol Ocul Trop Subtrop Sante Publique 1992; 69:147–165.
6. Mohan M, Pant CR, Angra SK, Mahajan VM. Berberine in trachoma. (A clinical trial). Indian J Ophthalmol 1982; 30:69–75.
7. Zeng X, Zeng X. Relationship between the clinical effects of berberine on severe congestive heart failure and its concentration in plasma studied by HPLC. Biomed Chromatogr 1999; 13:442–444.
8. Stermitz FR, Lorenz P, Tawara JN, Zenewicz LA, Lewis K. Synergy in a medicinal plant: anti-microbial action of berberine potentiated by 5′-methoxyhydnocarpin, a multidrug pump inhibitor. Proc Natl Acad Sci USA 2000; 97:1433–1437.
9. Stermitz FR, Tawara-Matsuda J, Lorenz P et al. 5′-Methoxyhydnocarpin-D and pheophorbide A: Berberis species components that potentiate berberine growth inhibition of resistant Staphylococcus aureus. J Nat Prod 2000; 63:1146–1149.
10. Mahady GB, Pendland SL, Stoia A, Chadwick LR. In vitro susceptibility of Helicobacter pylori to isoquinoline alkaloids from Sanguinaria canadensis and Hydrastis canadensis. Phytother Res 2003; 17:217–221.
11. Anis KV, Rajeshkumar NV, Kuttan R. Inhibition of chemical carcinogenesis by berberine in rats and mice. J Pharm Pharmacol 2001; 53:763–768.
12. Chung JG, Chen GW, Hung CF et al. Effects of berberine on arylamine N-acetyltransferase activity and 2-aminofluorene-DNA adduct formation in human leukemia cells. Am J Chin Med 2000; 28:227–238.
13. Fukuda K, Hibiya Y, Mutoh M et al. Inhibition by berberine of cyclooxygenase-2 transcriptional activity in human colon cancer cells. J Ethnopharmacol 1999; 66:227–233.
14. Chan E. Displacement of bilirubin from albumin by berberine. Biol Neonate 1993; 63:201–208.
15. McGuffin M, Hobbs C, Upton R, Goldberg A. American Herbal Products Association's Botanical Safety Handbook. Boca Raton, FL: CRC Press, 1997:231.
16. Farnsworth NR, Bingel AS, Cordell G, Crane FA, Fong HH. Potential value of plants as sources of new anti-fertility agents I. J Pharm Sci 1975; 64:535–598.

17. Brinker F. The Toxicology of Botanical Medicines. Sandy, OR: Eclectic Medical Publications, 2000:296.
18. Leung AY, Foster S. Encyclopedia of Common Natural Ingredients Used in Food, Drugs and Cosmetics, 2nd ed. New York, NY: John Wiley & Sons, 1996:649.
19. Abel G. [Chromosome-damaging effect of beta-asaron on human lymphocytes]. Planta Med 1987; 53:251–253.
20. Ghosh AK, Bhattacharyya FK, Ghosh DK. Leishmania donovani: amastigote inhibition and mode of action of berberine. Exp Parasitol 1985; 60:404–413.
21. Ghosh AK, Rakshit MM, Ghosh DK. Effect of berberine chloride on Leishmania donovani. Indian J Med Res 1983; 78:407–416.
22. Mahajan VM, Sharma A, Rattan A. Anti-mycotic activity of berberine sulphate: an alkaloid from an Indian medicinal herb. Sabouraudia 1982; 20:79–81.
23. Foster S, Tyler VE. Tyler's Honest Herbal. Binghamton, NY: Haworth Herbal Press, 1999.
24. Huang CG, Chu ZL, Wei SJ, Jiang H, Jiao BH. Effect of berberine on arachidonic acid metabolism in rabbit platelets and endothelial cells. Thromb Res 2002; 106:223–227.
25. Ivanovska N, Philipov S. Study on the anti-inflammatory action of Berberis vulgaris root extract, alkaloid fractions and pure alkaloids. Int J Immunopharmacol 1996; 18:553–561.
26. Ivanovska N, Philipov S, Hristova M. Influence of berberine on T-cell mediated immunity. Immunopharmacol Immunotoxicol 1999; 21:771–786.
27. Kupeli E, Kosar M, Yesilada E, Husnu K, Baser C. A comparative study on the anti-inflammatory, anti-nociceptive and anti-pyretic effects of isoquinoline alkaloids from the roots of Turkish Berberis species. Life Sci 2002; 72:645–657.
28. Yesilada E, Kupeli E. Berberis crataegina DC. root exhibits potent anti-inflammatory, analgesic and febrifuge effects in mice and rats. J Ethnopharmacol 2002; 79:237–248.
29. Zhang MF, Shen YQ. [Anti-diarrheal and anti-inflammatory effects of berberine]. Zhongguo Yao Li Xue Bao 1989; 10:174–176.
30. Li H, Miyahara T, Tezuka Y et al. The effect of kampo formulae on bone resorption in vitro and in vivo. II. Detailed study of berberine. Biol Pharm Bull 1999; 22:391–396.
31. Pan GY, Wang GJ, Liu XD, Fawcett JP, Xie YY. The involvement of P-glycoprotein in berberine absorption. Pharmacol Toxicol 2002; 91:193–197.

BLACK COHOSH
Cimicifuga racemosa

Synonyms/common names/related substances[1]

Baneberry, black snakeroot, bugbane, bugwort, cimicifuga, macrotys, phytoestrogen, rattle root, rattle snakeroot, rattle top, rattlesnake root, rattleweed, snakeroot, squaw root, squawroot

Indications

Menopausal symptoms:[2–4]	Evidence grade B1
Arthritis pain (with white willow bark, sarsaparilla, poplar bark and guaiacum resin):[5]	Evidence grade B2
Induction of labor:[6]	Evidence grade E

Pregnancy

Induces labor:[6]	Evidence level 4

A survey of midwives in the USA found that 45% use black cohosh to induce labor.[6] Black cohosh is part of a combination of herbal medicines that have been traditionally used in the third trimester to prepare a woman for delivery; this preparation is called 'mother's cordial' or 'partus preparatus'. In addition to black cohosh, mother's cordial contains: squaw vine *(Mitchella ripens)*, raspberry (*Rubus idaeus*), blue cohosh *(Caulophyllum thalictroides)* and false unicorn (*Chamaelirium luteum*).

Hormonal effect (potentially estrogenic and/or anti-estrogenic):[7]	Evidence level 4

It is unclear if black cohosh has an estrogenic and/or an anti-estrogenic effect.[7] Nonetheless, a review article recommended that black cohosh be avoided during pregnancy due to its potential hormonal effect.[7]

Emmenagogue (especially in first trimester):[8]	Evidence level 4

A herbal contraindication and drug interaction compendium reported that black cohosh was an emmenagogue and contraindicated during pregnancy, particularly in the first trimester.[8]

Anovulatory effects:[9]	Evidence level 4

A review article on the potential value of plants as sources of anti-fertility agents reported that black cohosh had anovulatory effects in vitro.[9]

Lactation

Hormonal effect (potentially estrogenic/anti-estrogenic):[7] Evidence level 4

It is unclear if black cohosh has an estrogenic and/or an anti-estrogenic effect.[7] Nonetheless, a review article recommended that black cohosh be avoided during lactation due to its potential hormonal effect.[7]

Constitutents

- Triterpene glycosides:[8] acetin, cimicifugoside, 27-deoxyacetin
- Organic acids: isoferulic acid,[8] cimicifugic acids (A, B, E and F), fukinolic acid,[1] caffeic acid,[1] salicylic acid[1]
- Cimicifugin[8]
- Tannins[8]
- Phytosterin[1]

Pharmacology

- In some studies, black cohosh constituents bind to estrogen receptors in vitro or have an estrogenic effect.[10–13] In other studies, black cohosh estrogenic or estrogen receptor-binding effects were not found.[14,15]
- Black cohosh antagonizes the proliferation of cells induced by estradiol in vitro, thereby having anti-estrogenic acitivity.[16]
- Black cohosh decreases luteinizing hormone (LH) levels, but has no effect on follicular stimulating hormone (FSH) levels.[12]
- Black cohosh inhibits the growth of human breast cancer cells in vitro.[17,18]
- Black cohosh has anti-inflammatory effects where the constituents caffeic acid, fukinolic acid and cimicifugic acids (A, B, E, F) were found to inhibit neutrophil elastase activity in vitro.[19]
- Black cohosh possesses a central activity instead of a hormonal effect.[20]

Drug interactions

Docetaxel[21]
Doxorubicin[21]

Parts used[8]

Roots, rhizome

References

1. Jellin JM, Batz F, Hitchens K. Natural Medicines Comprehensive Database. Stockton, CA: Therapeutic Research Faculty, 2004:1530.
2. Stoll W. [Phytopharmaceutical influences on atrophic vaginal epithelium. Double-blind study on Cimicifuga vs. an estrogen preparation]. Therapeutickon 1987; 1:23–32.
3. Warnecke G. Using phyto-treatment to influence menopause symptoms. Med Welt 1985; 36:871–874.

4. Lehmann-Willenbrock E, Riedel HH. [Clinical and endocrinologic studies of the treatment of ovarian insufficiency manifestations following hysterectomy with intact adnexa]. Zentralbl Gynakol 1988; 110:611–618.
5. Mills SY, Jacoby RK, Chacksfield M, Willoughby M. Effect of a proprietary herbal medicine on the relief of chronic arthritic pain: a double-blind study. Br J Rheumatol 1996; 35:874–878.
6. McFarlin BL, Gibson MH, O'Rear J, Harman P. A national survey of herbal preparation use by nurse-midwives for labor stimulation. Review of the literature and recommendations for practice. J Nurse Midwifery 1999; 44:205–216.
7. Mahady GB, Fabricant D, Chadwick LR, Dietz B. Black cohosh: an alternative therapy for menopause? Nutr Clin Care 2002; 5:283–289.
8. Brinker F. The Toxicology of Botanical Medicines. Sandy, OR: Eclectic Medical Publications, 2000:296.
9. Farnsworth NR, Bingel AS, Cordell GA, Crane FA, Fong HH. Potential value of plants as sources of new anti-fertility agents I. J Pharm Sci 1975; 64:535–598.
10. Jarry H, Harnischfeger G, Duker E. [The endocrine effects of constituents of Cimicifuga racemosa. 2. In vitro binding of constituents to estrogen receptors]. Planta Med 1985; 4:316–4319.
11. Liu Z, YZ, Zhu M, Huo J. [Estrogenicity of black cohosh (Cimicifuga racemosa) and its effect on estrogen receptor level in human breast cancer MCF-7 cells]. Wei Sheng Yan Jiu 2001; 30:77–80.
12. Duker EM, Kopanski L, Jarry H, Wuttke W. Effects of extracts from Cimicifuga racemosa on gonadotropin release in menopausal women and ovariectomized rats. Planta Med 1991; 57:420–424.
13. Kruse SO, Lohning A, Pauli GF, Winterhoff H, Nahrstedt A. Fukiic and piscidic acid esters from the rhizome of Cimicifuga racemosa and the in vitro estrogenic activity of fukinolic acid. Planta Med 1999; 65:763–764.
14. Liu J, Burdette J, Xu H et al. Evaluation of estrogenic activity of plant extracts for the potential treatment of menopausal symptoms. J Agric Food Chem 2001; 49:2472–2479.
15. Einer-Jensen N, Zhao J, Andersen KP, Kristoffersen K. Cimicifuga and Melbrosia lack oestrogenic effects in mice and rats. Maturitas 1996; 25:149–153.
16. Zierau O, Bodinet C, Kolba S, Wulf M, Vollmer G. Anti-estrogenic activities of Cimicifuga racemosa extracts. J Steroid Biochem Mol Biol 2002; 80:125–130.
17. Bodinet C, Freudenstein J. Influence of Cimicifuga racemosa on the proliferation of estrogen receptor-positive human breast cancer cells. Breast Cancer Res Treat 2002; 76:1–10.
18. Dixon-Shanies D, Shaikh N. Growth inhibition of human breast cancer cells by herbs and phytoestrogens. Oncol Rep 1999; 6:1383–1387.
19. Loser B, Kruse S, Melzig MF, Nahrstedt A. Inhibition of neutrophil elastase activity by cinnamic acid derivatives from Cimicifuga racemosa. Planta Med 2000; 66:751–753.
20. Borrelli F, Izzo A, Ernst E. Pharmacological effects of Cimicifuga racemosa. Life Sci 2003; 73:1215–1229.
21. Jellin JM, Batz F, Hitchens K. Natural Medicines Comprehensive Database, 3rd ed. Stockton, CA: Therapeutic Research Faculty, 2004:1530.

BLAZING STAR
Aletris farinosa

Synonyms/common names/related substances[1,2]
Ague grass, ague root, aloerot, colic root, crow corn, devil's-bit, stargrass, starwort, true-unicorn root, unicorn root, whitetube stargrass

Indications

Menstrual complaints:[3]	Evidence grade E

Pregnancy

Uterine stimulant:[4]	Evidence level 4

A review article on the potential value of plants as sources of anti-fertility agents reported that blazing star was a uterine stimulant.[4]

Uterine relaxant:[1,5]	Evidence level 4
Estrogenic:[6]	Evidence level 4

A herbal safety and drug interaction compendium reported that blazing star was a uterine relaxant.[1,5] A botanical safety compendium reported that blazing star has estrogenic and oxytoxic activity.[6] There are no reports in the medical literature of blazing star having estrogenic or oxytoxic activity nor are there reports that blazing star is contraindicated or safe during pregnancy.

Lactation

Oxytoxin antagonism:[6]	Evidence level 4

A botanical safety compendium reported that blazing star has estrogenic and oxytoxic activity.[6] There are no reports in the medical literature of blazing star having estrogenic or oxytoxic activity nor are there reports that blazing star is contraindicated or safe during lactation.

Contraindication
Infectious or inflammatory gastrointestinal conditions[5]

Caution
Hormone sensitive cancers (breast, uterine and ovarian)[3]
Endometriosis[3]
Uterine fibroids[3]

Constituents[1,3]

Diosgenin, volatile oils, and resin

Pharmacology

- Aletris was found to be estrogenic.[3]
- Diosgenin is one of the starting hormones use in the manufacture of steroid hormones.[3]
- Aletris may increase stomach acid secretion.[5]
- Aletris is an irritant to the gastrointestinal tract.[5]

Drug interactions

Oxytocin drugs[6]
Acid-inhibiting drugs[5]

Parts used[1]

Root

References

1. Brinker F. The Toxicology of Botanical Medicines. Sandy, OR: Eclectic Medical Publications, 2000:296.
2. Jellin JM, Batz F, Hitchens K. Natural Medicines Comprehensive Database, 3rd ed. Stockton, CA: Therapeutic Research Faculty, 2002:1530.
3. Leung AY, Foster S. Encyclopedia of Common Natural Ingredients Used in Food, Drugs and Cosmetics, 2nd ed. New York, NY: John Wiley & Sons, 1996:649.
4. Farnsworth NR, Bingel AS, Cordell G, Crane FA, Fong HH. Potential value of plants as sources of new anti-fertility agents I. J Pharm Sci 1975; 64:535–598.
5. Brinker F. Herb Contraindications and Drug Interactions, 3rd ed. Sandy, OR: Eclectic Medical Publications, 2001:432.
6. McGuffin M, Hobbs C, Upton R, Goldberg A. American Herbal Products Association's Botanical Safety Handbook. Boca Raton, FL: CRC Press, 1997:231.

BLUE COHOSH
Caulophyllum thalictroides

Synonyms/common names/related substances[1]
Blue ginseng, caulophyllum, papoose root, squaw root, yellow ginseng

Indications

Induction of labor:[2]	Evidence grade E

Pregnancy

Congestive heart failure:[3]	Evidence level 2

There is one report of a newborn infant whose mother ingested blue cohosh to promote uterine contractions. The newborn presented at birth with acute myocardial infarction associated with profound congestive heart failure and shock.[3] The infant remained critically ill for several weeks, although he eventually recovered.[3] The authors reported that all other causes of myocardial infarction were carefully excluded.[3] The authors believed that these observed effects were due to the vasoactive glycosides and an alkaloid of blue cohosh known to produce toxic effects on the myocardium.[3]

Severe multi-organ hypoxic injury:[4]	Evidence level 2

There is one report of severe multi-organ hypoxic injury in a child delivered 'naturally' with the aid of both blue and black cohosh (*Caulophyllum thalictroides*) who was not breathing at the time of birth.[4] The child survived with permanent central nervous system damage.[4] Blue cohosh possesses a vasoconstrictive glycoside which may have been responsible for the adverse effects.[4]

Abortifacient:[5–7]	Evidence level 2

Uterine stimulant:[5–7]	Evidence level 2

Emmenagogue:[7]	Evidence level 4

A 21-year-old woman developed signs of nicotinic toxicity, i.e. tachycardia, diaphoresis, abdominal pain, vomiting, and muscle weakness and fasciculations after using blue cohosh in an attempt to induce an abortion.[6] The saponins in blue cohosh are believed to be responsible for the uterine stimulant effect.[8] A review article on the potential value of plants as sources of anti-fertility agents also reported that blue cohosh was a potential abortifacient, emmenagogue, and uterine stimulant.[7]

Teratogenic:[8,9]	Evidence level 4

Embryotoxic:[9]	Evidence level 4

The alkaloid methylcytisine, a constituent of blue cohosh, was shown to be teratogenic in rats.[8,9] The alkaloid taspine, a constituent of blue cohosh, was shown to be highly embryotoxic in rats.[9]

Oxytocic:[10]	Evidence level 4

A compendium for medicinal plants reported that blue cohosh may have oxytocic effects.[10] Blue cohosh was not reported in the scientific literature as having an oxytocic effect.

Induces labor:[2]	Evidence level 4

A survey of midwives in the USA found that 64% use blue cohosh to induce labor.[2] Blue cohosh is part of a combination of herbal medicines that have been traditionally used in the third trimester to prepare a woman for delivery; this preparation is called 'mother's cordial' or 'partus preparatus'. In addition to blue cohosh, mother's cordial contains: squaw vine (*Mitchella ripens*), raspberry (*Rubus idaeus*), black cohosh (*Cimicifuga racemosa*) and false unicorn (*Chamaelirium luteum*).

Homeopathic blue cohosh (Caulophyllum)

Does not induce labor:[11,12]	Evidence level 1a

A systematic review concluded that there is insufficient evidence to recommend the use of homeopathic blue cohosh as a method of inducing of labor.[11,12] Although caulophyllum is a commonly used homeopathic therapy to induce labor, the treatment strategy used in this review may not reflect routine practice of homeopathy. A homeopathic preparation of *C. thalictroides,* called Caulophyllum, beyond the potency (dilution) of 12C, does not contain any molecules of the original substance.

Lactation

Possible cardiotoxic effects:[3]	Evidence level 4

Blue cohosh contains vasoactive glycosides and an alkaloid known to produce toxic effects on the myocardium of laboratory animals. Blue cohosh is not reported in the scientific literature as being either contraindicated or safe in lactation.

Constituents

- Triterpene saponins:[10,13] caulophyllogenin, hederagenin, caulosaponin
- Alkaloids:[9] thalictroidine, taspine, magnoflorine, anagyrine, baptifoline, 5,6-dehydro-α-isolupanine, α-isolupanine, lupanine, *N*-methylcytisine, sparteine

Toxicology

- Blue cohosh contains vasoactive glycosides and an alkaloid known to produce toxic effects on the myocardium of laboratory animals.
- Blue cohosh was reported to constrict coronary arteries and to decrease the flow of oxygen to the heart.[14]
- The alkaloid methylcytisine was shown to cause symptoms of nicotinic toxicity.[6]
- Methylcytisine was shown to be teratogenic in rats.[9]
- Taspine was shown to be embryotoxic in rats.[9]

Pharmacology

- Blue cohosh extract was shown to enhance estradiol binding to estrogen receptors and to increase estradiol-induced transcription activity in estrogen-responsive cells.[1]
- Blue cohosh was shown to decrease luteinizing hormone levels and to increase serum ceruloplasmin oxidase activity, which are measures of estrogenic activity in the liver.[1]

Drug interactions

Anti-diabetic drugs[1]
Cardiovascular drugs[3,10]
Nicotine[6]

Parts used[1]

Rhizome and root

References

1. Jellin JM, Batz F, Hitchens K. Natural Medicines Comprehensive Database. Stockton, CA: Therapeutic Research Faculty, 2002:1530.
2. McFarlin BL, Gibson MH, O'Rear J, Harman P. A national survey of herbal preparation use by nurse-midwives for labor stimulation. Review of the literature and recommendations for practice. J Nurse Midwifery 1999; 44:205–216.
3. Jones TK, Lawson B. Profound neonatal congestive heart failure caused by maternal consumption of blue cohosh herbal medication. J Pediatr 1998; 132(3 Pt 1):550–552.
4. Gunn TR, Wright IM. The use of black and blue cohosh in labour. N Z Med J 1996; 109:410–411.
5. McGuffin M, Hobbs C, Upton R, Goldberg A. American Herbal Products Association's Botanical Safety Handbook. Boca Raton, FL: CRC Press, 1997:231.
6. Rao RB, Hoffman R. Nicotinic toxicity from tincture of blue cohosh (Caulophyllum thalictroides) used as an abortifacient. Vet Hum Toxicol 2002; 44:221–222.
7. Farnsworth NR, Bingel AS, Cordell GA, Crane FA, Fong HH. Potential value of plants as sources of new antifertility agents I. J Pharm Sci 1975; 64:535–598.
8. Ganzera M, Dharmaratne H, Nanayakkara NP, Khan IA. Determination of saponins and alkaloids in Caulophyllum thalictroides (blue cohosh) by high-performance liquid chromatography and evaporative light scattering detection. Phytochem Anal 2003; 14:1–7.

9. Kennelly EJ, Flynn T, Mazzola EP et al. Detecting potential teratogenic alkaloids from blue cohosh rhizomes using an in vitro rat embryo culture. J Nat Prod 1999; 62:1385–1389.
10. Newall CA, Anderson LA, Phillipson JD. Herbal Medicines: A Guide for Health-care Professionals. London, UK: Pharmaceutical Press, 1996:296.
11. Smith CA. Homoeopathy for induction of labour. Cochrane Database Syst Rev 2001:CD003399.
12. Beer AM, Heiliger F. Randomized, double-blind trial of caulophyllum d4 for induction of labor after premature rupture of the membranes at term. Geburtshilfe und Frauenheilkunde 1999; 59:431–435.
13. Jhoo JW, Sang S, He K et al. Characterization of the triterpene saponins of the roots and rhizomes of blue cohosh (Caulophyllum thalictroides). J Agric Food Chem 2001; 49:5969–5974.
14. Edmunds J. Blue cohosh and newborn myocardial infarction? Midwifery Today Int Midwife 1999; Winter:34–35.

BORAGE
Borago officinalis

Synonyms/common names/related substances[1]

Borage oil, bugloss, burage, burrage, huile de bourrache, starflower

Indications

Oral

Rheumatoid arthritis:[2]	Evidence grade B1
*Atopic dermatitis:[3–6]	Evidence grade B1
Adult periodontitis:[7]	Evidence grade B1
Attenuates stress:[8]	Evidence grade B2
Hyperlipidemia:[9]	Evidence grade C
Atherosclerosis prevention:[9]	Evidence grade C
Skin irritation:[10]	Evidence grade C
Gastric cancer prevention:[11]	Evidence grade D
Hypertension:[12]	Evidence grade E

*One randomized controlled trial reported that several clinical symptoms of atopic dermatitis improved compared with placebo, but the overall response to borage oil did not reach statistical significance.[6] This study, however, found statistically significant benefits of borage oil on atopic dermatitis in a subgroup of the research subjects.[6]

Enteral

Acute respiratory distress syndrome (with eicosapentaenoic acid (EPA; fish oil) and antioxidants):[13]	Evidence grade B1

Topical

Infantile seborrheic dermatitis:[14]	Evidence grade B2

Pregnancy

Teratogenic and induces labor:[15]	Evidence level 1a

A review of randomized double-blind studies was conducted on the benefit of borage oil in the treatment of rheumatoid arthritis.[15] Evidence from published research indicated that the γ-linolenic acid (GLA) component of borage oil increases prostaglandin E levels.[15] It was recommended that borage oil be contraindicated in pregnancy given the teratogenic and labor-inducing effects of prostaglandin E agonists.[15]

Minimal risk:[16]	Evidence level 3

A study compared the effects of diets containing GLA from borage oil and other sources on reproduction, pup development and pup brain fatty acid composition in mice.[16] An increase in dietary GLA resulted in an increase in brain long chain n-6 fatty acids (20:4n-6 and 22:4n-6).[16] The authors did not report any adverse effects associated with the ingestion of borage oil.[16]

Fetotoxin:[17]	Evidence level 4
Mutagen:[17]	Evidence level 4
Hepatotoxic:[18,19]	Evidence level 4
Pneumotoxic:[18,19]	Evidence level 4
Genotoxic:[18,19]	Evidence level 4
Neurotoxic:[18,19]	Evidence level 4
Cytotoxic:[18,19]	Evidence level 4

Borage oil has been reported to contain small amounts of pyrrolizidine alkaloids.[20] Pyrrolizidine alkaloids are hepatotoxic, pneumotoxic, genotoxic, neurotoxic and cytotoxic, and may cause hepatic veno-occlusive disease.[18,19] A compendium on complementary and alternative medicine reported that therapeutic doses of borage seed oil can provide amounts of pyrrolizidine alkaloids that can reach toxic levels.[21] Borage seed oil containing pyrrolizidine alkaloids, dosed at 1–2 g/day, may provide approximately 10 μg of pyrrolizidine alkaloids, which exceeds the German Commission E recommendation by 10 times.[21,22]

Anti-gonadotrophic activity:[23]	Evidence level 4

A review article on the potential value of plants as sources of anti-fertility agents reported that borage had anti-gonadotrophic activity in rats.[23]

Lactation

Minimal risk:[24]	Evidence level 1b

A cross-sectional study was conducted on the effect of dietary supplementation of borage oil on the breast milk of atopic mothers.[24] Twenty atopic mothers received borage oil for 1 week (230 mg or 460 mg of GLA) and 20 non-atopic mothers received a placebo.[24] Arachidonic acid was found to be lower in breast milk of atopic mothers compared with non-atopic mothers.[24] Supplementation of the atopic mothers with borage oil significantly increased the levels of GLA and dihomo-GLA in breast milk in a dose-related way, but the level of arachidonic acid was not increased.[24] The authors did not report any adverse effects of borage oil supplementation on the mother or the infant.[24]

Mutagen:[17]	Evidence level 4

Hepatotoxic:[18,19]	Evidence level 4

Pneumotoxic:[18,19]	Evidence level 4

Genotoxic:[18,19]	Evidence level 4

Neurotoxic:[18,19]	Evidence level 4

Cytotoxic:[18,19]	Evidence level 4

Borage oil has been reported to contain small amounts of pyrrolizidine alkaloids.[20] Pyrrolizidine alkaloids are hepatotoxic, pneumotoxic, genotoxic, neurotoxic and cytotoxic, and may cause hepatic veno-occlusive disease.[18,19]

Constituents

GLA[15]
Pyrrolizidine alkaloids[20]

Pharmacology

- Diets rich in borage oil were shown to reduce systolic blood pressure, lower aldosterone, increase plasma renin and inhibit adrenal responsiveness to angiotensin II.[25]
- Borage oil alters stress reactivity in humans by attenuating blood pressure and heart rate responses to stress, increasing skin temperature, improving task performance, and augment the arterial baroreflex control of vascular resistance.[8,26]
- The borage oil constituent GLA increases prostaglandin E levels and reduces T cell proliferation in vivo.[15,27]
- Borage oil reverses epidermal hyperproliferation.[28]

- GLA supplementation was shown to decrease plasma triglyceride, increase high-density lipoprotein cholesterol, and significantly decrease total cholesterol and low-density lipoprotein cholesterol.[9]
- GLA supplementation was shown to decrease platelet aggregation and increase bleeding time by 40%.[9]
- Borage oil supplementation does not improve insulin sensitivity in vivo.[29]

Drug interactions

Anesthesia[30,31]
Anti-convulsant/anti-seizure drugs[31]
Anti-coagulant/anti-platelet drugs[9]
Nonsteroidal anti-inflammatory drugs[2,15]
Phenothiazines[32]

Parts used[17]

Seed and leaves

References

1. Jellin JM, Batz F, Hitchens K. Natural Medicines Comprehensive Database. Stockton, CA: Therapeutic Research Faculty, 2002:1530.
2. Leventhal LJ, Boyce EG, Zurier RB. Treatment of rheumatoid arthritis with gammalinolenic acid. Ann Intern Med 1993; 119:867–873.
3. van Gool CJ, Thijs C, Henquet CJ et al. Gamma-linolenic acid supplementation for prophylaxis of atopic dermatitis – a randomized controlled trial in infants at high familial risk. Am J Clin Nutr 2003; 77:943–951.
4. Buslau M, Thaci D. Atopic dermatitis: Borage oil for systemic therapy. Zeitschrift Fur Dermatologie 1996; 182:131–136.
5. Bahmer FA, Schafer J. [Treatment of atopic dermatitis with borage seed oil (Glandol)– a time series analytic study]. Kinderarztliche Praxis 1992; 60:199–202.
6. Henz BM, Jablonska S, van de Kerkhof PC et al. Double-blind, multicentre analysis of the efficacy of borage oil in patients with atopic eczema. Br J Dermatol 1999; 140:685–688.
7. Rosenstein ED, Kushner LJ, Kramer N, Kazandjian G. Pilot study of dietary fatty acid supplementation in the treatment of adult periodontitis. Prostaglandins Leukot Essent Fatty Acids 2003; 68:213–218.
8. Mills DE, Prkachin KM, Harvey KA, Ward RP. Dietary fatty acid supplementation alters stress reactivity and performance in man. J Hum Hypertens 1989; 3:111–116.
9. Guivernau M, Meza N, Barja P, Roman O. Clinical and experimental study on the long-term effect of dietary gamma-linolenic acid on plasma lipids, platelet aggregation, thromboxane formation, and prostacyclin production. Prostaglandins Leukot Essent Fatty Acids 1994; 51:311–316.
10. Loden M, Andersson AC. Effect of topically applied lipids on surfactant-irritated skin. Br J Dermatol 1996; 134:215–221.
11. Gonzalez CA, Sanz JM, Marcos G et al. Borage consumption as a possible gastric cancer protective factor. Cancer Epidemiol Biomarkers Prev 1993; 2:157–158.
12. Engler MM, Engler MB, Erickson SK, Paul SM. Dietary gamma-linolenic acid lowers blood pressure and alters aortic reactivity and cholesterol metabolism in hypertension. J Hypertens 1992; 10:1197–1204.

13. Gadek JE, DeMichele SJ, Karlstad MD et al. Effect of enteral feeding with eicosapentaenoic acid, gamma-linolenic acid, and antioxidants in patients with acute respiratory distress syndrome. Enteral Nutrition in ARDS Study Group. Crit Care Med 1999; 27:1409–1420.
14. Tollesson A, Frithz A. Transepidermal water loss and water content in the stratum corneum in infantile seborrhoeic dermatitis. Acta Derm Venereol 1993; 73:18–20.
15. Kast RE. Borage oil reduction of rheumatoid arthritis activity may be mediated by increased cAMP that suppresses tumor necrosis factor-alpha. Int Immunopharmacol 2001; 1:2197–2199.
16. Wainwright PE, Huang YS, DeMichele SJ et al. Effects of high-gamma-linolenic acid canola oil compared with borage oil on reproduction, growth, and brain and behavioral development in mice. Lipids 2003; 38:171–178.
17. Brinker F. Herb Contraindications and Drug Interactions. Sandy, OR: Eclectic Medical Publications, 2001:432.
18. Stickel F, Seitz HK, Hahn EG, Schuppan D. [Liver toxicity of drugs of plant origin]. Z Gastroenterol 2001; 39:225–232, 234–237.
19. Roeder E. Medicinal plants in China containing pyrrolizidine alkaloids. Pharmazie 2000; 55:711–726.
20. De Smet PAGM, Keller K, Hansel R, Chandler RF. Adverse Effects of Herbal Drugs. Vol. 1. New York, NY: Springer-Verlag, 1992.
21. Fetrow CW, Avala JR. Professional's Handbook of Complementary and Alternative Medicines. Philadelphia, PA: Springhouse Corporation, 2001:895.
22. Blumenthal M, Busse WR, Goldberg A et al. The Complete German Commission E Monographs: Therapeutic Guide to Herbal Medicines. Boston, MA: American Botanical Council, 1998.
23. Farnsworth NR, Bingel AS, Cordell GA, Crane FA, Fong HH. Potential value of plants as sources of new antifertility agents I. J Pharm Sci 1975; 64:535–598.
24. Thijs C, Houwelingen A, Poorterman I, Mordant A, van den Brandt P. Essential fatty acids in breast milk of atopic mothers: comparison with non-atopic mothers, and effect of borage oil supplementation. Eur J Clin Nutr 2000; 54:234–238.
25. Engler MM, Schambelan M, Engler MB, Ball DL, Goodfriend TL. Effects of dietary gamma-linolenic acid on blood pressure and adrenal angiotensin receptors in hypertensive rats. Proc Soc Exp Biol Med 1998; 218:234–237.
26. Mills DE, Mah M, Ward RP, Morris BL, Floras JS. Alteration of baroreflex control of forearm vascular resistance by dietary fatty acids. Am J Physiol 1990; 259:R1164–71.
27. Rossetti RG, Seiler CM, DeLuca P, Laposata M, Zurier RB. Oral administration of unsaturated fatty acids: effects on human peripheral blood T lymphocyte proliferation. J Leukoc Biol 1997; 62:438–443.
28. Chung S, Kong S, Seong K, Cho Y. Gamma-linolenic acid in borage oil reverses epidermal hyperproliferation in guinea pigs. J Nutr 2002; 132:3090–3097.
29. Simoncikova P, Wein S, Gasperikova D et al. Comparison of the extrapancreatic action of gamma-linolenic acid and n-3 PUFAs in the high fat diet-induced insulin resistance. Endocr Regul 2002; 36:143–149.
30. Shaw D, Leon C, Kolev S, Murray V. Traditional remedies and food supplements. A 5-year toxicological study (1991–1995). Drug Saf 1997; 17:342–356.
31. Miller LG. Herbal medicinals: selected clinical considerations focusing on known or potential drug–herb interactions. Arch Intern Med 1998; 158:2200–2211.
32. Newall CA, Anderson LA, Phillipson JD. Herbal Medicines: A Guide for Health-care Professionals. London, UK: Pharmaceutical Press, 1996:296.

CALAMUS
Acorus calamus

Synonyms/common names/related substances[1]
Cinnamon sedge, gladdon, grass myrtle, myrtle flag, myrtle sedge, sweet cane, sweet cinnamon, sweet flag, sweet grass, sweet myrtle, sweet root, sweet rush, sweet sedge

Indications

Urinary tract disorders, digestive stimulant:[2,3]	Evidence grade E

Pregnancy

Potentially hepatocarcinogenic:[4–8]	Evidence level 3

Calamus contains β-asarone, a volatile oil which has been shown to be hepatocarcinogenic in animal studies and in laboratory studies on human lymphocytes.[4–8]

Emmenagogue:[9]	Evidence level 4

Potential abortifiacient:[9]	Evidence level 4

A review article on the potential value of plants as sources of anti-fertility agents reported that calamus was an emmenagogue and a potential abortifiacient.[9]

Lactation

Potentially hepatocarcinogenic:[4–8]	Evidence level 3

Calamus contains β-asarone, a volatile oil which has been shown to be hepatocarcinogenic in animal studies and in laboratory studies on human lymphocytes.[4–8]

Constituents
Essential oils:[5,7,8,10] α- and β-asarone (volatile ethers)

Toxicology
LD_{50} of the tincture (1:2): 5 mL/kg[10]
Dietary levels of 500–5000 ppm of oil are carcinogenic in animals[10]

Pharmacology
- β-Asarone is potentially hepatocarcinogenic.[7] Once β-asarone has undergone metabolic 1′-hydroxylation in the liver, its carcinogenic potency is low

and its major metabolite (2,4,5-trimethoxycinnamic acid) was not reported as carcinogenic.[7,8,11]

- Calamus oil inhibits monoamine oxidase (MAO) activity and stimulates D- and L-amino oxidase.[12]
- β-Asarone has anti-spasmodic activity in vitro in the tracheal, intestinal, uterine, bronchial and vascular smooth muscle.[12,13]
- Calamus has a sedative effect and potentiates the barbiturate effect (increased sleeping time, reduction in body temperature).[12]
- α-Asarone decreases low-density lipoprotein cholesterol and triglycerides and increases high-density lipoproteins.[14,15]
- α-Asarone is non-mutagenic in mice.[16]

Drug interactions

Anti-coagulant drugs[17]
MOA inhibitor drugs[12]
Sedative/barbiturate drugs[12]

Part containing toxins[10,18]

Rhizome

References

1. Jellin JM, Batz F, Hitchens K. Natural Medicines Comprehensive Database. Stockton, CA: Therapeutic Research Faculty, 2002:1530.
2. Bruneton J. Pharmacognosy, Phytochemistry, Medicinal Plants. Secausus, NJ: Lavoisier Pub, 1999:1119.
3. Reynolds JEF, Parfitt K, Parsons AV. Martindale: The Extra Pharmacopoeia/The Royal Pharmaceutical Society, 31st ed. London, UK: Royal Pharmaceutical Society, 1996:2739.
4. Abel G. [Chromosome-damaging effect of beta-asaron on human lymphocytes]. Planta Med 1987; 53:251–253.
5. Goggelmann W, Schimmer O. Mutagenicity testing of beta-asarone and commercial calamus drugs with Salmonella typhimurium. Mutat Res 1983; 121:191–194.
6. Kevekordes S, Spielberger J, Burghaus CM et al. Micronucleus formation in human lymphocytes and in the metabolically competent human hepatoma cell line Hep-G2: results with 15 naturally occurring substances. Anticancer Res 2001; 21:461–469.
7. McGuffin M, Hobbs C, Upton R, Goldberg A. American Herbal Products Association's Botanical Safety Handbook. Boca Raton, FL: CRC Press, 1997:231.
8. Hasheminejad G, Caldwell J. Genotoxicity of the alkenylbenzenes alpha- and beta-asarone, myristicin and elimicin as determined by the UDS assay in cultured rat hepatocytes. Food Chem Toxicol 1994; 32:223–231.
9. Farnsworth NR, Bingel AS, Cordell GA, Crane FA, Fong HH. Potential value of plants as sources of new antifertility agents I. J Pharm Sci 1975; 64:535–598.
10. Brinker F. The Toxicology of Botanical Medicines. Sandy, OR: Eclectic Medical Publications, 2000:296.
11. Luo G, Qato MK, Guenthner TM. Hydrolysis of the 2′,3′-allylic epoxides of allylbenzene, estragole, eugenol, and safrole by both microsomal and cytosolic epoxide hydrolases. Drug Metab Dispos 1992; 20:440–445.

12. Newall CA, Anderson LA, Phillipson JD. Herbal Medicines: A Guide for Health-care Professionals. London, UK: Pharmaceutical Press, 1996:296.
13. Keller K, Odenthal KP, Leng-Peschlow E. [Spasmolytic effect of isoasaron free calamus]. Planta Med 1985:6–9.
14. Labarrios F, Garduno L, Vidal MR et al. Synthesis and hypolipidaemic evaluation of a series of alpha-asarone analogues related to clofibrate in mice. J Pharm Pharmacol 1999; 51:1–7.
15. Chamorro G, Salazar M, Salazar S, Mendoza T. [Pharmacology and toxicology of Guatteria gaumeri and alpha-asarone]. Rev Invest Clin 1993; 45:597–604.
16. Chamorro G, Salazar M, Tamariz J, Diaz F, Labarrios F. Dominant lethal study of alpha-asarone in male and female mice after sub-chronic treatment. Phytother Res 1999; 13:308–311.
17. Rubio-Poo C, Lemini C, Garcia-Mondragon J et al. The anticoagulant effect of beta-asarone in the mouse and the rat. Proc West Pharmacol Soc 1991; 34:107–112.
18. Wichtl M, Czygan FC, Frohne D et al. Herbal Drugs and Phytopharmaceuticals. Stuttgart, DE: Medpharm-CRC Press, 1994:566.

CALENDULA
Calendula officinalis

Synonyms/common names/related substances[1]
Garden marigold, gold-bloom, holligold, marigold, marybud, pot marigold

Indications

Topical

Burns:[2]	Evidence grade B2
Acute otitis media (with *Allium sativum*, *Verbascum thapsus*, and *Hypericum perforatum*):[3]	Evidence grade B2
Chronic colitis (with *Taraxacum officinale*, *Hypericum perforatum*, *Melissa officinalis*, and *Foeniculum vulgare*):[4]	Evidence grade C
Wound healing:[5]	Evidence grade D
Skin inflammation:[6]	Evidence grade E

Homeopathic C. officinalis *(Calendula)*

Wound healing:[7]	Evidence grade E

Pregnancy

Oral

Uterotonic effect:[8]	Evidence level 3

Calendula was shown to have a uterotonic effect when applied to isolated rabbit and guinea pig uterine horn.[8]

Potential abortifacient:[9]	Evidence level 4
Emmenagogue:[9]	Evidence level 4
Estrogenic:[10]	Evidence level 4

A review article on the potential value of plants as sources of anti-fertility agents reported that calendula was a potential abortifacient and an emmenagogue, and that it had estrogenic activity.[9,10]

Spermatocide:[1]	Evidence level 4

Anti-blastocyst:[1]	Evidence level 4

A compendium on herb toxicology and drug interactions reported that when taken orally, calendula may have spermatocide and anti-blastocyst activity.[11] Orally, calendula was not reported in the scientific literature as having spermatocide or anti-blastocyst activity.

Topical

Unknown:	Evidence level 5

Topically, calendula was not reported in the scientific literature as being either safe or contraindicated during pregnancy.

Homeopathic C. officinalis (Calendula)

Minimal risk:	Evidence level 5

A homeopathic preparation of *C. officinalis*, called Calendula, beyond the potency (dilution) of 12C, does not contain any molecules of the original substance. Homeopathic calendula is of minimal risk in pregnancy.

Lactation

Unknown:	Evidence level 5

Calendula was not reported in the scientific literature as being either safe or contraindicated during lactation.

Homeopathic C. officinalis (Calendula)

Minimal risk:	Evidence level 5

A homeopathic preparation of *C. officinalis*, called Calendula, beyond the potency (dilution) of 12C, does not contain any molecules of the original substance. Homeopathic calendula is of minimal risk in lactation.

Constituents

- Faradiol esters[12]
- Triterpene alcohols:[13] heliaol, taraxasterol, psi-taraxasterol, α-amyrin, β-amyrin, lupeol, taraxerol, cycloartenol, 24-methyl-enecycloartanol, tirucalla-7,24-dienol and dammaradienol
- Saponins[14]

Toxicity

- LD_{50} (intravenous):[15] 375 mg/kg to 526 mg/100 g
- LD_{50} (subcutaneous):[15] 45 mg/mouse
- LD_{100} (intraperitoneal):[15] 580 mg/kg

Pharmacology

- Calendula has anti-inflammatory and anti-edematous properties, and the faridol esters are believed to have the most pronounced anti-inflammatory effect.[6,12,16]
- Topically, the triterpene and flavonoid constituents were shown to have anti-inflammatory activity in vivo.[6,13,16]
- Topically, calendula increases physiologic regeneration and epitheliliazation of surgical wounds.[17]
- Calendula may have immune-stimulating activity in vitro.[18]
- Calendula has anti-bacterial and anti-viral activity.[19,20]
- Calendula has anti-mutagenic properties.[14]

Drug interactions

Barbiturates[21]
Drugs with sedative properties[21]

Part used[11]

Flowers

References

1. Jellin JM, Batz F, Hitchens K. Natural Medicines Comprehensive Database. Stockton, CA: Therapeutic Research Faculty, 2002:1530.
2. Lievre M, Marichy J, Baux S et al. Controlled study of three ointments for the local management of 2nd and 3rd degree burns. Clin Trials Metaanal 1992; 28:9–12.
3. Sarrell EM, Mandelberg A, Cohen HA. Efficacy of naturopathic extracts in the management of ear pain associated with acute otitis media. Arch Pediatr Adolesc Med 2001; 155:796–799.
4. Chakurski I, Matev M, Koichev A, Angelova I, Stefanov G. [Treatment of chronic colitis with an herbal combination of Taraxacum officinale, Hipericum perforatum, Melissa officinaliss, Calendula officinalis and Foeniculum vulgare]. Vutr Boles 1981; 20:51–54.
5. Neto JJ, Fracasso JF, Neves MD et al. Treatment of varicose ulcer and skin lesions with calendula. Revista de Ciencias Farm Sao Paulo 1996; 17:181–186.
6. Della Loggia R, Tubaro A, Sosa S et al. The role of triterpenoids in the topical anti-inflammatory activity of Calendula officinalis flowers. Planta Med 1994; 60:516–520.
7. Rao S, Udupa A, Udupa SL et al. Calendula and Hypericum: two homeopathic drugs promoting wound healing in rats. Fitoterapia 1991; 62:508–510.
8. Shipochliev T. [Uterotonic action of extracts from a group of medicinal plants]. Vet Med Nauki 1981; 18:94–98.

9. Farnsworth NR, Bingel AS, Cordell GA, Crane FA, Fong HH. Potential value of plants as sources of new antifertility agents I. J Pharm Sci 1975; 64:535–598.
10. Farnsworth NR, Bingel AS, Cordell GA, Crane FA, Fong HH. Potential value of plants as sources of new antifertility agents II. J Pharm Sci 1975; 64:717–753.
11. Brinker F. Herb Contraindications and Drug Interactions. Sandy, OR: Eclectic Medical Publications, 2001:432.
12. Zitterl-Eglseer K, Sosa S, Jurenitsch J et al. Anti-oedematous activities of the main triterpendiol esters of marigold (Calendula officinalis L). J Ethnopharmacol 1997; 57:139–144.
13. Akihisa T, Yasukawa K, Oinuma H et al. Triterpene alcohols from the flowers of compositae and their anti-inflammatory effects. Phytochemistry 1996; 43: 1255–1260.
14. Elias R, De Meo M V-OE, Laget M, Balansard G, Dumenil G. Antimutagenic activity of some saponins isolated from Calendula officinalis L., C. arvensis L. and Hedera helix L. Mutagenesis 1990; 5:327–331.
15. www.naturalstandard.com. Calendula (Calendula officinalis) Natural Standard Monograph: www.naturalstandard.com, 2004.
16. Bezakova L, Masterova I, Paulikova I, Psenak M. Inhibitory activity of isorhamnetin glycosides from Calendula officinalis L. on the activity of lipoxygenase. Pharmazie 1996; 51:126–127.
17. Newall CA, Anderson LA, Phillipson JD. Herbal Medicines: A Guide for Health-care Professionals. London, UK: Pharmaceutical Press, 1996:296.
18. Wagner H, Proksch A, Riess-Maurer I et al. [Immunostimulating action of polysaccharides (heteroglycans) from higher plants]. Arzneimittelforschung 1985; 35:1069–1075.
19. Boucaud-Maitre Y, Algernon O, Raynaud J. Cytotoxic and antitumoral activity of Calendula officinalis extracts. Pharmazie 1988; 43:220–221.
20. Dumenil G, Chemli R, Balansard C, Guiraud H, Lallemand M. [Evaluation of antibacterial properties of marigold flowers (Calendula officinalis L.) and mother homeopathic tinctures of C. officinalis L. and C. arvensis L]. Ann Pharm Fr 1980; 38:493–499.
21. Brinker F. Herb Contraindications and Drug Interactions. Sandy, OR: Eclectic Medical Publications, 1998.

CHASTETREE
Vitex agnus-castus

Synonyms/common names/related compounds[1]

Agnolyt, agnus castus, agnus-castus, chaste berry, chaste tree, chaste tree berry, chastetree, gattilier, hemp tree, monk's pepper, vitex, *Vitex agnus castus*

Indications

Premenstrual syndrome:[2–8]	Evidence grade B1
Cyclic mastalgia:[9,10]	Evidence grade B1
Hyperprolactinemia:[11]	Evidence grade B1
Infertility:[5,12,13]	Evidence grade B2
Acne:[5]	Evidence grade E
Menstrual disorders:[4,5]	Evidence grade E
Increases lactation:[5,12,14]	Evidence grade E

Homeopathic preparation

Infertility:[15]	Evidence grade B1

Pregnancy

Emmenagogue:[16]	Evidence level 4

A review article on the potential value of plants as sources of anti-fertility agents reported that chastetree was an emmenagogue.[17]

Uterine stimulant:[1]	Evidence level 4

Compendia on drug interactions and safety and on natural products reported that chastretree is a uterine stimulant.[1] There are no reports in the scientific literature of chastetree being a uterine stimulant or an emmenagogue.

Prevention of miscarriages:[5]	Evidence level 4

A compendium on herbal medicine reported that chastetree is used by some clinicians during the first trimester of pregnancy to prevent miscarriages in patients with progesterone deficiency.[5] There are no reports in the scientific literature that chastetree prevents miscarriages.

Hormonal activity:[18]	Evidence level 4

Chastetree may have estrogenic and progesterone activity.[18]

Homeopathic preparation

Increases progesterone:[15]	Evidence level 1a

A prospective, randomized, placebo-controlled, double-blind study was conducted on a homeopathic preparation of chastetree for women with fertility disorders.[15] The researchers observed a non-significant increase in fertility and a significant increase of progesterone during the luteal phase.[15]

Lactation

Conflicting evidence

Increases lactation:[5,12,14]	Evidence level 4
Decreases lactation:[4]	Evidence level 4

Compendia on herbal medicine and a plant monograph report that chastetree increases lactation.[5,12,14] Other sources report that chastetree decreases lactation as it suppresses prolactin release.[4] There are no reports in the scientific literature of chastetree either increasing or decreasing lactation.

Hormonal activity:[18]	Evidence level 4

Chastetree may have estrogenic and progesterone activity.[18]

Homeopathic preparation

Increases progesterone:[15]	Evidence level 1a

A prospective, randomized, placebo-controlled, double-blind study was conducted on a homeopathic preparation of chastetree for women with fertility disorders.[15] The researchers observed a non-significant increase in fertility and a significant increase of progesterone during the luteal phase.[15]

Constituents[1]

- Essential oils:[14] limonene, cineol, pinene, and sabinene
- Iridoid glycosides:[5,19] aucubin and agnoside
- Flavonoids:[5,14] casticin, kaempferol, quercetagetin, orientin, and isovitexin
- Diterpenes:[12,14,19,20] including vitexilactone, rotundifuran, and 6-β,7-β-diacetoxy-13-hydroxy-labda-8,14-dien
- Essential fatty acids:[12] oleic acid, linolenic acid, palmitic acid, and stearic acid

Toxicity

- No information available.[5]
- The LD_{50} of *Vitex leucoxylon* leaf, same genus as chastetree, was >3000 mg/kg (ethanol extract) and 800–1200 mg/kg (cold aqueous infusion).[21]

Pharmacology

- Chastetree may have estrogenic and progesterone activity.[18]
- Chastetree selectively binds to β-estrogen receptors (heart, vasculature, bone and bladder).[22]
- Chastetree may affect dopamine, acetylcholine, and opioid receptors.[20]
- In high doses, chastetree has agonist effects on pituitary dopamine (D2) receptors.[23,24]
- In women with hyperprolactinemia, chastetree appears to suppress prolactin release and normalize luteal phase defects in the menstrual cycle.[11]
- In men, lower doses of chastetree increase prolaction release while higher doses suppress prolaction release; chastetree does not appear to affect testosterone levels.[25]
- Chastetree may inhibit the growth of breast, ovarian, cervical, gastric, colon, and lung cancer cells.[26,27]
- Chasetree essential oils have anti-bacterial and anti-fungal properties.[5]

Drug interactions

Anti-psychotic drugs[23,24]
Dopamine agonists[20,23,24]
Oral contraceptives[28]
Hormone replacement therapy[28]

Part used[29]

Fruit

References

1. Jellin JM, Batz F, Hitchens K. Natural Medicines Comprehensive Database, 3rd ed. Stockton, CA: Therapeutic Research Faculty, 2002:1530.
2. Atmaca M, Kumru S, Tezcan E. Fluoxetine versus Vitex agnus castus extract in the treatment of premenstrual dysphoric disorder. Hum Psychopharmacol 2003; 18:191–195.
3. Schellenberg R. Treatment for the premenstrual syndrome with agnus castus fruit extract: prospective, randomised, placebo controlled study. BMJ 2001; 322:134–137.
4. McCaleb RS, Leigh E, Morien K. The Encyclopedia of Popular Herbs. Roseville, CA: Prima Health, 2000.
5. Mills S, Bone K. Principles and Practice of Phytotherapy: Modern Herbal Medicine. London: Churchill Livingstone, 2000.
6. Lauritzen CH, Reuter HD, Repges R et al. Treatment of premenstrual tension syndrome with Vitex agnus castus: controlled-double blind versus pyridoxine. Phytomedicine 1997; 4:183–189.

7. Berger D, Schaffner W, Schrader E, Meier B, Brattstrom A. Efficacy of Vitex agnus castus L. extract Ze 440 in patients with pre-menstrual syndrome (PMS). Arch Gynecol Obstet 2000; 264:150–153.
8. Loch EG, Selle H, Boblitz N. Treatment of premenstrual syndrome with a phytopharmaceutical formulation containing Vitex agnus castus. J Womens Health Gend Based Med 2000; 9:315–320.
9. Halaska M, Beles P, Gorkow C, Sieder C. Treatment of cyclical mastalgia with a solution containing a Vitex agnus castus extract: results of a placebo-controlled double-blind study. Breast 1999; 8:175–181.
10. Halaska M, Raus K, Beles P, Martan A, Paithner KG. [Treatment of cyclical mastodynia using an extract of Vitex agnus castus: results of a double-blind comparison with a placebo]. Ceska Gynekologie 1998; 63:388–392.
11. Milewicz A, Gejdel E, Sworen H et al. Vitex agnus castus extract in the treatment of luteal phase defects due to latent hyperprolactinemia. Results of a randomized placebo-controlled double-blind study. Arzneimittelforschung 1993; 43:752–756.
12. Du Mee C. Vitex agnus castus. Aust J Med Herb 1993; 5:63–65.
13. Gerhard II, Patek A, Monga B, Blank A, Gorkow C. Mastodynon(R) bei weiblicher Sterilitat. Forsch Komplementarmed 1998; 5:272–278.
14. Brown D. Vitex agnus castus clinical monograph. Qtrly Rev Natural Med 1994; 2:111–121.
15. Bergmann J, Luft B, Boehmann S, Runnebaum B, Gerhard I. [The efficacy of the complex medication Phyto-Hypophyson L in female, hormone-related sterility. A randomized, placebo-controlled clinical double-blind study]. Forsch Komplementarmed Klass Naturheilkd 2000; 7:190–199.
16. Brinker F. The Toxicology of Botanical Medicines. Sandy, OR: Eclectic Medical Publications, 2000:296.
17. Farnsworth NR, Bingel AS, Cordell G, Crane FA, Fong HH. Potential value of plants as sources of new antifertility agents I. J Pharm Sci 1975; 64:535–598.
18. Liu J, Burdette JE, Xu H et al. Evaluation of estrogenic activity of plant extracts for the potential treatment of menopausal symptoms. J Agric Food Chem 2001; 49:2472–2479.
19. Upton R. Chaste tree fruit. American Herbal Pharmacopoeia and Therapeutic Compendium. Santa Cruz, CA: American Herbal Pharmacopoeia, 2001:1–37.
20. Meier B, Berger D, Hoberg E et al. Pharmacological activities of Vitex agnuscastus extracts in vitro. Phytomedicine 2000; 7:373–381.
21. Makwana HG, Ravishankar B, Shakla VJ et al. General pharmacology of Vitex leucoxylon Linn leaves. Indian J Physiol Pharmacol 1994; 38:95–100.
22. Wuttke W, Jarry H, Christoffel V, Spengler B, Seidlova-Wuttke D. Chaste tree (Vitex agnus-castus) – pharmacology and clinical indications. Phytomedicine 2003; 10:348–357.
23. Wuttke W. Dopaminergic action of extracts of Agnus Castus. Forschende Komplementarmedizen 1996; 3:329–330.
24. Jarry H, Leonhardt S, Gorkow C, Wuttke W. In vitro prolactin but not LH and FSH release is inhibited by compounds in extracts of Agnus Castus: direct evidence for a dopaminergic principle by the dopamine receptor assay. Exp Clin Endocrinol 1994; 192:448–454.
25. Merz P, Gorkow C, Schroder A et al. The effects of a special Agnus castus extract (BP1095el) on prolactin secretion in healthy male subjects. Exp Clin Endocrinol Diabetes 1996; 104:447–453.

26. Dixon-Shanies D, Shaikh N. Growth inhibition of human breast cancer cells by herbs and phytoestrogens. Oncol Rep 1999; 6:1383–1387.
27. Ohyama K, Akaike T, Hirobe C, Yamakawa T. Cytotoxicity and apoptotic inducibility of Vitex agnus-castus fruit extract in cultured human normal and cancer cells and effect on growth. Biol Pharm Bull 2003; 26:10–18.
28. Brinker F. Herb Contraindications and Drug Interactions, 2nd ed. Sandy, OR: Eclectic Medical Publications, 1998.
29. Brinker F. Herb Contraindications and Drug Interactions, 3rd ed. Sandy, OR: Eclectic Medical Publications, 2001:432.

COFFEE

Coffea arabica, C. canephora, C. robusta, C. liberica

Synonyms/common names/related substances[1]

Cafe, caffea, espresso, java, mocha

Indications

Increases mental alertness and performance:[2,3]	Evidence grade B1
Decreases risk of Parkinson disease:[4,5]	Evidence grade C
Decreases risk of symptomatic gallbladder disease in men:[6]	Evidence grade C
Decreases risk of gallstones in women:[7]	Evidence grade C
Rectal cancer prevention:[8]	Evidence grade C

Pregnancy

Spontaneous abortion:[9,10]	Evidence level 1b

A case–control study of 3149 pregnant women reported that serum paraxanthine, a caffeine metabolite, concentration was higher in the women who had spontaneous abortions than in the controls.[9] Drinking more that six cups of coffee per day increases the risk of spontaneous abortions and that only extremely high serum paraxanthine concentrations are associated with spontaneous abortion.[9]

A case–control study of 1498 pregnant women reported that the consumption of 375 mg or more caffeine per day during pregnancy may increase the risk of spontaneous abortion.[10]

Increased risk of stillbirth:[11]	Evidence level 1b

A prospective follow-up study on 18 478 singleton pregnancies in women with valid information about coffee consumption during pregnancy[11] reported that pregnant women who drink eight or more cups of coffee per day have double the risk of stillbirth, when compared to women who do not drink coffee during pregnancy.[11]

Low birthweight infants:[12,13]	Evidence level 1b

A large prospective study on 2291 mothers reported that women consuming more than 600 mg of caffeine per day are at greater risk for having low birthweight infants.[13] A prospective study on 63 women reported that pregnant non-smokers consuming caffeine more than 300 mg/day had statistically significant lower weights of newborns and placentas ($p<0.05$).[12]

Teratogenic compounds:[14–17] Evidence level 3

Elevated caffeine intake causes histopathologically teratogenic effects on newborn rat cornea.[14] A study on the effects of coffee during pregnancy on mice reported long-term teratopharmacologic and behavioral alterations in the offspring of pregnant mice that consumed coffee.[15] A similar study on mice reported teratogenic effects associated with coffee ingestion during pregnancy.[17] A review study, however, reported that when caffeine is administered in fractioned quantities during the day, as it is the case with human caffeine intake, caffeine is no longer a teratogen in animals.[18]

Impairs trace mineral absorption in fetus:[19] Evidence level 3

A study on the effect of coffee consumption on pregnancy and lactation in mice[19] reported that maternal coffee intake may impair mobilization of trace elements from liver reserves in early life and that this may result in reduced hemoglobin synthesis.[19]

Harmful to the fetus:[20] Evidence level 4

Crosses the placenta:[20] Evidence level 4

A compendium on the safety of drugs in pregnancy and lactation reported that over three cups of coffee a day (300 mg of caffeine) may be harmful to the fetus.[20] The compendium also reported that caffeine crosses the human placenta where fetal blood and tissue levels are similar to maternal concentrations.[20]

Three cups of coffee throughout the day – possibly safe:[21,22] Evidence level 4

A drug compendium and a review study reported that three cups of coffee (approximately 300 mg of caffeine) consumed throughout the day seems safe during pregnancy.[21,22]

Estrogenic:[23] Evidence level 4

A review article on the potential value of plants as sources of anti-fertility agents reported that coffee has estrogenic activity.[23]

Lactation

Teratogenic compounds:[14–17] Evidence level 3

Two studies reported teratogenic and behavioral alterations in animals whose mothers were fed coffee.[14,15] A similar study on mice reported teratogenic effects associated with coffee ingestion during pregnancy.[17] Since caffeine appears in breast milk at half the concentration as in the mother's plasma, newborns may be exposed to teratogenic compounds.[24] A review study, however, reported that when caffeine is administered in fractioned quantities during the day, as it is the case with human caffeine intake, caffeine is no longer a teratogen in animals.[18]

Impairs trace mineral absorption in newborn:[19]	Evidence level 3

A study on the effects of coffee consumption on pregnancy and lactation in mice reported that maternal coffee intake may impair mobilization of trace elements from liver reserves in early life and that this may result in reduced hemoglobin synthesis.[19]

May cause sleeping disorders:[25]	Evidence level 4

A compendium on herbal medicine reported that nursing mothers who consume caffeine may have infants with sleeping disorders.[25]

Stimulates breast milk production:[22]	Evidence level 4

A review study reported that coffee consumption stimulates breast milk production in women and that it does not change breast milk composition.[22]

Contraindications

Cardiac problems[16]
Kidney disease[16]
Hyperthyroidism[16]

Caution

People who have a predisposition to convulsion or anxiety should not drink more than five cups or 500 mg of caffeine per day.[16]

Toxic constituents

Methylxanthine alkaloid: caffeine[16]
Polyphenolic acid: chlorogenic acid[16]
Caffeol[1]
Diterpenes[1]

Toxicity

- Toxic dose of caffeine: 1 g[16]
- Lethal dose of caffeine: 10 g (adult) and 5.3 g (child)[16,26]

Pharmacology

- Caffeine is a powerful stimulant of the central nervous system, respiration, and skeletal muscles.[16,26]
- Caffeine causes cardiac stimulation, coronary dilation, smooth muscle relaxation, increases blood pressure, increases heart rate and contractility, and diuresis.[1,26,27]

- Coffee stimulates gastric secretions.[28]
- Caffeine crosses the human placenta where fetal blood and tissue levels are similar to maternal concentrations.[20]
- Chlorogenic acid, a constituent in coffee, is reported to have stimulant, diuretic, choleretic properties and allergenic properties.[26,29]
- Chlorogenic acid may raise homocysteine levels.[30]
- Cafestol, a diterpene in unfiltered coffee, was shown to raise plasma triacylglycerol levels in humans.[31]
- Caffeine has anti-platelet activity.[32,33]

Drug interactions

Acetaminophen (paracetamol)[34]
Alendronate[35]
Anti-coagulant/anti-platelet drugs[32,33]
Anti-diabetic drugs[34]
Aspirin[32,33,36]
Benzodiazepines[35]
β-Adrenergic agonists[37]
Cimetidine[35]
Clozapine[38,39]
Central nervous system stimulants[38,40]
Disulfiram[37]
Ephedrine[34,41]
Ergotamine[37]
Estrogen[42]
Lithium[43,44]
Mexiletine[35]
Monoamine oxidase inhibitors[34]
Oral contraceptives[35]
Phenylpropanolamine[35]
Quinolones[45–47]
Riluzole[35]
Terbinafine[35]
Theophylline[35]
Verapamil[35]

Part used[16]

Dried ripe seed

References

1. Jellin JM, Batz F, Hitchens K. Natural Medicines Comprehensive Database, 3rd ed. Stockton, CA: Therapeutic Research Faculty, 2002:1530.
2. Yeomans MR, Ripley T, Davies L, Rusted JM, Rogers PJ. Effects of caffeine on performance and mood depend on the level of caffeine abstinence. Psychopharmacology (Berl) 2002; 164:241–249. Epub 2002 Sep 11.

3. Smith AP, Kendrick A, Maben AL. Effects of breakfast and caffeine on performance and mood in the late morning and after lunch. Neuropsychobiology 1992; 26:198–204.
4. Ross GW, Abbott RD, Petrovitch H et al. Association of coffee and caffeine intake with the risk of Parkinson disease. JAMA 2000; 283:2674–2679.
5. Ascherio A, Zhang SM, Hernan M et al. Prospective study of caffeine intake and risk of Parkinson's disease in men and women. Proceedings of the 125th Annual Meeting American Neurological Association, 15–18 October:42 (abstract 53). Boston, MA 2000.
6. Leitzmann MF, Willett WC, Rimm E, Stampfer MJ, Spiegelman D, Colditz GA, Giovannucci E. A prospective study of coffee consumption and the risk of symptomatic gallstone disease in men. JAMA 1999; 281:2106–2112.
7. Ruhl CE, Everhart JE. Association of coffee consumption with gallbladder disease. Am J Epidemiol 2000; 152:1034–1038.
8. Inoue M, Tajima K, Hirose K et al. Tea and coffee consumption and the risk of digestive tract cancers: data from a comparative case-referent study in Japan. Cancer Causes Control 1998; 9:209–216.
9. Klebanoff MA, Levine RJ, DerSimonian R, Clemens JD, Wilkins DG. Maternal serum paraxanthine, a caffeine metabolite, and the risk of spontaneous abortion. N Engl J Med 1999; 341:1639–1644.
10. Rasch V. Cigarette, alcohol, and caffeine consumption: risk factors for spontaneous abortion. Acta Obstet Gynecol Scand 2003; 82:182–188.
11. Wisborg K, Kesmodel U, Bech B, Hedegaard M, Henriksen TB. Maternal consumption of coffee during pregnancy and stillbirth and infant death in first year of life: prospective study. BMJ 2003; 326:420.
12. Balat O, Balat A, UM, Pence S. The effect of smoking and caffeine on the fetus and placenta in pregnancy. Clin Exp Obstet Gynecol 2003; 30:57–59.
13. Bracken MB, Triche EW, Belanger K, Hellenbrand K, Leaderer BP. Association of maternal caffeine consumption with decrements in fetal growth. Am J Epidemiol 2003; 157:456–466.
14. Everekliogiu C, Sari I, Alasehirli B et al. High dose of caffeine administered to pregnant rats causes histopathological changes in the cornea of newborn pups. Med Sci Monit 2003; 9:BR168–173.
15. Brinker F. The Toxicology of Botanical Medicines. Sandy, OR: Eclectic Medical Publications, 2000:296.
16. Ajarem JS, Ahmand M. Teratopharmacological and behavioral effects of coffee in mice. Acta Physiol Pharmacol Bulg 1996; 22:51–61.
17. Palm PE, Arnold EP, Nick M, Valentine JR, Doerfler TE. Two-year toxicity/carcinogenicity study of fresh-brewed coffee in rats initially exposed in utero. Toxicol Appl Pharmacol 1984; 74:364–382.
18. Nehlig A, Debry G. Consequences on the newborn of chronic maternal consumption of coffee during gestation and lactation: a review. J Am Coll Nutr 1994; 13:6–21.
19. Munoz L, Keen CL, Lonnerdal B, Dewey KG. Coffee intake during pregnancy and lactation in rats: maternal and pup hematological parameters and liver iron, zinc and copper concentration. J Nutr 1986; 116:1326–1333.
20. Briggs GB, Freeman RK, Yaffe SJ. Drugs in Pregnancy and Lactation. 5th ed. Philadelphia: Lippincott Williams & Wilkins, 1998.

21. McKevoy GK. Drug Information. Bethesda, MD: American Society of Health-System Pharmacists, 1998.
22. Nehlig A, Debry G. [Effects of coffee and caffeine on fertility, reproduction, lactation, and development. Review of human and animal data]. J Gynecol Obstet Biol Reprod (Paris) 1994; 23:241–256.
23. Farnsworth NR, Bingel AS, Cordell GA, Crane FA, Fong HH. Potential value of plants as sources of new antifertility agents II. J Pharm Sci 1975; 64:717–753.
24. Boyd JR. Facts and comparisons. St Louis, MI: J.B. Lippincott Co., 1985.
25. Gruenwald J, Brendler T, Jaenicke C. PDR for Herbal Medicines. Montvale, NJ: Medical Economics Company, 1998.
26. Leung AY, Foster S. Encyclopedia of Common Natural Ingredients Used in Food, Drugs and Cosmetics, 2nd ed. New York, NY: John Wiley & Sons, 1996:649.
27. Klag MJ, Wang NY, Meoni L et al. Coffee intake and risk of hypertension: the Johns Hopkins precursors study. Arch Intern Med 2002; 162:657–662.
28. Martindale: The Extra Pharmacopoeia. London: The Pharmaceutical Press, 1982.
29. Morton JF. Major Medicinal Plants: Botany, Culture, and Uses. Springfield, IL: Thomas, 1981.
30. Olthof MR, Hollman PC, Zock P, Katan MB. Consumption of high doses of chlorogenic acid, present in coffee, or of black tea increases plasma total homocysteine concentrations in humans. Am J Clin Nutr 2001; 73:532–538.
31. de Roos B, Caslake MJ, Stalenhoef A et al. The coffee diterpene cafestol increases plasma triacylglycerol by increasing the production rate of large VLDL apolipoprotein B in healthy normolipidemic subjects. Am J Clin Nutr 2001; 73:45–52.
32. Ali M, Afzal M. A potent inhibitor of thrombin stimulated platelet thromboxane formation from unprocessed tea. Prostaglandins Leukot Med 1987; 27:9–13.
33. Ardlie NG, Glew G, Schultz BG, Schwartz CJ. Inhibition and reversal of platelet aggregation by methyl xanthines. Thromb Diath Haemorrh 1967; 18:670–673.
34. Brinker F. Herb Contraindications and Drug Interactions, 2nd ed. Sandy, OR: Eclectic Medical Publications, 1998.
35. MICROMEDEX. Micromedex Healthcare Series. Englewood, CO: MICROMEDEX.
36. Robbers JE, Tyler VE. Tyler's Herbs of Choice: The Therapeutic Use of Phytomedicinals. New York, NY: The Haworth Herbal Press, 1999.
37. McKevoy GK. AHFS Drug Information. Bethesda, MD: American Society of Health-System Pharmacists, 1998.
38. Hagg S, Spigset O, Mjorndal T, Dahlqvist R. Effect of caffeine on clozapine pharmacokinetics in healthy volunteers. Br J Clin Pharmacol 2000; 49:59–63.
39. Sklar S et al. Drug therapy screening system. Indianapolis, IN: First Data Bank:99.
40. DiPiro JT, Talbert RL, Yee GC et al. Pharmacotherapy: A Pathophysiologic Approach, 4th ed. Stamford, CT: Appleton & Lange, 1999.
41. Schulz V, Hansel R, Tyler VE, Terry C. Rational Phytotherapy: A Physician's Guide to Herbal Medicine, 3rd ed. Berlin: Springer, 1998.
42. Pollock BG, Wylie M, Stack JA et al. Inhibition of caffeine metabolism by estrogen replacement therapy in postmenopausal women. J Clin Pharmacol 1999; 39:936–940.
43. Mester R, Toren P, Mizrachi I et al. Caffeine withdrawal increases lithium blood levels. Biol Psychiatry 1995; 37:348–350.

44. Jefferson JW. Lithium tremor and caffeine intake: two cases of drinking less and shaking more. J Clin Psychiatry 1988; 49:72–73.
45. Harder S, Fuhr U, Staib AH, Wolff T. Ciprofloxacin-caffeine: a drug interaction established using in vivo and in vitro investigations. Am J Med 1989; 87:89S–91S.
46. Carbo M, Segura J, De la Torre R et al. Effect of quinolones on caffeine disposition. Clin Pharmacol Ther 1989; 45:234–240.
47. Healy DP, Polk RE, Kanawati L et al. Interaction between oral ciprofloxacin and caffeine in normal volunteers. Antimicrob Agents Chemother 1989; 33:474–478.

CRANBERRY

Vaccinium macrocarpon, V. oxycoccos

Synonyms/common names/related compounds[1]

American cranberry, arandano Americano, arandano trepador, cranberries, European cranberry, grosse moosbeere, kranbeere, large cranberry, moosebeere, mossberry, ronce d'Amerique, small cranberry, trailing swamp cranberry, tsuru-kokemomo

Indications

Extract

Prevention of urinary tract infections:[2–4]	Evidence grade A

A systematic review concluded that the small number of poor-quality trials gives no reliable evidence of the effectiveness of cranberry juice for the prevention of urinary tract infections.[2] The systematic review also reported that other cranberry products such as cranberry capsules may be more acceptable.[2]

Juice

Prevention of urinary tract infections:[5,6]	Evidence grade B2
Urinary tract infections:[7,8]	Evidence grade E
Periodontal disease:[9]	Evidence grade E

A systematic review concluded that the small number of poor-quality trials gives no reliable evidence of the effectiveness of cranberry juice for the prevention of urinary tract infections.[2] The two studies above were not included in the systematic review.[5,6]

Pregnancy

Commonly used:[10,11]	Evidence level 1b

Safety

Unknown:	Evidence level 5

A survey was conducted on 400 Norwegian postpartum women.[11] The authors reported that cranberry was one of the most commonly used herbs during pregnancy, mostly for urinary tract infections.[11] This study did not evaluate the safety of cranberry during pregnancy.[11] There are no reports in the scientific literature of cranberry being either safe or contraindicated during pregnancy.

Food

Minimal risk:	Evidence level 4

A herbal compendium reported that cranberry is of minimal risk during pregnancy when consumed in food quantities.[12]

Lactation

Unknown:	Evidence level 5

There are no reports in the scientific literature of cranberry being either safe or contraindicated during lactation.

Food

Minimal risk:	Evidence level 4

A herbal compendium reported that cranberry is of minimal risk when consumed in food quantities.[12]

Caution
Kidney stones[13]

Constituents[14]
Proanthocyanidins
Triterpenoids
Lectins
Catechins
Ascorbic acid
Benzoic acid
Quinic acid
Citric acid
Malic acid

Toxicity
- Consuming up to 4 L/day of cranberry juice was shown to be non-toxic in healthy individuals.[15]
- Ingesting large amounts of cranberry juice (>3 L/day) may result in diarrhea, gastrointestinal distress, other gastrointestinal symptoms or toxicity in infants or young children.[16–18]

Pharmacology
- The proanthocyanidins in cranberry interfere with bacterial adherence to the urinary tract epithelial cells.[19–27]

- In the case of *Escherichia coli*, the cause of most urinary tract infections, proanthocyanidins were shown to wrap around these bacteria and prevent their adherence to the urinary tract wall.[7,28,29]
- Cranberry juice cocktail was shown to inhibit adherence in 77 clinical isolates of *E. coli* obtained from patients with diagnosed urinary tract infections and anti-adherence activity against Gram-negative rods.[7]
- The fructose in cranberries was shown to contribute to the anti-bacterial activity of cranberry.[25,29,30]
- Cranberry does not appear to have the ability to dislodge bacteria that have already adhered to the urinary tract epithelial cells.[31]
- Cranberry juice was shown to have anti-bacterial activity against *E. coli, Staphylococcus aureus, Klebsiella pneumoniae, Pseudomonas aeruginosa*, and *Proteus mirabilis*.[7,24,29]
- Cranberry was shown to have anti-viral action against the poliovirus type 1.[32]
- Cranberry may prevent the adherence of *Helicobacter pylori* in the stomach.[28]
- Cranberry may prevent adhesion of plaque bacteria that cause periodontal disease.[9]
- Cranberry may have anti-oxidant and anti-carcinogenic activity.[33,34]

Drug interactions[1]

Warfarin[35,36]

Drugs metabolized by cytochrome P450[9,35,36]

Part used

Fruit[1]

References

1. Jellin JM, Batz F, Hitchens K. Natural Medicines Comprehensive Database. Stockton, CA: Therapeutic Research Faculty, 2002:1530.
2. Jepson RG, Mihaljevic L, Craig J. Cranberries for preventing urinary tract infections. Cochrane Database Syst Rev 2000:CD001321.
3. Dignam R, Ahmed M, Denman S et al. The effect of cranberry juice on UTI rates in a long-term care facility. J Am Geriatr Soc 1997; 45:S53.
4. Walker EB, Barney DP, Mickelsen JN, Walton RJ, Mickelsen RAJ. Cranberry concentrate: UTI prophylaxis. J Fam Pract 1997; 45:167–168.
5. Kontiokari T, Sundqvist K, Nuutinen M et al. Randomised trial of cranberry-lingonberry juice and Lactobacillus GG drink for the prevention of urinary tract infections in women. BMJ 2001; 322:1571.
6. Foxman B, Geiger AM, Palin K, Gillespie B, Koopman JS. First-time urinary tract infection and sexual behavior. Epidemiology 1995; 6:162–168.
7. Schmidt DR, Sobota AE. An examination of the anti-adherence activity of cranberry juice on urinary and nonurinary bacterial isolates. Microbios 1988; 55:173–181.
8. Papas PN, Brusch CA, Ceresia GC. Cranberry juice in the treatment of urinary tract infections. Southwest Med 1966; 47:17–20.
9. Weiss EI, Lev-Dor R, Kashamn Y et al. Inhibiting interspecies coaggregation of plaque bacteria with a cranberry juice constituent. JADA 1998; 129:1719–1723.

10. Dwyer PL, O'Reilly M. Recurrent urinary tract infection in the female. Curr Opin Obstet Gynecol 2002; 14:537–543.
11. Nordeng H, Havnen GC. Use of herbal drugs in pregnancy: a survey among 400 Norwegian women. Pharmacoepidemiol Drug Saf 2004; 13:371–380.
12. Foster S, Tyler VE. Tyler's Honest Herbal: A Sensible Guide to the Use of Herbs and Related Remedies. Binghamton, NY: Haworth Herbal Press, 1993.
13. Terris MK, Issa MM, Tacker JR. Dietary supplementation with cranberry concentrate tablets may increase the risk of nephrolithiasis. Urology 2001; 57:26–29.
14. www.naturalstandard.com. Cranberry (Vaccinium macrocarpon) Natural Standard Monograph, 2003.
15. Bodel P, Cotran R, Kass E. Cranberry juice and the antibacterial action of hippuric acid. J Lab Clin Med 1959; 54:881–888.
16. Garcia-Calatayud S, Larreina Cordoba JJ, Lozano De La Torre MJ. [Severe cranberry juice poisoning]. An Esp Pediatr 2002; 56:72–73.
17. Johns Cupp M. Toxicology and Clinical Pharmacology of Herbal Products. Totowa, NJ: Humana Press, 2000.
18. Anonymous. Cranberry. Lawerence Review of Natural Products. St. Louis, MO: Facts and Comparisons, 1994.
19. Sobota AE. Inhibition of bacterial adherence by cranberry juice: potential use for the treatment of urinary tract infections. J Urol 1984; 131:1013–1016.
20. Ahuja S, Kaack B, Roberts J. Loss of fimbrial adhesion with the addition of Vaccinum macrocarpon to the growth medium of P-fimbriated Escherichia coli. J Urol 1998; 159:559–562.
21. Avorn J. The effect of cranberry juice on the presence of bacteria and white blood cells in the urine of elderly women. What is the role of bacterial adhesion? Adv Exp Med Biol 1996; 408:185–186.
22. Fleet JC. New support for a folk remedy: cranberry juice reduces bacteriuria and pyuria in elderly women. Nutr Rev 1994; 52:168–170.
23. Kinney AB, Blount M. Effect of cranberry juice on urinary pH. Nurs Res 1979; 28:287–290.
24. Lee YL, Owens J, Thrupp L, Cesario TC. Does cranberry juice have antibacterial activity? JAMA 2000; 283:1691.
25. Ofek I, Goldhar J, Zafriri D et al. Anti-Escherichia coli adhesin activity of cranberry and blueberry juices. N Engl J Med 1991; 324:1599.
26. Foo LY, Lu Y, Howell AB, Vorsa N. The structure of cranberry proanthocyanidins which inhibit adherence of uropathogenic P-fimbriated Escherichia coli in vitro. Phytochemistry 2000; 54:173–181.
27. Habash MB, Van der Mei HC, Busscher HJ, Reid G. The effect of water, ascorbic acid, and cranberry derived supplementation on human urine and uropathogen adhesion to silicone rubber. Can J Microbiol 1999; 45:691–694.
28. Burger O, Ofek I, Tabak M et al. A high molecular mass constituent of cranberry juice inhibits helicobacter pylori adhesion to human gastric mucus. FEMS Immunol Med Microbiol 2000; 29:295–301.
29. Harkins K. What's the use of cranberry juice? Age Ageing 2000; 29:9–12.
30. Howell AB, Vorsa N, Foo LY et al. Inhibition of the adherence of P-fimbriated Escherichia coli to uroepithelial-cell surfaces by proanthocyanidin extracts from cranberries (letter). N Engl J Med 1998; 339:1085–1086.
31. Lowe FC, Fagelman E. Cranberry juice and urinary tract infections: what is the evidence? Urology 2001; 57:407–413.

32. Konowalchuk J, Speirs JI. Antiviral effect of commercial juices and beverages. Appl Environ Microbiol 1978; 35:1219–1220.
33. Pedersen CB, Kyle J, Jenkinson AM et al. Effects of blueberry and cranberry juice consumption on the plasma antioxidant capacity of healthy female volunteers. Eur J Clin Nutr 2000; 54:405–408.
34. Bomser J, Madhavi DL, Singletary K, Smith MA. In vitro anticancer activity of fruit extracts from Vaccinium species. Planta Med 1996; 62:212–216.
35. Anon. Possible interaction between warfarin and cranberry juice. Curr Probl Pharmacovigilance 2003; 29:8.
36. Hodek P, Trefil P, Stiborova M. Flavonoids-potent and versatile biologically active compounds interacting with cytochromes P450. Chem Biol Interact 2002; 139:1–21.

DAMIANA
Turnera aphrodisiaca

Synonyms/common names/related compounds[1]

Damiana aphrodisiaca, damiana herb, damiana leaf, herba de la pastora, Mexican damiana, mizibcoc, old woman's broom, rosemary, Turnerae diffusae folium, Turnerae diffusae herba

Indications

Female sexual dysfunction (with ginseng, ginkgo, L-arginine, multivitamins and minerals):[2]	Evidence grade B1
Weight loss (with yerbe mate and guarana):[3]	Evidence grade B2
Sexual dysfunction:[4,5]	Evidence grade E

Pregnancy

Uterine stimulant:[6]	Evidence level 4

A review article on the potential value of plants as sources of anti-fertility agents reported that herbs from the *Turnera* spp., including damiana, are uterine stimulants.[6]

Lactation

Safety unknown:	Evidence level 5

There are no reports in the scientific literature of damiana being either safe or contraindicated during lactation.

Constituents

Arbutin[7]
Flavonoids[7]
Flavone glycosides [7]

Toxicity[8]

- An individual exhibited tetanus-like convulsions and paroxysms, similar to those of rabies or strychnine poisoning, following the ingestion of approximately 200 g of damiana.[8]
- High doses of arbutin (1 g) are considered toxic – 100 g of damiana plant material would have to be consumed to equal a dose of 1 g of arbutin.[8]

Pharmacology

- Damiana contains high levels of phyto-progestins, which may increase the progestin activity of saliva.[9]
- Progesterone-binding herbs, such as damiana, were shown to have neutral or antagonist effects on breast cancer cell lines.[9]
- Damiana extracts are reported to have central nervous system depressant activity.[8]
- Damiana was shown not to have hypoglycemic effects.[10]
- Arbutin may have anti-bacterial properties.[8]

Drug interactions

Diabetic drugs (when using non-water extract or whole herb)[8]

Parts used[1]

Leaf and stem

References

1. Jellin JM, Batz F, Hitchens K. Natural Medicines Comprehensive Database. Stockton, CA: Therapeutic Research Faculty, 2002:1530.
2. Ito TY, Trant AS, Polan ML. A double-blind placebo-controlled study of ArginMax, a nutritional supplement for enhancement of female sexual function. J Sex Marital Ther 2001; 27:541–549.
3. Andersen T, Fogh J. Weight loss and delayed gastric emptying following a South American herbal preparation in overweight patients. J Hum Nutr Diet 2001; 14:243–250.
4. Cohen AJ. Using natural products to treat sexual dysfunction, 152nd Annual Meeting of the American Psychiatric Association, Washington DC, USA, May 15–20, 1999.
5. Rowland DL, Tai W. A review of plant-derived and herbal approaches to the treatment of sexual dysfunctions. J Sex Marital Ther 2003; 29:185–205.
6. Farnsworth NR, Bingel AS, Cordell GA, Crane FA, Fong HH. Potential value of plants as sources of new antifertility agents I. J Pharm Sci 1975; 64:535–598.
7. Piacente S, Camargo EE, Zampelli A et al. Flavonoids and arbutin from Turnera diffusa. Z Naturforsch [C] 2002; 57:983–985.
8. Newall CA, Anderson LA, Phillipson JD. Herbal Medicines: A Guide for Health-care Professionals. London, UK: Pharmaceutical Press, 1996:296.
9. Zava DT, Dollbaum CM, Blen M. Estrogen and progestin bioactivity of foods, herbs, and spices. Proc Soc Exp Biol Med 1998; 217:369–378.
10. Alarcon-Aguilar FJ, Roman-Ramos R, Flores-Saenz JL, Aguirre-Garcia F. Investigation on the hypoglycaemic effects of extracts of four Mexican medicinal plants in normal and alloxan-diabetic mice. Phytother Res 2002; 16:383–386.

DANDELION
Taraxacum officinale

Synonyms/common names/related compounds[1]

Blowball, cankerwort, common dandelion, dandelion herb, dandelion root, lion's tooth, pissenlit, priest's crown, swine snout, *T. herba,* taraxacum, wild endive.

Indications

Hepatitis B (multiple herb combination Jiedu Yanggan Gao):[2]	Evidence grade B2
Urinary tract infections (with uva ursi):[3]	Evidence grade C
Non-specific colitis (with St. John's wort, lemon balm, calendula and fennel):[4]	Evidence grade C
Diabetes:[5]	Evidence grade E
Anti-inflammatory effects:[6]	Evidence grade E
Diuretic:[7]	Evidence grade E

Pregnancy

Unknown:	Evidence level 5

There are no reports in the scientific literature of dandelion being either safe or contraindicated during pregnancy.

Food amounts

Minimal risk:[8]	Evidence level 4

A herbal medicine compendium reported that dandelion is of minimal risk during pregnancy when consumed in food amounts.[8]

Lactation

Unknown:	Evidence level 5

There are no reports in the scientific literature of dandelion being either safe or contraindicated during lactation.

Caution
Bile duct and intestinal obstruction[9]
Kidney disease[9]

Constituents

Root
Eudesmanolide and germacranolide sesquiterpene lactones[10]
Triterpene alcohols and phytosterols[10,11]
γ-Butyrolactone glycoside[12]: taraxacoside
Caffeic acid and p-hydroxyphenylacetic acid[13]
Potassium[14]
Inulin[14,15]

Leaf
Germacranolide sesquiterpene lactones[10,16]
Triterpenes:[17] cycloartenol
Phytosterols[16,17]
p-Hydroxyphenylacetic acid[10,16]
Flavonoids:[15] apigenin-7-glucoside, luteolin-7-glucoside
Furan fatty acids[18]
Potassium[19–21]

Toxicity

Root
LD_{50} (intraperitoneally): 36.6 g/kg[19]

Above ground parts
LD_{50} (intraperitoneally): 28.8 g/kg[19]

Pharmacology
- The bitter constituents in dandelion root increase bile flow.[22]
- Dandelion was shown to have diuretic and anti-inflammatory effects.[8]
- Dandelion may have some hypoglycemic activity.[8]
- The constituent taraxacin (eudesmanolides) is an appetite stimulant.[23]
- Dandelion may have a mild laxative effect.[24]
- Dandelion has been shown to have anti-tumor activity in vitro.[8]

Drug interactions[1]
Antacids[25]
Anti-diabetic drugs[25]

H2-blockers[25]
Lithium[25]
Potassium-sparing diuretics[8]
Proton pump inhibitors[25]

Part used

Whole plant[1]

References

1. Jellin JM, Batz F, Hitchens K. Natural Medicines Comprehensive Database, 3rd ed. Stockton, CA: Therapeutic Research Faculty, 2002:1530.
2. Chen Z. [Clinical study of 96 cases with chronic hepatitis B treated with jiedu yang-gan gao by a double-blind method]. Zhong Xi Yi Jie He Za Zhi 1990; 10:71–74, 67.
3. Larsson B, Jonasson A, Fianu S. Prophylactic effect of UVA-E in women with recurrent cystitis: a preliminary report. Curr Ther Res 1993; 53:441–443.
4. Chakurski I, Matev M, Koichev A, Angelova I, Stefanov G. [Treatment of chronic colitis with an herbal combination of Taraxacum officinale, Hipericum perforatum, Melissa officinaliss, Calendula officinalis and Foeniculum vulgare]. Vutr Boles 1981; 20:51–54.
5. Akhtar MS, Khan QM, Khaliq T. Effects of Portulaca oleracae (Kulfa) and Taraxacum officinale (Dhudhal) in normoglycaemic and alloxan-treated hyperglycaemic rabbits. J Pak Med Assoc 1985; 35:207–210.
6. Mascolo N, Autore G, Capasso G, et al. Biological screening of Italian medicinal plants for anti-inflammatory activity. Phytother Res 1987; 1:28–31.
7. Racz-Kotilla E, Racz G, Soloman A. The action of Taraxacum officinale extracts on the body weight and diuresis of laboratory animals. Planta Med 1974; 26:212–217.
8. Newall CA, Anderson LA, Phillipson JD. Herbal Medicines: A Guide for Health-care Professionals. London, UK: Pharmaceutical Press, 1996:296.
9. www.naturalstandard.com. Dandelion (Taraxacum officinale) Natural Standard Monograph, 2004.
10. Hansel R, Kartarahardja M, Huang JT, Bohlmann F. Sesquiterpenlacton-beta-D-glucopyranoside sowie ein neues Eudesmanolid aus Taraxacum officinale. Phytochemistry 1980; 19:857–861.
11. Burrows S, Simpson JCE. The triterpene group. Part IV. The triterpene alcohols of Taraxacum root. J Chem Soc 1938:2042–2047.
12. Rauwald H-W, Huang JT. Taraxacoside, a type of acylated gamma-butyrolactone glycoside from Taraxacum officinale. Phytochemistry 1985; 24:1557–1559.
13. Faber K. Der Lowenzahn – Taraxacum officinale weber. Pharmazie 1958; 13:423–436.
14. Vogl HH, Schaette R. Phytotherapeutische Reflexionen. Betrachtungen uber Silybum marianum (Carduus marianus), Taraxacum officinale, Cichorium intybus, Bryonia alba et dioica, Viscum album und ihre Beziehungen zur Leber. Erfahrungsheilkunde 1977; 26:247–255.
15. List PH, Horhammer L, eds. Taraxacum. Hagers Handbuch der pharmazeutischen Praxis, Band VI, C. Berlin-Heidelberg: Springer-Verlag, 1979:16–21.
16. Kuusi T, Pyysalo H, Autio K. The bitterness properties of dandelion II. Chemical investigations. Lebensm-Wiss Technol 1985; 18:347–349.
17. Westerman L, Roddick JG. Annual variations in sterol levels in leaves of Taraxacum officinale Weber. Plant Physiol 1981; 68:872–875.

18. Hanneman K, Puchta V, Simon E et al. The common occurrence of furan fatty acids in plants. Lipids 1989; 24:296–298.
19. Racz-Kotilla E, Racz G, Solomon A. The action of Taraxacum officinale extracts on the body weight and diuresis of laboratory animals. Planta Med 1974; 26:212–217.
20. Racz G, Bodon J, Tolgyesi G. Determination of the mineral content of 41 medicinal plant species by chemotaxonomical and biochemical observations. Herba Hung 1978; 17:43–54.
21. Hook I, McGee A, Henman M. Evaluation of dandelion for diuretic activity and variation in potassium content. Int J Pharmacog 1993; 31:29–34.
22. Schulz V, Hansel R, Tyler VE, Terry C. Rational Phytotherapy: A Physician's Guide to Herbal Medicine, 3rd ed. Berlin: Springer, 1998.
23. The Review of Natural Products by Facts and Comparisons. St. Louis, MO: Wolters Kluwer Co., 1999.
24. Foster S, Tyler VE. Tyler's Honest Herbal: A Sensible Guide to the Use of Herbs and Related Remedies, 3rd ed. Binghamton, NY: Haworth Herbal Press, 1993.
25. Brinker F. Herb Contraindications and Drug Interactions, 2nd ed. Sandy, OR: Eclectic Medical Publications, 1998.

DEADLY NIGHTSHADE
Atropa belladonna

Synonyms/common names/related substances[1]
Belladonna, dwale, devil's cherries, poison black cherry, devil's herb, divale, dwayberry, great morel, naughty man's cherries

Indications

A. belladonna *herbal or pharmaceutical preparations*

Irritable bowel syndrome[2,3] (in combination with other drugs):	Evidence grade B1
Migraine headaches[4,5] (in combination with other drugs):	Evidence grade B1
Premenstrual syndrome:[6]	Evidence grade B1
Autonomic nervous system conditions:[7,8]	Evidence grade B2
Airway obstruction:[9]	Evidence grade C

Homeopathic A. belladonna *(Belladonna)*

Migraine headaches:[10]	Evidence grade B1
Otitis media:[11]	Evidence grade C

Pregnancy

Drug derivative – minimal side-effects during labor:[12,13]	Evidence level 1a

Drugs derived from *Atropa* are sometimes used during labor or abortions.[12,13] Prifinium bromide, an atropine drug, was administered to women in labor as part of a controlled trial.[12] The atropine administered led to a shorter period of labor, normal intra-partum hemorrhage and normal amniotic fluid.[12] The atropine had no effect on fetal heart rate or AGPAR score.[12]

Teratogenic – potential birth defects:[14,15]	Evidence level 2
Teratogenic – potential eye malformation:[16]	Evidence level 3
Teratogenic – potential respiratory abnormalities:[17]	Evidence level 4

Teratogenic – potential penile abnormalities (hypospadia):[17]	Evidence level 4

Teratogenic – potential ear malformations:[17]	Evidence level 4

Although no direct relationship between first trimester use of atropine and birth defects was found, a study reported an increase in birth defects in the offspring of mothers who had taken belladonna.[14] Scopolamine and hyoscyamine were found to have teratogenic effects in animals.[15] The eyes of atropine-exposed chicken embryos were found to have abnormal features and appearance.[16] An evidenced-based compendium on natural health products reported that there are anecdotal reports that the use of belladonna during pregnancy may increase the risk of respiratory abnormalities, hypospadias (penile urethral malformation in males), and ear malformation.[17]

No adverse effect with phenothiazine – first trimester:[18]	Evidence level 2

A case report in the scientific literature reported that belladonna supplementation, along with phenothiazine, to two pregnant women with sialorrhea and hyperemesis resulted in no side effects in the women or in the newborn.[18]

Temporary mydriasis:[19]	Evidence level 2

A neonate whose mother had recently taken the anti-depressant amitriptyline developed fixed dilated pupils after a modest dose of intravenous atropine.[19] The neonate's pupils became reactive again after 7 hours and there were no neurological sequelae.[19]

Homeopathic A. belladonna *(Belladonna)*

Minimal risk:[20,21]	Evidence level 1a

A homeopathic preparation of *A. belladonna*, called Belladonna, beyond the potency (dilution) of 12C, does not contain any molecules of the original substance. A randomized controlled trial found that Belladonna did not produce any significant symptoms that were different to placebo.[20]

Lactation

Potentially unsafe – caution:[1]	Evidence level 4

A compendium on natural health products reported that *Atropa* decreases the production of breast milk due to its anti-cholinergic properties and that it is secreted in breast milk.[1] *Atropa* was not reported in the scientific literature as either being safe or causing harm to the nursing infant.

Contraindications

Glaucoma[22]

Constituents

Alkaloids:[22] atropine (hyoscyamine), scopolamine (hyoscine)

Toxicology

Lethal dose (children): 10–100 mg of atropine, 5–50 g of powdered deadly nightshade, more than three berries[22]

Pharmacology

- Atropine acts on the muscarinic receptors where it blocks the parasympathetic effects on smooth muscle, cardiac muscle, and glandular cells.[23]
- Atropine blocks the activity of the vagus nerve, thereby increasing the firing rate of the sinoatrial node.[23]
- Atropine reduces heart rate and peristalsis, increases bladder pressure, relaxes the bile duct, reduces the production of saliva and gastric fluids, and reduces the secretions from the pancreas, eye, and bronchi.[23]
- Deadly nightshade is believed to have no or very little effect on blood pressure control.[7]

Drug interactions

Anti-cholinergic drugs[24]

Parts containing toxins[22]

Roots, leaves, berries, flowers

References

1. Jellin JM, Batz F, Hitchens K. Natural Medicines Comprehensive Database. Stockton, CA: Therapeutic Research Faculty, 2002:1530.
2. Rhodes JB, Abrams JH, Manning RT. Controlled clinical trial of sedative-anticholinergic drugs in patients with the irritable bowel syndrome. J Clin Pharmacol 1978; 18:340–345.
3. Ritchie JA, Truelove SC. Treatment of irritable bowel syndrome with lorazepam, hyoscine butylbromide, and ispaghula husk. Br Med J 1979; 1:376–378.
4. Friedman AP, Di SFJ, Hwang DS. Symptomatic relief of migraine: multicenter comparison of Cafergot((R)) P-B, Cafergot((R)), and placebo. Clin Ther 1989; 11:170–182.
5. Stieg RL. Double-blind study of belladonna-ergotamine-phenobarbital for interval treatment of recurrent throbbing headache. Headache 1977; 17:120–124.
6. Robinson K, Huntington KM, Wallace MG. Treatment of the premenstrual syndrome. Br J Obstet Gynaecol 1977; 84:784–788.
7. Bettermann H, Cysarz D, Portsteffen A, Kummell HC. Bimodal dose-dependent effect on autonomic, cardiac control after oral administration of Atropa belladonna. Auton Neurosci 2001; 90:132–137.

8. Dobrescu DI. Propranolol in the treatment of disturbances of the autonomic nervous system. Curr Ther Res Clin Exper 1971; 13:69–73.
9. Kahn A, Rebuffat E, Sottiaux M et al. Prevention of airway obstructions during sleep in infants with breath-holding spells by means of oral belladonna: a prospective double-blind crossover evaluation. Sleep 1991; 14:432–438.
10. Brigo B, Serpelloni G. Homeopathic treatment of migraines: a randomized double-blind controlled study of sixty cases (homeopathic remedy versus placebo). Berlin J Res Homoeopath 1991; 1:98–106.
11. Friese KH, Kruse S, Ludtke R, Moeller H. The homoeopathic treatment of otitis media in children – comparisons with conventional therapy. Int J Clin Pharmacol Ther 1997; 35:296–301.
12. Tolino A, Cardone A, Iervolino P, Granata P. The effect of an atropine-like parasympathologic drug on labour. Minerva Ginecol 1980; 32:655–662.
13. Krumholz W, Stoyanov M, Kothe M, Hempelmann G. [Influence of various premedication agents, inhalation anesthetics and adjuvants on anesthesia with an opioid, alfentanyl]. Anasth Intensivther Notfallmed 1985; 20:171–174.
14. Diaz DM, Diaz SF, Marx GF. Cardiovascular effects of glycopyrrolate and belladonna derivatives in obstetric patients. Bull N Y Acad Med 1980; 56:245–248.
15. Magras IN, Kotsaki-Kovatsi VP, Kovatsis A, Adamidou L. Teratogenic effects of a mixture of scopolamine and hyoscyamine in chick embryos. Vet Hum Toxicol 1993; 35:434–435.
16. Angelini C, Costa M, Morescalchi F et al. Muscarinic drugs affect cholinesterase activity and development of eye structures during early chick development. Eur J Histochem 1998; 42:309–320.
17. http://www.naturalstandard.com.
18. Freeman JJ, Altier RH, Baptiste HJ et al. Evaluation and management of sialorrhea of pregnancy with concomitant hyperemesis. J Natl Med Assoc 1994; 86:704–708.
19. Yung M, Herrema I. Persistent mydriasis following intravenous atropine in a neonate. Paediatr Anaesth 2000; 10:438–440.
20. Walach H. Does a highly diluted homoeopathic drug act as a placebo in healthy volunteers? Experimental study of Belladonna 30C in double-blind crossover design – a pilot study. J Psychosom Res 1993; 37:851–860.
21. Walach H, Koster H, Hennig T, Haag G. The effects of homeopathic belladonna 30CH in healthy volunteers – a randomized, double-blind experiment. J Psychosom Res 2001; 50:155–160.
22. Brinker F. The Toxicology of Botanical Medicines. Sandy, OR: Eclectic Medical Publications, 2000:296.
23. McGuffin M, Hobbs C, Upton R, Goldberg A. American Herbal Products Association's Botanical Safety Handbook. Boca Raton, FL: CRC Press, 1997:231.
24. Blumenthal M, Busse WR, Goldberg A et al. The Complete German Commission E Monographs: Therapeutic Guide to Herbal Medicines. Boston, MA: American Botanical Council, 1998.

DONG QUAI
Angelica sinensis

Synonyms/common names/related substances[1]

Chinese angelica, dang gui, danggui, dong qua, dong-quai, ligustilides, phyto-estrogen, tan kue bai zhi, tang kuei

Indications

Premenstrual syndrome (within a multiple herb Chinese formula):[2]	Evidence grade A
Abdominal pain:[3]	Evidence grade B2
Pulmonary hypertension in patients with chronic obstructivepulmonary disease (COPD) (with nifedipine):[4]	Evidence grade B2
Cerebral thrombosis (within a multiple herb Chinese formula):[5]	Evidence grade C
Cirrhosis:[6]	Evidence grade C
Coronary heart disease:[7]	Evidence grade C
Idiopathic thrombocytopenic purpura (within a multiple herb Chinese formula):[8]	Evidence grade D

Pregnancy

No estrogenic effects:[9]	Evidence level 1a

A randomized placebo-controlled trial on postmenopausal women was conducted in order to evaluate the estrogenic effects of dong quai.[9] It was concluded that dong quai does not produce estrogen-like responses in endometrial thickness or in vaginal maturation and that it was no more helpful than placebo in relieving menopausal symptoms.[9]

Uterine stimulant:[10,11]	Evidence level 3
Uterine relaxant:[10,12]	Evidence level 3

In mice, decoctions of dong quai were found to have a stimulating effect on the uterus in vitro.[11] The stimulating action of dong quai was related to its stimulation of H1 receptors in the uterus.[11] Ferulic acid, a constituent of dong quai, was found to inhibit uterine contraction in rats.[12]

Lactation

Unknown:	Evidence level 5

Dong quai was not reported in the evidence-based medicine literature as being safe or contraindicated in lactation.

Contraindications

Warfarin therapy[13,14]

Caution

Menorrhagia
Metrorrhagia

Constituents[1,12,15]

Coumarins: osthol, psoralen, bergapten
Butylidene phthalide
Ligustilide
n-Butylidene-phthalide
Sesquiterpenes
Carvacrol
Dihydrophthalic anhydride
Ferulic acid

Pharmacology

- Dong quai has anti-inflammatory effects where it lowered plasma prostaglandin F2α (PGF2 α) and menstrual blood PGF2 α in patients with dysmenorrhea.[16]
- Dong quai was found to stimulate the growth of human breast cancer cell lines independently of estrogenic activity.[17]
- The coumarin constituent bergapten is believed to be carcinogenic.[1]
- The coumarin constituent osthol has a stimulant effect on the central nervous system.[1]
- Dong quai appears to potentiate the effect of warfarin and thereby increase prothrombin time.[13,14,18,19]
- Intravenous administration of dong quai decreased serum gastrin levels of inferior vena cava, hepatic and peripheral veins in patients with liver cirrhosis[6]
- Dong quai has an analgesic and anti-septic effect in abdominal pain.
- Dong quai administered with nifedipine was shown to decrease mean pulmonary arterial pressure and increase cardiac output and PaO_2 in COPD.[4]
- In combination with ginseng and astragalus, dong quai was found to improve many symptoms of coronary artery disease.[7]
- The coumarins psoralen and bergapten are photosensitizing and may cause photodermatitis.[1]

Drugs interactions

Anti-coagulant/anti-platelet drugs[1]
Warfarin[13,14,18,19]

Part used[10]

Root

References

1. Jellin JM, Batz F, Hitchens K. Natural Medicines Comprehensive Database. Stockton, CA: Therapeutic Research Faculty, 2002:1530.
2. Hardy ML. Herbs of special interest to women. J Am Pharm Assoc (Wash) 2000; 40:234–242.
3. Sun SW, Wang JF. [Efficacy of danggui funing pill in treating 162 cases of abdominal pain]. Zhongguo Zhong Xi Yi Jie He Za Zhi 1992; 12:531–532, 517.
4. Xu JY, Li BX, Cheng SY. [Short-term effects of Angelica sinensis and nifedipine on chronic obstructive pulmonary disease in patients with pulmonary hypertension]. Zhongguo Zhong Xi Yi Jie He Za Zhi 1992; 12:716–718, 707.
5. Zhao L, Zhang Y, Xu ZX. [Clinical effect and experimental study of xijian tong-shuan pill]. Zhongguo Zhong Xi Yi Jie He Za Zhi 1994; 14:71–73, 67.
6. Huang ZP, Liang KH. [Effect of radix Angelicae sinensis on serum gastrin levels in patients with cirrhosis]. Zhonghua Nei Ke Za Zhi 1994; 33:373–375.
7. Liao JZ, Chen JJ, Wu ZM et al. Clinical and experimental studies of coronary heart disease treated with yi-qi huo-xue injection. J Tradit Chin Med 1989; 9:193–198.
8. Shi YM, Wu QZ. [Idiopathic thrombocytopenic purpura in children treated with replenishing qi and tonifying kidney and the changes in thrombocyte aggregative function]. Zhong Xi Yi Jie He Za Zhi 1991; 11:14–16, 3.
9. Hirata JD, Swiersz LM, Zell B, Small R, Ettinger B. Does dong quai have estrogenic effects in postmenopausal women? A double-blind, placebo-controlled trial. Fertil Steril 1997; 68:981–986.
10. Brinker F. Herb Contraindications and Drug Interactions. Sandy, OR: Eclectic Medical Publications, 2001:432.
11. Shi M, Chang L, He G. [Stimulating action of Carthamus tinctorius L., Angelica sinensis (Oliv.) Diels and Leonurus sibiricus L. on the uterus]. Zhongguo Zhong Yao Za Zhi 1995; 20:173–175, 192.
12. Ozaki Y, Ma JP. Inhibitory effects of tetramethylpyrazine and ferulic acid on spontaneous movement of rat uterus in situ. Chem Pharm Bull (Tokyo) 1990; 38:1620–1623.
13. Page RLN, Lawrence JD. Potentiation of warfarin by dong quai. Pharmacotherapy 1999; 19:870–876.
14. Smolinske SC. Dietary supplement–drug interactions. J Am Med Womens Assoc 1999; 54:191–192, 195.
15. Bensky D, Gamble A, Kaptchuk TJ. Chinese Herbal Medcine: Materia Medica. Seattle, WA: Eastland Press, 1993:556.
16. Xie C. [Effects of danggui shaoyao powder on blood rheological indexes and prostaglandin F2 alpha in dysmenorrhea patients]. Zhong Xi Yi Jie He Za Zhi 1990; 10:410–412, 389.
17. Amato P, Christophe S, Mellon PL. Estrogenic activity of herbs commonly used as remedies for menopausal symptoms. Menopause 2002; 9:145–150.

18. Chan K, Lo AC, Yeung JH, Woo KS. The effects of Danshen (Salvia miltiorrhiza) on warfarin pharmacodynamics and pharmacokinetics of warfarin enantiomers in rats. J Pharm Pharmacol 1995; 47:402–406.
19. Lo AC, Chan K, Yeung JH, Woo KS. Danggui (Angelica sinensis) affects the pharmacodynamics but not the pharmacokinetics of warfarin in rabbits. Eur J Drug Metab Pharmacokinet 1995; 20:55–60.

ECHINACEA
Echinacea angustifolia, E. pallida, E. purpurea

Synonyms/common names/related substances[1]

American cone flower, black Sampson, black Susan, *Brauneria angustifolia*, *B. pallida*, comb flower, coneflower, echinaceawurzel, hedgehog, igelkopfwurzel, Indian head, Kansas snakeroot, narrow-leaved purple cone flower, pale coneflower, purple cone flower, purpursonnenhutkraut, purpursonnenhutwurzel, racine d'echininacea, red sunflower, rock-up-hat, roter sonnenhut, schmallblaettrige kegelblumenwurzel, schmallblaettriger sonnenhut, scurvy root, snakeroot, sonnenhutwurzel

Indications

Upper respiratory tract infection – treatment:[2–4]	Evidence grade A
Upper respiratory tract infection – prevention:[5–7]	Evidence grade B2
Radiation associated leukopenia:[8–10]	Evidence grade B2
Cancer survival time:[11,12]	Evidence grade C

Pregnancy

Minimal risk:[13,14]	Evidence level 1b

A prospective follow-up study on 206 pregnant women, 112 of whom had used echinacea in the first trimester of pregnancy reported that gestational use of echinacea during the first trimester (organogenesis) is not associated with an increased risk for major malformations.[13] The German Commission E compendium, produced by an expert panel on botanical medicine, considers oral echinacea in recommended doses safe for use during pregnancy.[14] Echinacea was not reported in the scientific literature as being contraindicated during pregnancy.

Lactation

Minimal risk:[14]	Evidence level 4

The German Commission E compendium, produced by an expert panel on botanical medicine, considers oral echinacea in recommended doses safe for use during lactation.[14] Echinacea was not reported in the scientific literature as being either safe or contraindicated during lactation.

Constituents[15]

Caffeic acid derivatives: echinocoside, cichoric acid, cynarin
Polysaccharides

Glycoproteins
Alkamides

Toxicity

- LD_{50} in mice: >2500 mg/kg[16]
- LD_{50} of intravenous echinacea juice: 50 mL/kg[17]

Pharmacology

- The immunostimulatory effects of echinacea have not been attributed to any single compound.[18]
- Echinacea increases the proliferation of phagocytes in spleen and bone marrow, stimulates monocytes to produce cytokines (interleukin (IL)-1, IL-6, tumor necrosis factor), increases the number of polymorphonuclear leukocytes (PMN), activates macrophages, and promotes the adherence of PMN to endothelial cells.[19–22]
- Echinacea was shown to inhibit hyaluronidase production in vitro and in vivo.[18,23,24]
- Echinacea has anti-viral, anti-bacterial and anti-fungal properties.[15, 25–27]
- Echinacea was shown to inhibit the influenza virus and the herpes simplex virus (I and II).[26, 27]
- Topically, echinacea has anti-inflammatory properties where it inhibits edema.[28, 29]
- Echinacea may interfere with cytochrome P450 (CYP) 3A4 (CYP3A4) enzyme.[30]

Drug interactions

Immunosuppressant drugs[31]
Drugs metabolized by the cytochrome P450 (CYP) 3A4 (CYP3A4) enzyme[30]

Parts used[32]

Roots, stems, and leaves

References

1. Jellin JM, Batz F, Hitchens K. Natural Medicines Comprehensive Database. Stockton, CA: Therapeutic Research Faculty, 2002:1530.
2. Barrett B, Vohmann M, Calabrese C. Echinacea for upper respiratory infection. J Fam Pract 1999; 48:628–635.
3. Henneicke-von Zepelin H, Hentschel C, Schnitker J et al. Efficacy and safety of a fixed combination phytomedicine in the treatment of the common cold (acute viral respiratory tract infection): results of a randomised, double blind, placebo controlled, multicentre study. Curr Med Res Opin 1999; 15:214–227.
4. Melchart D, Linde K, Fischer P, Kaesmayr J. Echinacea for preventing and treating the common cold. Cochrane Database Syst Rev 2000:CD000530.
5. Turner RB, Riker DK, Gangemi J. Ineffectiveness of echinacea for prevention of experimental rhinovirus colds. Antimicrob Agents Chemother 2000; 44:1708–1709.

6. Melchart D, Walther E, Linde K, Brandmaier R, Lersch C. Echinacea root extracts for the prevention of upper respiratory tract infections: a double-blind, placebo-controlled randomized trial. Arch Fam Med 1998; 7:541–545.
7. Forth H, Beuscher N. [Effect on the frequency of banal cold infections by esberitox]. ZFA (Stuttgart) 1981; 57:2272–2275.
8. Sartor KJ. [Efficacy of Esberitox in the treatment of radiation-induced leukopenia]. Ther Ggw 1972; 111:1147–1150.
9. Pohl P. [Treatment of radiation-induced leukopenia with Esberitox]. Ther Ggw 1970; 109:902 passim.
10. Bendel R, Bendel V, Renner K, Carstens V, Stolze K. [Additional treatment with Esberitox N in patients with chemo-radiotherapy treatment of advanced breast cancer]. Onkologie 1989; 12(Suppl 3):32–38.
11. Lersch C, Zeuner M, Bauer A et al. Nonspecific immunostimulation with low doses of cyclophosphamide (LDCY), thymostimulin, and Echinacea purpurea extracts (echinacin) in patients with far advanced colorectal cancers: preliminary results. Cancer Invest 1992; 10:343–348.
12. Lersch C, Zeuner M, Bauer A et al. Stimulation of the immune response in outpatients with hepatocellular carcinomas by low doses of cyclophosphamide (LDCY), echinacea purpurea extracts (Echinacin) and thymostimulin. Arch Geschwulstforsch 1990; 60:379–383.
13. Gallo M, Sarkar M, Au W, Pietrzak K, Comas B, Smith M, Jaeger TV, Einarson A, Koren G. Pregnancy outcome following gestational exposure to echinacea: a prospective controlled study. Arch Intern Med 2000; 160:3141–3143.
14. Blumenthal M, Busse WR, Goldberg A et al. The Complete German Commission E Monographs: Therapeutic Guide to Herbal Medicines. Boston, MA: American Botanical Council, 1998.
15. Boon H, Smith M. The Botanical Pharmacy: The Pharmacology of 47 Common Herbs. Kingston, ON: Quarry Health Books/CCNM, 1999:320.
16. Lenk M. Acute toxicity if various polysaccharides from Echinacea purpurea in the mouse. Zeitschrift Fur Phytotherapie 1989; 10:49–52.
17. Mengs U, Clare CB, Poiley JA. Toxicity of Echinacea purpurea. Acute, subacute and genotoxicity studies. Arzneimittelforschung 1991; 41:1076–1081.
18. Bauer R, Wagner H. Echinacea species as potential immunostimulatory drugs. Econ Med Plant Res 1991; 5:253–321.
19. Roesler J, Steinmuller C, Kiderlen A et al. Application of purified polysaccharides from cell cultures of the plant Echinacea purpurea to mice mediates protection against systemic infections with Listeria monocytogenes and Candida albicans. Int J Immunopharmacol 1991; 13:27–37.
20. Mose JR. Effect of echinacin on phagocytosis and natural killer cells. Medizinische Welt 1983; 34:1463–1467.
21. Stimpel M, Proksch A, Wagner H, Lohmann-Matthes ML. Macrophage activation and induction of macrophage cytotoxicity by purified polysaccharide fractions from the plant Echinacea purpurea. Infect Immun 1984; 46:845–849.
22. Burger RA, Torres AR, Warren R, Caldwell VD, Hughes BG. Echinacea-induced cytokine production by human macrophages. Int J Immunopharmacol 1997; 19:371–379.
23. Busing KH. Inhibition of hyaluronidase by Echinacin. Arzneimittelforschung 1952; 2:467–472.

24. Korting GW, Born W. Beeinflusseng des trypanociden salvason-effekts durch hyaluronidase und einen hyaluronidase-inhibitor (Echinacin). Arzneimittelforschung 1954; 4:424–426.
25. Steinmuller C, Roesler J, Grottrup E, Franke G, Wagner H, Lohmann-Matthes ML. Polysaccharides isolated from plant cell cultures of Echinacea purpurea enhance the resistance of immunosuppressed mice against systemic infections with Candida albicans and Listeria monocytogenes. Int J Immunopharmacol 1993; 15:605–614.
26. Thompson KD. Antiviral activity of Viracea against acyclovir susceptible and acyclovir resistant strains of herpes simplex virus. Antiviral Res 1998; 39:55–61.
27. Wacker A, W. [Virus-inhibition by echinacea purpurea (author's transl)]. Planta Med 1978; 33:89–102.
28. Tragni E, Tubaro A, Melis S, Galli CL. Evidence from two classical irritation tests for an anti-inflammatory action of a natural extract, echinacea B. Food Chem Toxicol 1985; 23:317–319.
29. Tubaro A, Tragni E, Del Negro P et al. Anti-inflammatory activity of a polysaccharide fraction of Echinacea angustifolia. J Pharm Pharmacol 1987; 39:567–569.
30. Budzinski JW, Foster BC, Vandenhoek S, Arnason JT. An in vitro evaluation of human cytochrome P450 3A4 inhibition by selected commercial herbal extracts and tinctures. Phytomedicine 2000; 7:273–282.
31. Chavez ML, Chavez PI. Echinacea. Hosp Pharm 1998; 33:180–188.
32. Brinker F. The Toxicology of Botanical Medicines. Sandy, OR: Eclectic Medical Publications, 2000:296.

EPHEDRA

Ephedra vulgaris, E. distachya, E. equisetina, E. shennungiana, E. gerardiana, E. intermedia, E. sinica

Synonyms/common names/related compounds[1]

Cao mahuang, Chinese ephedra, Chinese joint-fir, cao ma-huang, desert herb, *Ephedrae herba*, *E. sinensis*, herbal ecstasy, Indian jointfir, joint fir, mahuang, ma huang, ma-huang, mahuanggen (ma huang root), Mongolian ephedra, muzei ma huang, Pakistani ephedra, popotillo, sea grape, shuang sui ma huang, teamster's tea, yellow astringent, yellow horse, zhong mahuang

Indications

Hypotension during spinal anesthesia for cesarean delivery:[2]	Evidence grade A
Weight loss (with caffeine):[3–5]	Evidence grade B1
Allergic rhinitis:[6]	Evidence grade B1
Weight loss:[7,8]	Evidence grade B2
Asthmatic bronchoconstriction:[9,10]	Evidence grade B2
Hypotension (with caffeine):[11]	Evidence grade B2
Sexual arousal in women:[12]	Evidence grade B2
Hypotension during epidural block:[13]	Evidence grade C

Pregnancy

Crosses the placenta:[14]	Evidence level 1a
Does not affect fetal wellbeing or neonatal outcome:[14]	Evidence level 1a

A randomized controlled trial on 40 pregnant women undergoing elective cesarean reported that ephedrine crosses the placenta where the fetal blood level is approximately 70% of the maternal level.[14] The presence of ephedrine in the fetal circulation did not seem to have any deleterious effects on fetal wellbeing or neonatal outcome.[14]

Increases neonatal heart rate:[15]	Evidence level 1a

A study of fetal heart rate changes during epidural anesthesia in 71 patients found that ephedrine administration was associated with significant increases in fetal hear rate and beat-to-beat variability.[15] The authors reported that the fetal heart rate changes were dose related and were not associated with fetal asphyxia as judged by measurement of fetal scalp blood pH or APGAR scores.[15] A randomized controlled trial on 40 pregnant women undergoing elective cesarean reported that ephedrine increased fetal heart rate for 40–50 minutes after intramuscular injection to the mother.[14] Ephedrine did not adversely affect the fetus.[14]

Uterine stimulant:[16]	Evidence level 4

A review article on the potential value of plants as sources of anti-fertility agents reported that ephedra is a uterine stimulant and that its constituents ephedrine and pseudoephedrine are uterine stimulants.[16]

Ephedrine

May cause hypertension in the mother:[17,18]	Evidence level 1a

A systematic review on the dose–response characteristics of prophylactic intravenous ephedrine for the prevention of hypotension during spinal anesthesia for cesarean delivery found that at larger doses of ephedrine, the likelihood of causing hypertension was actually more than that of preventing hypotension and there was also a minor decrease in umbilical arterial pH.[17] As such, the authors did not recommend prophylactic ephedrine.[17] A previous systematic review in 2002 also found similar results.[18]

Increases blood flow to the uterus:[19]	Evidence level 1b

An outcome study in order to assess the effects of ephedrine on uterine artery velocities and resistance index using the Doppler technique during the active phase of labor found that a bolus administration of intravenous ephedrine may increase uterine perfusion pressure during labor and restore uterine blood flow to the placenta during uterine contractions, thereby preventing fetal asphyxia.[19]

Teratogenic – limb defects (with theophylline and phenobarbital):[20]	Evidence level 2

Two cases were observed of severe limb defects in infants following the use of sympathomimetic drugs during pregnancy.[20] The mother of one infant had taken large doses of Primatene (ephedrine, theophylline, phenobarbital) as tablets and mist throughout pregnancy, where her baby was born with oligoectrosyndactyly.[20] The authors also reported that studies in pregnant rabbits using Primatene in both low and high dosage resulted in limb reduction defects and other malformations in a significant number of the offspring compared with controls.[20]

Potential abortifacient (with theophylline and phenobarbital):[21] Evidence level 2

A case was reported of an aborted human embryo from a mother who had taken four tablets of Tedral (130 mg theophylline, 25 mg ephedrine, 8 mg phenobabital) for an upper respiratory tract infection when the embryo was at approximately 30 days of development.[21]

Avoid in pregnancy-induced hypertension:[22] Evidence level 4

A review study on the influence of epidural analgesia on fetal and neonatal well-being reported that epidural analgesia-containing ephedrine should be avoided in women with pregnancy-induced hypertension.[22]

Uterine stimulant:[16] Evidence level 4

A review article on the potential value of plants as sources of anti-fertility agents reported that ephedrine is a uterine stimulant.[16]

Pseudoephedrine

Causes birth defects (gastroschisis and small intestine atresia [SIA]):[23–25] Evidence level 1b

A retrospective cohort study was conducted on the relationship between maternal use of cough/cold/analgesic medications containing pseudoephedrine and risks of gastroschisis and SIA.[23] The authors examined the mothers of 206 gastroschisis cases, 126 SIA cases, and 798 controls.[23] The risk of gastroschisis was elevated for use of pseudoephedrine and pseudoephedrine combined with acetaminophen (paracetamol).[23] The risk of SIA was increased for use of pseudoephedrine and for use of pseudoephedrine in combination with acetaminophen.[23]

A case–control study of gastroschisis where they evaluated the risks associated with mother's first-trimester use of medications found an elevated risk of gastroschisis with maternal use of pseudoephedrine.[24] Another study found the same association between pseudoephedrine use during pregnancy and the increased risk of gastroschisis.[25]

Teratogenic – limb defects (with phenylephrine and phenylpropanolamine):[20] Evidence level 2

Two cases were observed of severe limb defects in infants following the use of sympathomimetic drugs during pregnancy.[20] The mother of one infant had taken Triaminic (pseudoephedrine, phenylephrine, phenylpropanolamine) during preganancy where her baby was born with distal limb defects.[20]

Uterine stimulant:[16]	Evidence level 4

A review article on the potential value of plants as sources of anti-fertility agents reported that pseudoephedrine is a uterine stimulant.[16]

Lactation

May cross into breast milk:[26]	Evidence level 2

A case was reported of a 3-month-old child with irritability, excessive crying, and disturbed sleep patterns for 5 days.[26] Further investigation led to the discovery that the mother was taking a long-acting nasal decongestant, containing dexbrompheniramine and d-isoephedrine, for allergic rhinitis.[26] Symptoms subsided after the mother discontinued the decongestant.[26] The author reported that it was not possible to prove conclusively that ephedrine (d-isoephedrine) crosses into breast milk.[26]

Pseudoephedrine

Decreases milk production:[27]	Evidence level 1a
Unlikely to affect the infant:[27]	Evidence level 1a

A randomized crossover study was conducted on eight lactating women to assess the effects of pseudoephedrine on breast blood flow, temperature and milk production, and to estimate the likely infant dose during breast-feeding.[27] Pseudoephedrine was found to significantly reduce milk production, where the depression of prolactin secretion may be a contributing factor.[27] The authors reported that at the maximum recommended pseudoephedrine doses, the calculated infant dose delivered via milk was <10% of the maternal dose, and is unlikely to affect the infant adversely.[27]

Contraindications

Pregnancy-induced hypertension[22]
Enlarged prostate[28]
Organic heart disease[28]
Hypertension[28]
Diabetes[28]
Anxiety/restlessness[28]
Closed-angle glaucoma[28]
Impaired cerebral circulation[28]
Pheochromocytoma[28]
Hyperthyroidism[28]

Caution[28]

Anorexia
Insomnia
Suicidal persons
Concomitant use with caffeine

Constituents

Alkaloids:[28–31] ephedrine, pseudoephedrine, phenylpropanolamine, norpseudoephedrine, methylephedrine, norephedrine

Toxicity

- Ephedrine is toxic >300 mg per day.[28]
- Lethal dose: 1–2 g of ephedrine.[28]
- In dogs, the minimum dose at which death was reported was 5.8 mg/kg (2.6 mg/lb).[32]

Pharmacology

- Ephedrine decreases direct uterine arterial vasoconstriction during pregnancy by increasing the release of an endogenous vasodilator (nitrous oxide), either from the vascular endothelium or the vessel wall.[33]
- Ephedrine can stimulate uterine contractions, and theoretically, can be catabolized to mutagenic nitrosamines.[34]
- The sympathomimetics ephedrine and pseudoephedrine can directly and indirectly stimulate the sympathetic nervous system.[35]
- Ephedra alkaloids have been linked to myocarditis, myocardial infarction, coronary artery vasoconstriction, cardiac arrhythmia, cerebral hemorrhage, cerebral vasculitis, and ischemic stroke.[1,36]
- Ephedrine and pseudoephedrine can increase systolic and diastolic blood pressure, heart rate and cardiac contractility, and cause peripheral vasoconstriction, bronchodilation and central nervous system stimulation.[30]
- Ephedrine causes thermogenesis and modest weight loss, possibly by stimulating norepinephrine release.[37]
- Ephedrine appears to have anti-tussive, bacteriostatic and anti-inflammatory properties.[34,38,39]
- Ephedrine may exacerbate urinary retention, but can also have diuretic effects.[40]
- Ephedrine relaxes the smooth muscle in the gastrointestinal and urinary tract.[41]
- Ephedrine causes catecholamine release and increases central nervous system stimulation, which may lead to better anaerobic exercise performance.[42]

Drug interactions

Caffeine[43]
Dexamethasone (Decadron)[44]

Diabetic drugs[44]
Ergotamine[45]
Monoamine oxidase inhibitors[45]
Oxytocin[45]
QT-interval prolonging drugs[46]
Reserpine[44]
Theophylline[44]
Urinary acidifiers[30]
Urinary alkalinizers[30]

Parts used[28]

Stems, twigs; root and fruits (lesser extent)

References

1. Jellin JM, Batz F, Hitchens K. Natural Medicines Comprehensive Database. Stockton, CA: Therapeutic Research Faculty, 2002:1530.
2. Lee A, Ngan Kee WD, Gin T. A quantitative, systematic review of randomized controlled trials of ephedrine versus phenylephrine for the management of hypotension during spinal anesthesia for cesarean delivery. Anesth Analg 2002; 94:920–926.
3. Astrup A, Breum L, Toubro S, Hein P, Quaade F. The effect and safety of an ephedrine/caffeine compound compared to ephedrine, caffeine and placebo in obese subjects on an energy restricted diet. A double blind trial. Int J Obes Relat Metab Disord 1992; 16:269–277.
4. Boozer CN, Nasser JA, Heymsfield SB et al. An herbal supplement containing Ma Huang-Guarana for weight loss: a randomized, double-blind trial. Int J Obes Relat Metab Disord 2001; 25:316–324.
5. Breum L, Pedersen JK, Ahlstrom F, Frimodt-Moller J. Comparison of an ephedrine/caffeine combination and dexfenfluramine in the treatment of obesity. A double-blind multi-centre trial in general practice. Int J Obes Relat Metab Disord 1994; 18:99–103.
6. Shaikh WA. Ephedrine-saline nasal wash in allergic rhinitis. J Allergy Clin Immunol 1995; 96:597–600.
7. Pasquali R, Cesari MP, Melchionda N et al. Does ephedrine promote weight loss in low-energy-adapted obese women? Int J Obes 1987; 11:163–168.
8. Astrup A, Lundsgaard C, Madsen J, Christensen NJ. Enhanced thermogenic responsiveness during chronic ephedrine treatment in man. Am J Clin Nutr 1985; 41:83–94.
9. Tinkelman DG, Avner SE. Ephedrine therapy in asthmatic children. Clinical tolerance and absence of side effects. JAMA 1977; 237:553–557.
10. McLaughlin ET, Bethea LH, Wittig HJ. Comparison of the bronchodilator effect of oral fenoterol and ephedrine in asthmatic children. Ann Allergy 1982; 49:191–195.
11. Astrup A, Toubro S, Cannon S, Hein P, Madsen J. Thermogenic synergism between ephedrine and caffeine in healthy volunteers: a double-blind, placebo-controlled study. Metabolism 1991; 40:323–329.
12. Meston CM, Heiman JR. Ephedrine-activated physiological sexual arousal in women. Arch Gen Psychiatry 1998; 55:652–656.
13. Ueda W, Kataoka Y, Takimoto E et al. Ephedrine-induced increases in arterial blood pressure accelerate regression of epidural block. Anesth Analg 1995; 81:703–705.

14. Hughes SC, Ward MG, Levinson G et al. Placental transfer of ephedrine does not affect neonatal outcome. Anesthesiology 1985; 63:217–219.
15. Wright RG, Shnider SM, Levinson G, Rolbin SH, Parer JT. The effect of maternal administration of ephedrine on fetal heart rate and variability. Obstet Gynecol 1981; 57:734–738.
16. Farnsworth NR, Bingel AS, Cordell GA, Crane FA, Fong HH. Potential value of plants as sources of new antifertility agents I. J Pharm Sci 1975; 64:535–598.
17. Lee A, Ngan Kee WD, Gin T. A dose-response meta-analysis of prophylactic intravenous ephedrine for the prevention of hypotension during spinal anesthesia for elective cesarean delivery. Anesth Analg 2004; 98:483–490.
18. Lee A, Ngan Kee WD, Gin T. Prophylactic ephedrine prevents hypotension during spinal anesthesia for Cesarean delivery but does not improve neonatal outcome: a quantitative systematic review. Can J Anaesth 2002; 49:588–599.
19. Ducros L, Bonnin P, Cholley BP et al. Increasing maternal blood pressure with ephedrine increases uterine artery blood flow velocity during uterine contraction. Anesthesiology 2002; 96:612–616.
20. Gilbert-Barness E, Drut RM. Association of sympathomimetic drugs with malformations. Vet Hum Toxicol 2000; 42:168–171.
21. Matsuoka R, Gilbert EF, Bruyers HJ, Optiz JM. An aborted human fetus with truncus arteriosus communis – possible teratogenic effect of Tedral. Heart Vessels 1985; 1:176–178.
22. Scherer R, Holzgreve W. Influence of epidural analgesia on fetal and neonatal well-being. Eur J Obstet Gynecol Reprod Biol 1995; 59:S17–29.
23. Werler MM, Sheehan JE, Mitchell AA. Maternal medication use and risks of gastroschisis and small intestinal atresia. Am J Epidemiol 2002; 155:26–31.
24. Torfs CP, Katz EA, Bateson TF, Lam PK, Curry CJ. Maternal medications and environmental exposures as risk factors for gastroschisis. Teratology 1996; 54:84–92.
25. Werler MM, Mitchell AA, Shapiro S. First trimester maternal medication use in relation to gastroschisis. Teratology 1992; 45:361–367.
26. Mortimer EAJ. Drug toxicity from breast milk? Pediatrics 1977; 60:780–781.
27. Aljazaf K, Hale TW, Ilett KF et al. Pseudoephedrine: effects on milk production in women and estimation of infant exposure via breastmilk. Br J Clin Pharmacol 2003; 56:18–24.
28. Brinker F. The Toxicology of Botanical Medicines. Sandy, OR: Eclectic Medical Publications, 2000:296.
29. Gurley BJ, Gardner SF, Hubbard MA. Content versus label claims in ephedra-containing dietary supplements. Am J Health Syst Pharm 2000; 57:963–969.
30. Haller CA, Jacob P, Benowitz NL. Pharmacology of ephedra alkaloids and caffeine after single-dose dietary supplement use. Clin Pharmacol Ther 2002; 71:421–432.
31. White LM, Gardner SF, Gurley BJ et al. Pharmacokinetics and cardiovascular effects of ma-huang (Ephedra sinica) in normotensive adults. J Clin Pharmacol 1997; 37:116–122.
32. Ooms TG, Khan SA, Means C. Suspected caffeine and ephedrine toxicosis resulting from ingestion of an herbal supplement containing guarana and ma huang in dogs: 47 cases (1997–1999). J Am Vet Med Assoc 2001; 218:225–229.
33. Li P, Tong C, Eisenach JC. Pregnancy and ephedrine increase the release of nitric oxide in ovine uterine arteries. Anesth Analg 1996; 82:288–293.
34. Leung AY, Foster S. Encyclopedia of Common Natural Ingredients Used in Food, Drugs and Cosmetics. New York, NY: John Wiley & Sons, 1996:649.

35. Martindale W. Martindale: The Extra Pharmacopoeia. London: The Pharmaceutical Press, 1982.
36. Haller CA, Benowitz NL. Adverse cardiovascular and central nervous system events associated with dietary supplements containing ephedra alkaloids. N Engl J Med 2000; 343:1833–1838.
37. Horton TJ, Geissler CA. Aspirin potentiates the effect of ephedrine on the thermogenic response to a meal in obese but not lean women. Int J Obes 1991; 15:359–366.
38. Schulz V, Hansel R, Tyler VE, Terry C. Rational Phytotherapy: A Physician's Guide to Herbal Medicine. Berlin: Springer, 1998.
39. Blumenthal M, Busse WR, Goldberg A et al. The Complete German Commission E Monographs: Therapeutic Guide to Herbal Medicines. Boston, MA: American Botanical Council, 1998.
40. Robbers JE, Tyler VE. Tyler's Herbs of Choice: The Therapeutic Use of Phytomedicinals. New York, NY: The Haworth Herbal Press, 1999.
41. McKevoy GK. AHFS drug information. Bethesda, MD: American Society of Health-System Pharmacists, 1998.
42. Bell DG, Jacobs I, Ellerington K. Effect of caffeine and ephedrine ingestion on anaerobic exercise performance. Med Sci Sports Exerc 2001; 33:1399–1403.
43. Dulloo AG. Herbal simulation of ephedrine and caffeine in treatment of obesity. Int J Obes Relat Metab Disord 2002; 26:590–592.
44. Brinker F. Herb Contraindications and Drug Interactions. Sandy, OR: Eclectic Medical Publications, 1998.
45. White LM, Gardner SF, Gurley BJ et al. Pharmacokinetics and cardiovascular effects of ma-huang (Ephedra sinica) in normotensive adults. J Clin Pharmacol 1997; 37:116–122.
46. McBride BF, Karapanos AK, Krudysz A et al. Electrocardiographic and hemodynamic effects of a multicomponent dietary supplement containing ephedra and caffeine: a randomized controlled trial. JAMA 2004; 291:216–221.

EVENING PRIMROSE
Oenothera biennis

Synonyms/common names/related compounds[1]
EPO, fever plant, huile d'onagre, king's cureall, night willow-herb, primrose, scabish, sun drop

Indications

Atopic dermatitis and eczema:[2–5]	Evidence grade A
Diabetic peripheral neuropathy:[6]	Evidence grade B1
Diabetes:[7]	Evidence grade B1
Rheumatoid arthritis:[8]	Evidence grade B2
Breast cysts:[9]	Evidence grade B2
Pregnancy-induced hypertension and preeclampsia:[10–12]	Evidence grade B2
Raynaud's phenomenon:[13]	Evidence grade B2
Post-viral fatigue syndrome:[14]	Evidence grade B2
Breast cancer (with tamoxifen):[15]	Evidence grade B2
Breast pain (mastalgia):[16]	Evidence grade C
Multiple sclerosis:[17]	Evidence grade C
Pre-menstrual syndrome:[18]	Evidence grade E

Pregnancy

Minimal risk:[10–12,19,20]	Evidence level 1a

A randomized controlled trial was conducted on the effects of evening primrose oil (EPO) supplementation of vasodilatory prostacyclin (PGI2) and vasoconstrictor thromboxane A2 in 18 preeclamptic women between 31 and 26 weeks of gestation.[19] The authors did not report any adverse effects on the women, the pregnancy outcome, and any malformations in the newborns.[19] Another study conducted on prostaglandin pathways in women with preeclampsia did not report any risk in pregnancy associated with EPO.[20]

A placebo-controlled, partially double-blinded, clinical trial on the effects of EPO and fish oil in preventing preeclampsia of pregnancy did not report any adverse effects on the women, the pregnancy outcome, and any malformations in the newborns.[10]

A comparative study on the vascular sensitivity to angiotensin II in the midtrimester of pregnancy in women after taking EPO did not report any adverse effects on the women, the pregnancy outcome, and any malformations in the newborns.[11] A comparative study on EPO and co-factors for prostaglandin synthesis in 10 pregnant and 10 non-pregnant women did not report any adverse effects on the women, the pregnancy outcome, and any malformations in the newborns.[12]

Teratogenic and induces labor:[15]	Evidence level 1a

A review of randomized double-blind studies reported that γ-linolenic acid (GLA) increases prostaglandin E levels.[15] It was recommended that GLA be avoided in pregnancy given the teratogenic and labor-inducing effects of prostaglandin E agonists.[15]

May induce labor but effectiveness is unclear:[21,22]	Evidence level 1b

EPO is widely used by many midwives to hasten cervical ripening, to shorten labor and to decrease the incidence of post-date pregnancies.[21] A survey of midwives in the USA found that 60% used EPO to induce labor.[22] A two-group retrospective quasi-experimental design on a sample of women, where selected outcomes in 54 women taking EPO in their pregnancy were compared with outcomes in 54 women who did not showed that the oral administration of EPO from the 37th week of gestation until birth did not shorten gestation or decrease the overall length of labor.[21]

Increased risk of pregnancy complications (prolonged rupture of membranes, oxytocin and augmentation, arrest of descent, vacuum extraction):[21]	Evidence level 1b

A two-group retrospective quasi-experimental design reported that orally administered EPO may be associated with an increase in the incidence of prolonged rupture of membranes, oxytocin augmentation, arrest of descent, and vacuum extraction.[21]

Lactation

Minimal risk:[10–12]	Evidence level 1a

A randomized controlled trial on the total fat and essential fatty acid content of breast milk following EPO and placebo supplementation in 39 women for a period of 8 months starting between the second and sixth months of lactation reported an increase in fatty acids in breast milk, but did not report any adverse effects in the infants or mothers.[23] A study was conducted on whether formulae with EPO and fish oils raise long-chain polyunsaturated fatty acids in plasma cholesterol esters, erythrocytes, and platelets to levels encountered in breast-fed infants.[24] The authors did not report any adverse effects in the infants.[24]

Constituents[25,26]

2–16% GLA
65–80% linolenic acid
Vitamin E

Pharmacology

- EOP has anti-inflammatory activity where it blocks the transformation of arachidonic acid to leukotrienes, increases the production of 1-series prostaglandins and acts as a competitive inhibitor of 2-series prostaglandins and 4-series leukotrienes.[25]
- EPO may help women with PMS who have lower levels of GLA, possibly due to a defect in the conversion of linoleic acid to GLA.[27]
- EPO may help children with attention-deficit hyperactivity disorder who have lower levels of GLA.[28]
- EPO may lower levels of plasma lipids and inhibit platelet aggregation.[29]
- EPO may improve neuronal blood supply and possibly prevent diabetic neuropathy.[30]
- EPO was found to reverse epidermal hyperproliferation in guinea pigs.[31]

Drug interactions[1]

Anesthesia[32]
Anti-convulsant/anti-seizure drugs[33]
Anti-coagulant/anti-platelet drugs[29]
Phenothiazines[1]

Part used[1]

Seed

References

1. Jellin JM, Batz F, Hitchens K. Natural Medicines Comprehensive Database, 3rd ed. Stockton, CA: Therapeutic Research Faculty, 2002:1530.
2. Morse PF, Horrobin DF, Manku MS et al. Meta-analysis of placebo-controlled studies of the efficacy of Epogam in the treatment of atopic eczema. Relationship between plasma essential fatty acid changes and clinical response. Br J Dermatol 1989; 121:75–90.
3. Wright S, Burton JL. Oral evening-primrose-seed oil improves atopic eczema. Lancet 1982; ii:1120–1122.
4. Schalin-Karrila M, Mattila L, Jansen CT, Uotila P. Evening primrose oil in the treatment of atopic eczema: effect on clinical status, plasma phospholipid fatty acids and circulating blood prostaglandins. Br J Dermatol 1987; 117:11–19.

5. Biagi PL, Bordoni A, Hrelia S. The effect of gamma-linolenic acid on clinical status, red cell fatty acid composition and membrane microviscosity in infants with atopic dermatitis. Drugs Exp Clin Res 1994; 20:77–84.
6. Keen H, Payan J, Allawi J. Treatment of diabetic neuropathy with gamma-linolenic acid. The gamma-Linolenic Acid Multicenter Trial Group. Diabetes Care 1993; 16:8–15.
7. Arisaka M, Arisaka O, Yamashiro Y. Fatty acid and prostaglandin metabolism in children with diabetes mellitus. II. The effect of evening primrose oil supplementation on serum fatty acid and plasma prostaglandin levels. Prostaglandins Leukot Essent Fatty Acids 1991; 43:197–201.
8. Belch JJ, Ansell D, Madhok R, O'Dowd A, Sturrock RD. Effects of altering dietary essential fatty acids on requirements for non-steroidal anti-inflammatory drugs in patients with rheumatoid arthritis: a double blind placebo controlled study. Ann Rheum Dis 1988; 47:96–104.
9. Mansel RE, Harrison BJ, Melhuish J et al. A randomized trial of dietary intervention with essential fatty acids in patients with categorized cysts. Ann N Y Acad Sci 1990; 586:288–294.
10. D'Almeida A, Carter JP, Anatol A, Prost C. Effects of a combination of evening primrose oil (gamma linolenic acid) and fish oil (eicosapentaenoic + docahexaenoic acid) versus magnesium, and versus placebo in preventing pre-eclampsia. Women Health 1992; 19:117–131.
11. O'Brien PM, Pipkin FB. The effect of essential fatty acid and specific vitamin supplements on vascular snesitivity in the mid-trimester of human pregnancy. Clin Exp Hypertens B 1983; 2:247–254.
12. O'Brien PM, Morrison R, Broughton Pipkin F. The effect of dietary supplementation with linoleic and gammalinolenic acids on the pressor response to angiotensin II – a possible role in pregnancy-induced hypertension? Br J Clin Pharmacol 1985; 19:335–342.
13. Belch JJ, Shaw B, O'Dowd A et al. Evening primrose oil (Efamol) in the treatment of Raynaud's phenomenon: a double blind study. Thromb Haemost 1985; 54:490–494.
14. Behan PO, Behan WM, Horrobin D. Effect of high doses of essential fatty acids on the postviral fatigue syndrome. Acta Neurol Scand 1990; 82:209–216.
15. Kenny JS, Pinder SE, Ellis O et al. Gamma linolenic acid with tamoxifen as primary therapy in breast cancer. Int J Cancer 2000; 85:643–648.
16. Pye JK, Mansel RE, Hughes LE. Clinical experience of drug treatments for mastalgia. Lancet 1985; ii:373–377.
17. Horrobin DS. Multiple sclerosis: a rational basis for the treatment with colchicine and evening primrose oil. Med Hypotheses 1979; 5:365–378.
18. Campbell EM, Peterkin D, O'Grady K, Sanson-Fisher R. Premenstrual symptoms in general practice patients. Prevalence and treatment. J Reprod Med 1997; 42:637–646.
19. Laivuori H, Hovatta O, Viinikka L, Ylikorkala O. Dietary supplementation with primrose oil or fish oil does not change urinary excretion of prostacyclin and thromboxane metabolites in pre-eclamptic women. Prostaglandins Leukot Essent Fatty Acids 1993; 49:691–694.
20. Moodley J, Norman RJ. Attempts at dietary alteration of prostaglandin pathways in the management of pre-eclampsia. Prostaglandins Leukot Essent Fatty Acids 1989; 37:145–147.

21. Dove D, Johnson P. Oral evening primrose oil: its effect on length of pregnancy and selected intrapartum outcomes in low-risk nulliparous women. J Nurse Midwifery 1999; 44:320–324.
22. McFarlin BL, Gibson MH, O'Rear J, Harman P. A national survey of herbal preparation use by nurse-midwives for labor stimulation. Review of the literature and recommendations for practice. J Nurse Midwifery 1999; 44:205–216.
23. Cant A, Shay J, Horrobin DF. The effect of maternal supplementation with linoleic and gamma-linolenic acids on the fat composition and content of human milk: a placebo-controlled trial. J Nutr Sci Vitaminol (Tokyo) 1991; 37:573–579.
24. Woltil HA, van Beusekom CM, Schaafsma A, Okken A, Muskiet FA. Does supplementation of formula with evening primrose and fish oils augment long chain polyunsaturated fatty acid status of low birthweight infants to that of breast-fed counterparts? 1999; 60:199–208.
25. Belch JJ, Hill A. Evening primrose oil and borage oil in rheumatologic conditions. Am J Clin Nutr 2000; 71:352S–356S.
26. Kleijnen J. Evening primrose oil. BMJ 1994; 309:824–825.
27. Hardy ML. Herbs of special interest to women. J Am Pharm Assoc (Wash) 2000; 40:234–242.
28. Aman MG, Mitchell EA, Turbott SH. The effects of essential fatty acid supplementation by Efamol in hyperactive children. J Abnorm Child Psychol 1987; 15:75–90.
29. Guivernau M, Meza N, Barja P, Roman O. Clinical and experimental study on the long-term effect of dietary gamma-linolenic acid on plasma lipids, platelet aggregation, thromboxane formation, and prostacyclin production. Prostaglandins Leukot Essent Fatty Acids 1994; 51:311–316.
30. Head RJ, McLennan PL, Raederstorff D et al. Prevention of nerve conduction deficit in diabetic rats by polyunsaturated fatty acids. Am J Clin Nutr 2000; 71:386S–392S.
31. Chung S, Kong S, Seong K, Cho Y. Gamma-linolenic acid in borage oil reverses epidermal hyperproliferation in guinea pigs. J Nutr 2002; 132;3090–3097.
32. Shaw D, Leon C, Kolev S, Murray V. Traditional remedies and food supplements. A 5-year toxicological study (1991–1995). Drug Saf 1997; 17:342–356.
33. Miller LG. Herbal medicines: selected clinical considerations focusing on known or potential drug–herb interactions. Arch Intern Med 1998; 158:2200–2211.

FALSE UNICORN
Chamaelirium luteum

Synonyms/common names/related substances[1]
Blazing star, fairywand, helonias, starwort

Indications

Menstrual complaints:[2]	Evidence grade E
Diuretic:[3]	Evidence grade E

Pregnancy

Induces labor:[4]	Evidence level 4

False unicorn is part of a combination of herbal medicines that have been traditionally used in the third trimester to prepare a woman for delivery; this preparation is called 'mother's cordial' or 'partus preparatus'. In addition to false unicorn, mother's cordial contains: squaw vine *(Mitchella ripens)*, raspberry (*Rubus idaeus*), blue cohosh *(Caulophyllum thalictroides)* and black cohosh (*Cimicifuga racemosa*).

Uterine stimulant:[2,3]	Evidence level 4
Emmenagogue:[5]	Evidence level 4

A compendium for medicinal plants reported that false unicorn may have a uterine stimulant effect.[2,3] A herbal contraindication and drug interaction compendium reported that false unicorn was an emmenagogue and contraindicated during pregnancy.[5] False unicorn was not reported in the scientific literature as having a uterine stimulant effect or being an emmenagogue, nor was it reported as being contraindicated or safe in pregnancy.

Anti-gonadotrophic activity:[6]	Evidence level 4
Estrogenic:[7]	Evidence level 4

A review article on the potential value of plants as sources of anti-fertility agents reported that false unicorn had anti-gonadotrophic activity in rats and has estrogenic activity.[6,7]

Constituents
No available information

Pharmacology

False unicorn is reported to have anthelmintic, diuretic, uterine stimulant and menstruation stimulant activity.[3,8]

Drug interactions

None reported

Parts used[1]

Root and rhizome

References

1. Jellin JM, Batz F, Hitchens K. Natural Medicines Comprehensive Database, 3rd ed. Stockton, CA: Therapeutic Research Faculty, 2002:1530.
2. McGuffin M, Hobbs C, Upton R, Goldberg A. American Herbal Products Association's Botanical Safety Handbook. Boca Raton, FL: CRC Press, 1997:231.
3. Gruenwald J, Brendler T, Jaenicke C. PDR for Herbal Medicines. Montvale, NJ: Medical Economics Company, 1998.
4. Blumenthal M, Busse WR, Goldberg A et al. The Complete German Commission E Monographs: Therapeutic Guide to Herbal Medicines. Boston, MA: American Botanical Council, 1998.
5. Brinker F. The Toxicology of Botanical Medicines. Sandy, OR: Eclectic Medical Publications, 2000:296.
6. Farnsworth NR, Bingel AS, Cordell G, Crane FA, Fong HH. Potential value of plants as sources of new antifertility agents I. J Pharm Sci 1975; 64:535–598.
7. Farnsworth NR, Bingel AS, Cordell GA, Crane FA, Fong HH. Potential value of plants as sources of new antifertility agents II. J Pharm Sci 1975; 64:717–753.
8. Newall CA, Anderson LA, Phillipson JD. Herbal Medicines: A Guide for Health-care Professionals. London, UK: Pharmaceutical Press, 1996:296.

FENNEL
Foeniculum vulgare

Synonyms/common names/related compounds[1]

Bitter fennel, carosella, common fennel, finnochio, Florence fennel, garden fennel, large fennel, phytoestrogen, sweet fennel, wild fennel

Indications

Oil

Infant colic:[2] — Evidence grade B1

Chronic colitis (with Taraxacum *officinale, Hypericum perforatum, Calendula officinalis* and *Melissa officinalis*):[3] — Evidence grade C

Digestive complaints:[4] — Evidence grade F

Pregnancy

Oil

Decreases uterine contractions:[5] — Evidence level 3

A study on the effects of fennel essential oil on the rat uterus reported that fennel essential oil significantly reduced the intensity of oxytocin and PGE2-induced contractions in the rat uterus and reduced the frequency of contractions induced by PGE2.[5]

Potential abortifacient:[6] — Evidence level 4

Emmenagogue:[6] — Evidence level 4

A review article on the potential value of plants as sources of anti-fertility agents reported that fennel was a potential abortifacient and an emmenagogue.[6]

Hormonal effects: — Evidence level 4

A herbal toxicology and drug interaction compendium reported that fennel may have hormonal effects.[7]

Seed

Emmenagogue:[6] — Evidence level 4

Estrogenic:[8]	Evidence level 4

A review article on the potential value of plants as sources of anti-fertility agents reported that fennel seeds are an emmenagogue and have estrogenic activity.[6,8]

Food amounts

Likely safe:[1]	Evidence level 4

A natural product database reported that fennel is likely safe when consumed in food amounts.[1]

Lactation

Avoid:[7]	Evidence level 4

A toxicology and drug interaction compendium reported that fennel oil should be avoided while breast-feeding.[7] There are no reports in the scientific literature of fennel oil being either safe or contraindicated during lactation.

Cautions

- Avoid long term use as estragole is a procarcinogen.[9]
- Avoid oral use in liver disease or alcoholism, and during use of acetaminophen (paracetamol).[7]
- Infants or toddlers[4,5]

Constituents

Seed[10,11]

β-Carotene
Vitamin C
Calcium
Magnesium
Iron

Oil[1,7]

Anethole
Fenchone
Estragole

Toxicity

Oil

Oral LD_{50}: 1.3 g/kg to 4.5 g/kg[5,7,12]

Anethole
Oral LD_{50}: 2.09 g/kg[13]

Pharmacology

- Anethole has estrogenic activity and may deplete liver glutathione.[7,14]
- Anethole and fenchone reduce upper respiratory tract secretions.[14]
- Anethole may be insecticidal and toxic.[1]
- Aqueous fennel extract might increase mucociliary activity.[14]
- Fennel seed can promote gastrointestinal motility, and in higher concentrations, can act as an anti-spasmodic.[4]
- Fennel may be allergenic.[15]
- Estragole is a procarcinogen that is not directly hepatotoxic or hepatocarcinogenic as it requires activation by liver enzymes to reach full toxicity.[9]

Drug interactions

Ciprofloxacin (Cipro)[11]

Parts used[1]

Seed, oil

References

1. Jellin JM, Batz F, Hitchens K. Natural Medicines Comprehensive Database. Stockton, CA: Therapeutic Research Faculty, 2002:1530.
2. Alexandrovich I, Rakovitskaya O, Kolmo E, Sidorova T, Sushunov S. The effect of fennel (Foeniculum Vulgare) seed oil emulsion in infantile colic: a randomized, placebo-controlled study. Altern Ther Health Med 2003; 9:58–61.
3. Chakurski I, Matev M, Koichev A, Angelova I, Stefanov G. [Treatment of chronic colitis with an herbal combination of Taraxacum officinale, Hipericum perforatum, Melissa officinaliss, Calendula officinalis and Foeniculum vulgare]. Vutr Boles 1981; 20:51–54.
4. Blumenthal M, Busse WR, Goldberg A et al. The Complete German Commission E Monographs: Therapeutic Guide to Herbal Medicines. Boston, MA: American Botanical Council, 1998.
5. Ostad SN, Soodi M, Shariffzadeh M, Khorshidi N, Marzban H. The effect of fennel essential oil on uterine contraction as a model for dysmenorrhea, pharmacology and toxicology study. J Ethnopharmacol 2001; 76:299–304.
6. Farnsworth NR, Bingel AS, Cordell GA, Crane FA, Fong HH. Potential value of plants as sources of new antifertility agents I. J Pharm Sci 1975; 64:535–598.
7. Brinker F. The Toxicology of Botanical Medicines. Sandy, OR: Eclectic Medical Publications, 2000:296.
8. Farnsworth NR, Bingel AS, Cordell GA, Crane FA, Fong HH. Potential value of plants as sources of new antifertility agents II. J Pharm Sci 1975; 64:717–753.
9. McGuffin M, Hobbs C, Upton R, Goldberg A. American Herbal Products Association's Botanical Safety Handbook. Boca Raton, FL: CRC Press, 1997:231.
10. Brinker F. Herb Contraindications and Drug Interactions. Sandy, OR: Eclectic Medical Publications, 1998.

11. Zhu M, Wong PY, Li RC. Effect of oral administration of fennel (Foeniculum vulgare) on ciprofloxacin absorption and disposition in the rat. J Pharm Pharmacol 1999; 51:1391–1396.
12. De Smat PAGM, Keller K, Hansel R, Chandler RF. Adverse Effects of Herbal Drugs, vol 1. Berlin: Springer-Verlag, 1992.
13. Albert-Puleo M. Fennel and anise as estrogenic agents. J Ethnopharmacol 1980; 2:337–344.
14. Leung AY, Foster S. Encyclopedia of Common Natural Ingredients Used in Food, Drugs and Cosmetics. New York, NY: John Wiley & Sons, 1996:649.
15. Garcia-Gonzalez JJ, Bartolome-Zavala B, Fernandez-Melendez S et al. Occupational rhinoconjunctivitis and food allergy because of aniseed sensitization. Ann Allergy Asthma Immunol 2002; 88:518–522.

FENUGREEK

Trigonella foenum-graecum, T. foenugraecum

Synonyms/common names/related compounds[1]

Alholva, bird's foot, bockshornklee, bockshornsame, foenugraeci semen, foenugreek, Greek clover, Greek hay, Greek hay seed, hu lu ba, methi, trigonella

Indications

Type 2 diabetes:[2–5]	Evidence grade B2
Type 1 diabetes:[6]	Evidence grade B2
Hyperlipidemia:[2,6,7]	Evidence grade B2

Pregnancy

Pseudo-maple syrup urine disease:[8,9]	Evidence level 2

There are case reports of neonates being born with a peculiar odor following maternal consumption of fenugreek just before delivery.[8,9] In one study, the authors reported that the odor should not be confused with maple syrup urine disease and that there were no long-term effects.[8] The odor is believed to originate from the fenugreek constituent sotolone.[9]

Potential abortifacient:[10,11]	Evidence level 3
Uterine stimulant:[10,11]	Evidence level 3
Emmenagogue:[11]	Evidence level 4

Fenugreek extracts, both aqueous and alcoholic, have been shown to have a stimulating effect on the guinea pig uterus, especially during late pregnancy.[10] A review article on the potential value of plants as sources of anti-fertility agents reported that fenugreek is a potential abortifacient, emmanogogue, and uterine stimulant.[11]

Food

Minimal risk:[11]	Evidence level 4

Fenugreek is reported to have minimal risk when taken in food amounts during pregnancy.[11]

Lactation

Galactogogue:[12,13]	Evidence level 4

A review article on fenugreek reports that there is anecdotal evidence that it stimulate lactation.[13] A clinical trial compared fenugreek versus torbangun, a plant used traditionally in Indonesia for lactation, and reported that fenugreek is frequently used by women to promote lactation.[13]

Potential oxytocic activity:[14]	Evidence level 4

A herbal medicine compendium reported that fenugreek has potential oxytocic activity.[14]

Caution

Do not take with drugs as the mucilage content may decrease or delay drug absorption[14]

Constituents

Trigonelline[14]
4-Hydroxyisoleucine[14]
Fenugreekine[14]

Toxicity

Oral LD_{50}: 10 g/kg[15]
Acute oral LD_{50}: >5 g/kg[16]
Intra-peritoneal LD_{50}: 1.9 g/kg[15]
Acute dermal LD_{50}: >2 g/kg[16]

Pharmacology

- Fenugreek slows glucose absorption in the gastrointestinal tract.[17]
- Fenugreek and its constituent trigonelline have hypoglycemic activity.[14]
- The constituent 4-hydroxyisoleucine may directly stimulate insulin.[17]
- In patients with type 2 diabetes, fenugreek has been shown to increase beta-cell secretion, improve insulin resistance, significantly decrease triglyceride levels and increase high-density lipoproteins.[2]
- Fenugreek seed consumption may decrease calcium oxalate deposition in the kidneys.[18]
- The constituent fenugreekine may have cardiotonic, hypoglycemic, diuretic, anti-inflammatory, anti-hypertensive, and anti-viral properties.[14]

Drug interactions[1]

Diabetic drugs[5,19]
Corticosteroids[14]
Hormone therapy[14]
Monoamine oxidase inhibitors[14]

Part used

Seeds[1]

References

1. Jellin JM, Batz F, Hitchens K. Natural Medicines Comprehensive Database, 3rd ed. Stockton, CA: Therapeutic Research Faculty, 2002:1530.
2. Gupta A, Gupta R, Lal B. Effect of Trigonella foenum-graecum (fenugreek) seeds on glycaemic control and insulin resistance in type 2 diabetes mellitus: a double blind placebo controlled study. J Assoc Physicians India 2001; 49:1057–1061.
3. Raghuram TC, Sharma RD, Sivakumar B, et al. Effect of fenugreek seeds on intravenous glucose disposition in non-insulin dependent diabetic patients. Phytother Res 1994; 8:83–86.
4. Sharma RD, Raghuram TC. Hypoglycaemic effect of fenugreek seeds in non-insulin dependent diabetic subjects. Nutr Res 1990; 10:731–739.
5. Madar Z, Abel R, Samish S, Arad J. Glucose-lowering effect of fenugreek in non-insulin dependent diabetics. Eur J Clin Nutr 1988; 42:51–54.
6. Sharma RD, Raghuram TC, Rao N. Effect of fenugreek seeds on blood glucose and serum lipids in type I diabetes. Eur J Clin Nutrit 1990; 44:301–306.
7. Sharma RD, Raghuram TC, Dayasagar Rao V. Hypolipidaemic effect of fenugreek seeds. A clinical study. Phytother Res 1991; 3:145–147.
8. Yalcin SS, Tekinalp G, Ozalp I. Peculiar odor of traditional food and maple syrup urine disease. Pediatr Int 1999; 41:108–109.
9. Korman SH, Cohen E, Preminger A. Pseudo-maple syrup urine disease due to maternal prenatal ingestion of fenugreek. J Paediatr Child Health 2001; 37:403–404.
10. Abdo MS, al-Kafawi AA. Experimental studies on the effect of Trigonella foenum-graecum. Planta Med 1969; 17:14–18.
11. Farnsworth NR, Bingel AS, Cordell G, Crane FA, Fong HH. Potential value of plants as sources of new antifertility agents I. J Pharm Sci 1975; 64:535–598.
12. Gabay MP. Galactogogues: medications that induce lactation. J Hum Lact 2002; 18:274–279.
13. Damanik R, Wahlqvist ML, Wattanapenpaiboon N. The use of a putative lactagogue plant on breast milk production in Simalungun, North Sumatra, Indonesia. Asia Pac J Clin Nutr 2004; 13 (Suppl):S118.
14. Newall CA, Anderson LA, Phillipson JD. Herbal Medicines: A Guide for Health-care Professionals. London, UK: Pharmaceutical Press, 1996:296.
15. Abdel-Barry JA, Abdel-Hassan IA, Al-Hakiem MH. Hypoglycaemic and antihyperglycaemic effects of Trigonella foenum-graecum leaf in normal and alloxan induced diabetic rats. J Ethnopharmacol 1997; 58:149–155.
16. Opdyke DL. Fenugreek absolute. Food Cosmet Toxicol 1978; 16:755–756.
17. Broca C, Manteghetti M, Gross R et al. 4-Hydroxyisoleucine: effects of synthetic and natural analogues on insulin secretion. Eur J Pharmacol 2000; 390:339–345.
18. Ahsan SK,Tariq M, Ageel AM, al-Yahya MA, Shah AH. Effect of Trigonella foenum-graecum and Ammi majus on calcium oxalate urolithiasis in rats. J Ethnopharmacol 1989; 26:249–254.
19. Bhardwaj PK, Dasgupta DJ, Prashar BS, Kaushal SS. Control of hyperglycaemia and hyperlipidaemia by plant product. J Assoc Physicians India 1994; 42:33–35.

FEVERFEW
Tanacetum parthenium

Synonyms/common names/related compounds[1]
Altamisa, bachelor's buttons, featerfoiul, featherfew, featherfoil, fever few, flirtwort midsummer daisy, santa maria, *Tanaceti parthenii*

Indications

Migraine headaches:[2,3]	Evidence grade A

Pregnancy

Emmenagogue:[4]	Evidence level 4
Safety unknown:	Evidence level 5

A herbal medicine compendium reported that feverfew is an emmenagogue.[4] There are no reports in the scientific literature of feverfew being either safe or contraindicated during pregnancy.

Lactation

Safety unknown:	Evidence level 5

There are no reports in the scientific literature of feverfew being either safe or contraindicated during lactation.

Constituents
- Sesquiterpene lactone:[5] parthenolide
- Flavonoid glycoside:[6,7] tanetin, apigenin, luteolin 7-glucuronides, quercetagetin, 6-hydroxykaempferol
- Oil:[8] chrysanthenyl acetate
- Monoterpenes[5]
- Tannins[5]
- Melatonin[9]

Toxicity
- A LD_{50} value has not been estimated for feverfew.[4]
- Detailed blood analysis of 60 feverfew users (some >1 year) did not show any significant differences when compared with that of controls.[10]
- Rats and guinea pigs fed feverfew (>100 times the human daily dose for 5 weeks, and >150 times the human daily dose for 7 weeks, respectively) were identical to control animals, especially with regard to appetite and weight gain, and no adverse effects were reported.[11]

- Parthenolide at concentrations up to 800 mmol was found to be non-mutagenic.[12]
- Sesquiterpene lactones that contain an α-methylene butyrolactone ring are known to cause allergic reaction.[13,14] Compounds with this structure are present in feverfew and reports of contact dermatitis have been documented.[15–18]

Pharmacology

- The constituent parthenolide was widely believed to be the active constituent in feverfew.[19,20] It is now believed that other constituents are necessary in the prevention and treatment of migraines.[8,20–22]
- Feverfew may inhibit platelet aggregation and inhibit serotonin release from platelets and leukocytes.[20,23–27]
- Feverfew appears to block prostaglandin synthesis by inhibiting phospholipase, thereby preventing the release of arachidonic acid.[25,28,29]
- Feverfew may inhibit inflammation and pain transmission, and have an analgesic effect.[6,30–32]
- Feverfew leaves and parthenolide may cause irreversible inhibition of vascular muscle contraction.[33,34]
- The melatonin in feverfew may contribute to its pharmacological effect where migraines have been associated with decreased melatonin secretion.[9,35] Fresh or dried leaves contain significantly more melatonin than commercially prepared standardized feverfew tablets.[9]
- Feverfew has a cytostatic effect on tumor cell growth.[36]

Drug interactions[1]

Anti-coagulant/anti-platelet drugs[20,23–27,37]
Nonsteroidal anti-inflammatory drugs[38,39]

Part used

Leaf[1]

References

1. Jellin JM, Batz F, Hitchens K. Natural Medicines Comprehensive Database. Stockton, CA: Therapeutic Research Faculty, 2002:1530.
2. Vogler BK, Pittler MH, Ernst E. Feverfew as a preventive treatment for migraine: a systematic review. Cephalalgia 1998; 18:704–708.
3. Ernst E, Pittler MH. The efficacy and safety of feverfew (Tanacetum parthenium L.): an update of a systematic review. Public Health Nutr 2000; 3:509–514.
4. Newall CA, Anderson LA, Phillipson JD. Herbal Medicines: A Guide for Health-care Professionals. London, UK: Pharmaceutical Press, 1996:296.
5. www.naturalstandard.com. Feverfew (Tanacetum parthenium L. Schultz-Bip.) Natural Standard Monograph.
6. Williams CA, Hoult JR, Harborne JB et al. A biologically active lipophilic flavonol from Tanacetum parthenium. Phytochemistry 1995; 38:267–270.
7. Williams CA, Harborne JB, Geiger H, Hoult JR. The flavonoids of Tanacetum parthenium and T. vulgare and their anti-inflammatory properties. Phytochemistry 1999; 51:417–423.

8. de Weerdt GJ, Bootsman HPR, Hendriks H. Herbal medicines in migraine prevention. Randomized double-blind, placebo-controlled, crossover trial of a feverfew preparation. Phytomedicine 1996; 3:225–230.
9. Murch SJ, Simmons CB, Saxena PK. Melatonin in feverfew and other medicinal plants. Lancet 1997; 350:1598–1599.
10. Baldwin CA, Anderson LA, Phillipson JD. What pharmacists should know about feverfew. Pharm J 1987; 239:237–238.
11. Johnson ES. Feverfew (overcoming common problems). London: Sheldon Press, 1984:78.
12. Marles RJ, Pazos-Sanou L, Compadre CM et al. Sesquiterpene lactones revisited. In: Arnason JT, Mata R, Romeo JT, eds. Recent Advances in Phytochemistry, Vol 29, Phytochemistry of Medicinal Plants. New York, NY: Plenum Press, 1995:333–356.
13. Rodriguez E, Epstein WL, Mitchell JC. The role of sesquiterpene lactones in contact hypersensitivity to some North and South American species of feverfew (Parthenium–Compositae). Contact Dermatitis 1977; 3:155–162.
14. Mitchell J, Rook A. Botanical Dermatology – Plants and Plant Products Injurious to the Skin. Vancouver: Greengrass, 1979.
15. Burry J. Compositae dermatitis in South Australia: contact dermatitis from Chrysanthemum parthenium. Contact Dermatitis 1980; 6:445.
16. Mitchell JC, Geissman TA, Dupuis G, Towers GH. Allergic contact dermatitis caused by Artemisia and Chrysanthemum species. The role of sesquiterpene lactones. J Invest Dermatol 1971; 56:98–101.
17. Schmidt RJ, Kingston T. Chrysanthemum dermatitis in South Wales; diagnosis by patch testing with feverfew (Tanacetum parthenium) extract. Contact Dermatitis 1985; 13:120–127.
18. Mensing H, Kimmig W, Hausen BM. Airborne contact dermatitis. Der Hautarzt 1985; 36:398–402.
19. Tyler VE. Herbs of Choice. Binghamton, NY: Pharmaceutical Products Press, 1994.
20. Awang DVC. Prescribing therapeutic feverfew [Tancetum pathrnium (L.) Schultz Bip., syn. Chrysanthemumparthenium (L.) Bernh.]. Int Med 1998; 1:11–13.
21. Awang DV. Parthenocide: demise of a facile theory of feverfew activity. J Herbs Spices Med Plants 1998; 5:95–98.
22. Robbers JE, Tyler VE. Tyler's Herbs of Choice: The Therapeutic Use of Phytomedicinals. New York, NY: The Haworth Herbal Press, 1999.
23. Heptinstall S, Groenewegen WA, Spangenberg P, Loesche W. Extracts of feverfew may inhibit platelet behaviour via neutralization of sulphydryl groups. J Pharm Pharmacol 1987; 39:459–465.
24. Heptinstall S, White A, Williamson L, Mitchell JR. Extracts of feverfew inhibit granule secretion in blood platelets and polymorphonuclear leucocytes. Lancet 1985; 1:1071–1074.
25. Makheja AN, Bailey JM. A platelet phospholipase inhibitor from the medicinal herb feverfew (Tanacetum parthenium). Prostaglandins Leukot Med 1982; 8:653–660.
26. Groenewegen WA, Heptinstall S. A comparison of the effects of an extract of feverfew and parthenolide, a component of feverfew, on human platelet activity in-vitro. J Pharm Pharmacol 1990; 42:553–557.
27. Heptinstall S, Groenewegen WA, Spangenberg P, Losche W. Inhibition of platelet behaviour by feverfew: a mechanism of action involving sulphydryl groups. Folia Haematol Int Mag Klin Morphol Blutforsch 1988; 115:447–449.
28. Makheja AN, Bailey JM. The active principle in feverfew. Lancet 1981; 2:1054.

29. Collier HO, Butt NM, McDonald-Gibson WJ, Saeed SA. Extract of feverfew inhibits prostaglandin biosynthesis. Lancet 1980; 2:922–923.
30. Jain NK, Kulkarni SK. Antinociceptive and anti-inflammatory effects of Tanacetum parthenium L. extract in mice and rats. J Ethnopharmacol 1999; 68:251–259.
31. Pittler MH, Vogler BK, Ernst E. Feverfew for preventing migraine. Cochrane Database Syst Rev 2000; 3:CD002286.
32. Pugh WJ, Sambo K. Prostaglandin synthetase inhibitors in feverfew. J Pharm Pharmacol 1988; 40:743–745.
33. Barsby R, Salan U, Knight DW, Hoult JR. Irreversible inhibition of vascular reactivity by feverfew. Lancet 1991; 338:1015.
34. Barsby RW, Salan U, Knight DW, Hoult JR. Feverfew extracts and parthenolide irreversibly inhibit vascular responses of the rabbit aorta. J Pharm Pharmacol 1992; 44:737–740.
35. Brun J, Claustrat B, Saddier P, Chazot G. Nocturnal melatonin excretion is decreased in patients with migraine without aura attacks associated with menses. Cephalalgia 1995; 15:136–139.
36. Ross JJ, Arnason JT, Birnboim HC. Low concentrations of the feverfew component parthenolide inhibit in vitro growth of tumor lines in a cytostatic fashion. Planta Med 1999; 65:126–129.
37. Biggs MJ, Johnson ES, Persaud NP, Ratcliffe DM. Platelet aggregation in patients using feverfew for migraine. Lancet 1982; 2:776.
38. The Review of Natural Products by Facts and Comparisons. St. Louis, MO: Wolters Kluwer Co., 1999.
39. Miller LG. Herbal medicinals: selected clinical considerations focusing on known or potential drug–herb interactions. Arch Intern Med 1998; 158:2200–2211.

FLAX
Linum usitatissimum

Synonyms/common names/related compounds[1]
Flax seed, graine de lin, leinsamen, lini semen, linseed, lint bells, linum, phytoestrogen, winterlien

Indications

Flaxseed

Hyperlipidemia:[2,3]	Evidence grade B1
Breast cancer prevention:[4–10]	Evidence grade B1
Constipation:[11]	Evidence grade B2
Menopausal symptoms:[12]	Evidence grade B2
Diabetes:[12–14]	Evidence grade B2
Hypertension:[15,16]	Evidence grade B2
Coronary artery disease/atherosclerosis:[17]	Evidence grade C
Cyclic mastalgia:[10,18]	Evidence grade C
Lupus nephritis:[19,20]	Evidence grade C
HIV/AIDS (with arginine and yeast RNA):[21]	Evidence grade C
Prostate cancer:[22]	Evidence grade D

Oil

Hyperlipidemia:[15]	Evidence grade B1
Hypertension:[15,16]	Evidence grade B2
Coronary artery disease/atherosclerosis:[17,23]	Evidence grade C
Diabetes:[14]	Evidence grade C

Pregnancy

Flaxseed

Estrogenic/anti-estrogenic effects:[24–27]	Evidence level 3
Lowers birthweight:[24]	Evidence level 3

Flaxseeds consumed during pregnancy were shown to have estrogenic and anti-estrogenic effects on newborn rats.[24] Flaxseed had no effect on pregnancy outcome except that a 10% flaxseed diet lowered birthweight.[24] A review article on the potential value of plants as sources of anti-fertility agents reported that flax has estrogenic activity.[27]

Conflicting evidence

Does not affect fetal development:[25]	Evidence level 3
Does affect fetal development:[24,25]	Evidence level 3
May alter reproduction:[26]	Evidence level 3
May affect estrous cycle:[25]	Evidence level 3

Female rat offspring from mothers fed flaxseed during pregnancy had shortened anogenital distance, greater uterine and ovarian relative weights, earlier age and lighter body weight at puberty, lengthened estrous cycle and persistent estrus.[24] The male rat offspring from mothers fed flaxseed during pregnancy had reduced postnatal weight gain and had greater sex gland and prostate relative weights.[24] Another study reported that flaxseed can potentially alter reproduction, depending on the dose and timing of exposure.[26] Another study, however, reported that flaxseed ingestion during pregnancy did not affect fetal development but did affect indices of postnatal development such as the estrous cycle.[25]

Increases essential fatty acids in offspring serum and tissue:[28]	Evidence level 3

Flaxseed increased α-linolenic acid (ALA) and eicosapentaenoic acid (EPA) and decreased arachidonic acid in serum and tissues of rat dams and offspring.[28]

Not embryotoxic:[29]	Evidence level 3

A study of the effect of flaxseed on rat embryos concluded that diets high in flaxseed or flaxseed meal do not result in serum factors that are directly embryotoxic to organogenesis-staged rat embryos.[29]

Strengthens bones prior to adulthood:[30]	Evidence level 3

Female rat bone is more sensitive to the estrogen-like action of flaxseed lignans during early life when endogenous levels of sex hormones are low.[31] By adulthood, however, the improved bone strength does not persist.[31] Exposure to purified lignan does not have negative effects on bone strength.[31]

Does not affect spermatogenesis or testis development:[31,32]	Evidence level 3

Quantitative information was collected on male reproductive effects in the rat of maternal and postnatal dietary exposure to flaxseed.[31] It was reported that exposure to flaxseed does not adversely affect testis structure or spermatogenesis.[31] A similar study also found that spermatogenesis was unaffected by flaxseed consumption.[32]

Potential abortifacient:[33]	Evidence level 4

Emmenagogue:[33]	Evidence level 4

A review article on the potential value of plants as sources of anti-fertility agents reported that flax was a potential abortifacient and an emmenagogue.[33]

Oil

Unknown:	Evidence level 5

There are no reports in the scientific literature of flax oil being either safe or contraindicated during pregnancy.

Food amounts

Minimal risk:[1]	Evidence level 4

A natural product compendium reported that flaxseed and flax oil pose minimal risk during pregnancy if taken in food amounts.[1]

Lactation

Flaxseed

Minimal risk:[30]	Evidence level 3

A study on the effect of flaxseed supplementation during pregnancy and lactation reported that there were no significant effects of exposing male or female offspring to flaxseed during lactation.[31] They reported that their findings are in contrast to the estrogenic effects observed in male and female offspring exposed to flaxseed during fetal life and suggest that fetal life is a more hormone-sensitive period of development.[31] Although maternal feeding of flaxseed during lactation appears to be safe with respect to reproductive indices among offspring, the authors reported that future investigation is required to elucidate whether there are any long-term implications with respect to fertility.[31]

Estrogenic/anti-estrogenic effects:[24]	Evidence level 3

Flaxseeds consumed during pregnancy have estrogenic and anti-estrogenic effects on newborn rats.[24] As such, flaxseed was not recommended during lactation as its hormonal effect may have an impact on the developing infant.[24]

Crosses into breast milk:[24,34]	Evidence level 3

Through radioactive labeling, a study reported that flax lignans were transferred to the offspring via rat dam's milk.[24] Another study found that nervonic acid, found in flaxseed, is not readily transferred across the placental barrier but does readily cross the mammary epithelium and is incorporated into milk.[34]

Increases essential fatty acid content in breast milk:[35,36]	Evidence level 3

Flaxseed in the diet of lactating cows increased the beneficial fatty acids in milk without depressing nutrient digestibility.[35] Flaxseed fed to cows increased milk protein percentage and its n-6 to n-3 fatty acids ratio.[36]

Does not affect bone strength in men:[37]	Evidence level 3

Exposing male rats to a diet containing flaxseed either during lactation or through to early adulthood is safe with respect to bone health, as measured by bone mass and strength.[37]

Oil

Unknown:	Evidence level 5

There are no reports in the scientific literature of flax oil being either safe or contraindicated during lactation.

Food amounts

Minimal risk:[1]	Evidence level 4

A natural product compendium reported that flaxseed and flax oil pose minimal risk during lactation if taken in food amounts.[1]

Contraindications

Intestinal obstruction[38]
Esophageal or gastrointestinal stricture[38]
Acute gastroenteritis[38]
Esophagitis[38]

Caution

Large quantities of flaxseed can lead to intestinal obstruction if not taken with sufficient fluid.[38]

Constituents

Seed[39,40]

ALA
Cyanogenic glycosides (linamarin, linustatin, neolinustatin)
Lignan (secoisolariciresinol diglycoside)
Glutamic acid derivative (linatine)
Unsaturated fatty acids (linolenic acid, linoleic acid, oleic acid)
Soluble fiber mucilage (D-xylose, L-galactose, L-rhamnose, D-galacturonic acid)
Monoglycerides
Triglycerides
Sterols
Phenylpropane derivatives

Oil[39]

ALA
Unsaturated fatty acids (linolenic acid, linoleic acid, oleic acid)

Toxicity

LD_{50} of linatine: 2 mg (intraperitoneal)[38]

Pharmacology

Flaxseed

- Flaxseed is a bulk-forming fiber that stimulates intestinal peristalsis, thereby producing a laxative effect.[41]
- Flaxseed supplementation significantly increases n-3 polyunsaturated fatty acids in plasma and erythrocytes.[13,42]
- Since flaxseed reduces platelet aggregation and serum cholesterol, flaxseed thereby reduces the risk of atherosclerosis.[43–47]
- Flaxseed may have hypoglycemic activity and lower insulin levels in postmenopausal women.[12,13]
- Flaxseed is an abundant indirect food source of lignans, where lignans may have estrogenic and anti-estrogenic effects.[48,49]
- The lignans in flaxseed inhibit the growth of hormone-dependent breast cancer cells, inhibit mammary tumor growth in vitro, decrease cellular proliferation in mammary glands, increase mammary gland differentiation and reduce endogenous estrogen binding to estrogen receptors in breast cancer cells.[40,48,50–59]

- ALA was shown to reduce the growth of established tumors and have an anti-inflammatory effect.[45,60]
- The enzyme linamarase releases cyanide from linamarin, but linamarase is deactivated in normal gastric acid.[38]
- Grinding the seeds into a fine powder makes the cyanogenic glycosides more liable to hydrolysis and enhances the absorption of cyanide.[38]

Oil

- Flaxseed oil is among the best sources of ALA.[43]
- ALA raises serum n-3 polyunsaturated fatty acids, including EPA and docosahexaenoic acid (DHA).[42,61]
- Flaxseed oil may lower triglyceride levels, increase systemic arterial elasticity and protect against ischemic stroke and lacunar infarction.[62–64]
- Flaxseed oil may decrease platelet aggregation.[45,61]

Drug interactions[1]

Anti-coagulant/anti-platelet drugs[65]
Anti-diabetic drugs[12,13]
Oral drugs[66]

Parts used[1]

Seed and oil

References

1. Jellin JM, Batz F, Hitchens K. Natural Medicines Comprehensive Database. Stockton, CA: Therapeutic Research Faculty, 2002:1530.
2. Lucas EA, Wild RD, Hammond LJ et al. Flaxseed improves lipid profile without altering biomarkers of bone metabolism in postmenopausal women. J Clin Endocrinol Metab 2002; 87:1527–1532.
3. Jenkins DJ, Kendall CW, Vidgen E et al. Health aspects of partially defatted flaxseed, including effects on serum lipids, oxidative measures, and ex vivo androgen and progestin activity: a controlled crossover trial. Am J Clin Nutr 1999; 69:395–402.
4. Hutchins AM, Martini MC, Olson BA et al. Flaxseed consumption influences endogenous hormone concentrations in postmenopausal women. Nutr Cancer 2001; 39:58–65.
5. Haggans CJ, Travelli EJ, Thomas W et al. The effect of flaxseed and wheat bran consumption on urinary estrogen metabolites in premenopausal women. Cancer Epidemiol Biomarker Prev 2000; 9:719–725.
6. Haggans CJ, Hutchins AM, Olson BA et al. Effect of flaxseed consumption on urinary estrogen metabolites in postmenopausal women. Nutr Cancer 1999; 33:188–195.
7. Phipps WR, Martini MC, Lampe JW, Slavin JL, Kurzer MS. Effect of flax seed ingestion on the menstrual cycle. J Clin Endocrinol Metab 1993; 77:1215–1219.
8. Kurzer MS, Lampe JW, Martini MC, Adlercreutz H. Fecal lignan and isoflavonoid excretion in premenopausal women consuming flaxseed powder. Cancer Epidemiol Biomarkers Prev 1995; 4:353–358.

9. Bougnoux P, Koscielny S, Chajes V et al. alpha-Linolenic acid content of adipose breast tissue: a host determinant of the risk of early metastasis in breast cancer. Br J Cancer 1994; 70:330–334.
10. Plu-Bureau G, Thalabard JC, Sitruk-Ware R, Asselain B, Mauvais-Jarvis P. Cyclical mastalgia as a marker of breast cancer susceptibility: results of a case-control study among French women. Br J Cancer 1992; 65:945–949.
11. Tarpila S, Kivinen A. Ground flaxseed is an effective hypolipidemic bulk laxative [published abstract]. Gastroenterology 1997; 112:A836.
12. Lemay A, Dodin S, Kadri N et al. Flaxseed dietary supplement versus hormone replacement therapy in hypercholesterolemic menopausal women. Obstet Gynecol 2002; 100:495–504.
13. Cunnane SC, Ganguli S, Menard C et al. High alpha-linolenic acid flaxseed (Linum usitatissimum): some nutritional properties in humans. Br J Nutr 1993; 69:443–453.
14. Glauber H, Wallace P, Griver K, Brechtel G. Adverse metabolic effect of omega-3 fatty acids in non-insulin-dependent diabetes mellitus. Ann Intern Med 1988; 108:663–668.
15. Singer P, Jaeger W, Berger I et al. Effects of dietary oleic, linoleic and alpha-linolenic acids on blood pressure, serum lipids, lipoproteins and the formation of eicosanoid precursors in patients with mild essential hypertension. J Hum Hypertens 1990; 4:227–233.
16. Berry EM, Hirsch J. Does dietary linolenic acid influence blood pressure? Am J Clin Nutr 1986; 44:336–340.
17. Hu FB, Stampfer MJ, Manson JE et al. Dietary intake of alpha-linolenic acid and risk of fatal ischemic heart disease among women. Am J Clin Nutr 1999; 69:890–897.
18. Goss PE, Li T, Theriault M et al. Effects of dietary flaxseed in women with cyclical mastalgia. Breast Cancer Res Treat 2000; 64:49.
19. Clark WF, Kortas C, Heidenheim AP et al. Flaxseed in lupus nephritis: a two-year nonplacebo-controlled crossover study. J Am Coll Nutr 2001; 20:143–148.
20. Clark WF, Parbtani A, Huff MW et al. Flaxseed: a potential treatment for lupus nephritis. Kidney Int 1995; 48:475–480.
21. Suttmann U, Ockenga J, Schneider H et al. Weight gain and increased concentrations of receptor proteins for tumor necrosis factor after patients with symptomatic HIV infection received fortified nutrition support. J Am Diet Assoc 1996; 96:565–569.
22. Demark-Wahnefried W, Price DT, Polascik TJ et al. Pilot study of dietary fat restriction and flaxseed supplementation in men with prostate cancer before surgery: exploring the effects on hormonal levels, prostate-specific antigen, and histopathologic features. Urology 2001; 58:47–52.
23. Anonymous. Dietary supplementation with n-3 polyunsaturated fatty acids and vitamin E after myocardial infarction: results of the GISSI-Prevenzione trial. Gruppo Italiano per lo Studio della Sopravvivenza nell'Infarto miocardico. Lancet 1999; 354:447–455.
24. Tou JC, Chen J, Thompson LU. Flaxseed and its lignan precursor, secoisolariciresinol diglycoside, affect pregnancy outcome and reproductive development in rats. J Nutr 1998; 128:1861–1868.
25. Collins TF, Sprando RL, Black TN et al. Effects of flaxseed and defatted flaxseed meal on reproduction and development in rats. Food Chem Toxicol 2003; 41:819–834.

26. Tou JC, Chen J, Thompson LU. Dose, timing, and duration of flaxseed exposure affect reproductive indices and sex hormone levels in rats. J Toxicol Environ Health A 1999; 56:555–570.
27. Farnsworth NR, Bingel AS, Cordell GA, Crane FA, Fong HH. Potential value of plants as sources of new antifertility agents II. J Pharm Sci 1975; 64:717–753.
28. Wiesenfeld PW, Babu US, Collins TF et al. Flaxseed increased alpha-linolenic and eicosapentaenoic acid and decreased arachidonic acid in serum and tissues of rat dams and offspring. Food Chem Toxicol 2003; 41:841–855.
29. Flynn TJ, Collins TF, Sprando RL et al. Developmental effects of serum from flaxseed-fed rats on cultured rat embryos. Food Chem Toxicol 2003; 41:835–840.
30. Ward WE, Chen J, Thompson LU. Exposure to flaxseed or its purified lignan during suckling only or continuously does not alter reproductive indices in male and female offspring. J Toxicol Environ Health A 2001; 64:567–577.
31. Sprando RL, Collins TF, Wiesenfeld P et al. Testing the potential of flaxseed to affect spermatogenesis: morphometry. Food Chem Toxicol 2000; 38:887–892.
32. Sprando RL, Collins TF, Black TN et al. The effect of maternal exposure to flaxseed on spermatogenesis in F generation rats. Food Chem Toxicol 2000; 38:325–334.
33. Farnsworth NR, Bingel AS, Cordell GA, Crane FA, Fong HH. Potential value of plants as sources of new antifertility agents I. J Pharm Sci 1975; 64:535–598.
34. Bettger WJ, DiMichelle-Ranalli E, Dillingham B, Blackadar CB. Nervonic acid is transferred from the maternal diet to milk and tissues of suckling rat pups. J Nutr Biochem 2003; 14:160–165.
35. Soita HW, Meier JA, Fehr M et al. Effects of flaxseed supplementation on milk production, milk fatty acid composition and nutrient utilization by lactating dairy cows. Arch Tierernahr 2003; 57:107–116.
36. Petit HV. Digestion, milk production, milk composition, and blood composition of dairy cows fed whole flaxseed. J Dairy Sci 2002; 85:1482–1490.
37. Ward WE, Yuan YV, Cheung AM, Thompson LU. Exposure to flaxseed and its purified lignan reduces bone strength in young but not older male rats. J Toxicol Environ Health A 2001; 63:53–65.
38. Brinker F. The Toxicology of Botanical Medicines. Sandy, OR: Eclectic Medical Publications, 2000:296.
39. www.naturalstandard.com. Flaxseed and Flaxseed Oil (Linum usitatissimum) Natural Standard Monograph.
40. Tan KP, Chen J, Ward WE, Thompson LU. Mammary gland morphogenesis is enhanced by exposure to flaxseed or its major lignan during suckling in rats. Exp Biol Med (Maywood) 2004; 229:147–157.
41. Gruenwald J, Brendler T, Jaenicke C. PDR for Herbal Medicines. Montvale, NJ: Medical Economics Company, 1998.
42. Cunnane SC, Hamadeh MJ, Liede AC et al. Nutritional attributes of traditional flaxseed in healthy young adults. Am J Clin Nutr 1995; 61:62–68.
43. The Review of Natural Products by Facts and Comparisons. St. Louis, MO: Wolters Kluwer Co., 1999.
44. Jenkins DJ, Kendall CWC, Vidgen E et al. Health aspects of partially defatted flaxseed, including effects on serum lipids, oxidative measures, and ex vivo androgen and progestin activity: a controlled, crossover trial. Am J Clin Nutr 1999; 69:395–402.

45. Prasad K. Dietary flax seed in prevention of hypercholesterolemic atherosclerosis. Atherosclerosis 1997; 132:69–76.
46. Prasad K, Mantha SV, Muir AD, Westcott ND. Reduction of hypercholesterolemic atherosclerosis by CDC-flaxseed with very low alpha-linolenic acid. Atherosclerosis 1998; 136:367–375.
47. Bierenbaum ML, Reichstein R, Watkins TR. Reducing atherogenic risk in hyperlipemic humans with flaxseed supplementation: a preliminary report. J Am Coll Nutr 1993; 12:501–504.
48. Thompson LU, Rickard SE, Cheung F et al. Variability in anticancer lignan levels in flaxseed. Nutr Cancer 1997; 27:26–30.
49. Kilkkinen A, Stumpf K, Pietinen P et al. Determinants of serum enterolactone concentration. Am J Clin Nutr 2001; 73:1094–1100.
50. Rose DP. Dietary fiber and breast cancer. Nutr Cancer 1990; 13:1–8.
51. Mousavi Y, Adlercreutz H. Enterolactone and estradiol inhibit each other's proliferative effect on MCF-7 breast cancer cells in culture. J Steroid Biochem Mol Biol 1992; 41:615–619.
52. Sung MK, Lautens M, Thompson LU. Mammalian lignans inhibit the growth of estrogen-independent human colon tumor cells. Anticancer Res 1998; 18:1405–1408.
53. Serraino M, Thompson LU. The effect of flaxseed supplementation on the initiation and promotional stages of mammary tumorigenesis. Nutr Cancer 1992; 17:153–159.
54. Lampe JW, Martini MC, Kurzer MS et al. Urinary lignan and isoflavonoid excretion in premenopausal women consuming flaxseed powder. Am J Clin Nutr 1994; 60:122–128.
55. Adlercreutz H, Fotsis T, Bannwart C et al. Determination of urinary lignans and phytoestrogen metabolites, potential antiestrogens and anticarcinogens, in urine of women on various habitual diets. J Steroid Biochem 1986; 25:791–797.
56. Adlercreutz H. Diet, breast cancer, and sex hormone metabolism. Ann N Y Acad Sci 1990; 595:281–290.
57. Wang C, Makela T, Hase T et al. Lignans and flavonoids inhibit aromatase enzyme in human preadipocytes. J Steroid Biochem Mol Biol 1994; 50:205–212.
58. Serraino M, Thompson LU. The effect of flaxseed supplementation on early risk markers for mammary carcinogenesis. Cancer Lett 1991; 60:135–142.
59. Rickard SE, Yuan YV, Thompson LU. Plasma insulin-like growth factor I levels in rats are reduced by dietary supplementation of flaxseed or its lignan secoisolariciresinol diglycoside. Cancer Lett 2000; 161:47–55.
60. Thompson LU, Rickard SE, Orcheson LJ, Seidl MM. Flaxseed and its lignan and oil components reduce mammary tumor growth at a late stage of carcinogenesis. Carcinogenesis 1996; 17:1373–1376.
61. Allman MA, Pena MM, Pang D. Supplementation with flaxseed oil versus sunflower seed oil in healthy young men consuming a low fat diet: effects on platelet composition and function. Eur J Clin Nutr 1995; 49:169–178.
62. Singer P, Wirth M, Berger I. A possible contribution of decrease in free fatty acids to low serum triglyceride levels after diets supplemented with n-6 and n-3 polyunsaturated fatty acids. Atherosclerosis 1990; 83:167–175.
63. Nestel PJ, Pomeroy SE, Sasahara T et al. Arterial compliance in obese subjects is improved with dietary plant n-3 fatty acid from flaxseed oil despite increased LDL oxidizability. Arterioscler Thromb Vasc Biol 1997; 17:1163–1170.
64. Iso H, Sato S, Umemura U et al. Linoleic acid, other fatty acids, and the risk of stroke. Stroke 2002; 33:2086–2093.

65. Nordstrom DC, Honkanen VE, Nasu Y et al. Alpha-linolenic acid in the treatment of rheumatoid arthritis. A double-blind, placebo-controlled and randomized study: flaxseed vs. safflower seed. Rheumatol Int 1995; 14:231–234.
66. Brinker F. Herb Contraindications and Drug Interactions. Sandy, OR: Eclectic Medical Publications, 1998.

FOXGLOVE
Digitalis lanata, D. purpurea

Synonyms/common names/related substances[1]

Dead man's bells, fairy cap, fairy finger, foxglove, lady's thimble, lion's mouth, purple foxglove, Scotch mercury, throatwort, witch's bells, wolly foxglove

Indications

Congestive heart failure:[2]	Evidence grade A

Pregnancy

Musculoskeletal malformations:[3]	Evidence level 1b

A serial examination of 20 248 livebirths, stillbirths and abortions to assess correlations between drug exposure and major malformations found a statistically significant association between digitalis and anomalies of the musculoskeletal system.

Treatment of hydrops fetalis:[4–6]	Evidence level 2

There are a few cases in the scientific literature of digitalis being used to treat hydrops fetalis.[4–6] The treatment outcomes were successful in some cases and unsuccessful in others.[4–6]

Treatment of fetal cardiac disorders:[7–10]	Evidence level 2

There are cases in the scientific literature where digitalis was used to treat fetal cardiac disorders, such as fetal tachycardia and fetal atrial flutter.[7–10] The treatment outcomes were successful in some cases and unsuccessful in others.[7–10]

Can be prescribed during pregnancy:[11,12]	Evidence level 4

Two review articles report that digitalis drug preparations can be prescribed during pregnancy.[11,12]

Cytotoxic:[13]	Evidence level 4

A review article on the potential value of plants as sources of anti-fertility agents reported that foxglove has cytotoxic activity.[13]

Unsafe:[14]	Evidence level 4

A botanical safety compendium reports that digitalis is unsafe during pregnancy.[14]

Crosses the placenta:[15]	Evidence level 4

A review article in the scientific literature reported that digoxin rapidly crosses the placenta and reaches equilibrium with maternal and fetal serum having equal concentrations.[15]

Lactation

Unsafe:[14]	Evidence level 4

A botanical safety compendium reports that digitalis is unsafe during lactation.[14] There are no reports in the scientific literature of digitalis being either safe or contraindicated during lactation.

Contraindications

Second- or third-degree atrioventricular blocks[16]
Hypercalcemia[16]
Hypertrophic cardiomyopathy[16]
Carotid sinus syndrome[16]
Ventricular tachycardia[16]
Thoracic aortic aneurysm[16]
Wolff–Parkinson–White syndrome[16]

Toxicity

- Toxic dose: 520 mg of powder[16]
- Lethal dose: 2 g of powder[16]

Constituents

- Cardiac (steroidal) glycosides:[16] digitoxin (glycoside A), gitoxin (glycoside B), gitaloxin, digitonin (*D. purpurea*), digoxin, digitalin, gitaloxin, lanatosides A, B, C, D and E (*D. lanata*)
- Cardelonides[16]

Pharmacology

- Cardiac glycosides in digitalis increase cardiac contractility, decrease heart rate and reduce atrioventricular node conduction.[17]
- Digitalis increases cardiac output.[17]
- Digitalis relieves pulmonary congestion and peripheral edema.[17]

Drug interactions

Digoxin (Lanoxin)[18]
Potassium-depleting diuretics, quinine[18,19]
Stimulant laxatives[18,19]
Tetracyclines and macrolide antibiotics (erythromycin-like drugs)[20]

Parts used

Leaves, seeds, flowers[16]

References

1. Jellin JM, Batz F, Hitchens K. Natural Medicines Comprehensive Database. Stockton, CA: Therapeutic Research Faculty, 2002:1530.
2. Hood WBJ, Dans AL, Guyatt GH, Jaeschke R, McMurray JJV. Digitalis for treatment of congestive heart failure in patients in sinus rhythm. Cochrane Database Syst Rev, 2001.
3. Queisser-Luft A, Eggers I, Stolz G, Kieninger-Baum D, Schlaefer K. Serial examination of 20,248 newborn fetuses and infants: correlations between drug exposure and major malformations. Am J Med Genet 1996; 63:268–276.
4. Nagashima M, Asai T, Suzuki C, Matsushima M, Ogawa A. Intrauterine supraventricular tachyarrhythmias and transplacental digitalisation. Arch Dis Child 1986; 61:996–1000.
5. Kovats-Szabo E, Horvath I, Nagy M, Kadar K. [Intrauterine treatment of fetal tachycardia causing circulatory failure]. Orv Hetil 1990; 131:807–809.
6. Koike T, Minakami H, Shiraishi H et al. Digitalization of the mother in treating hydrops fetalis in monochorionic twin with Ebstein's anomaly. Case report. J Perinat Med 1997; 25:295–297.
7. Auzelle MP, Mensire A, Lachassine E et al. [In utero treatment of fetal tachycardias with a digitalis-beta blocker combination. Apropos of 2 cases]. J Gynecol Obstet Biol Reprod (Paris) 1987; 16:383–391.
8. Oberhaensli I, Extermann P, Friedli B, Beguin F. Ultrasound screening for congenital cardiac malformations in the fetus. Its importance for peri- and postnatal care. Pediatr Radiol 1989; 19:94–99.
9. Pal A, Gembruch U, Hansmann M. [Practical importance of the exact diagnosis of fetal arrhythmias]. Orv Hetil 1991; 132:1359–1362.
10. Stavem K, Steen T. [Atrial fibrillation during pregnancy]. Tidsskr Nor Laegeforen 1993; 113:2405.
11. Grand A. [Pregnancy and cardiac drugs]. Rev Fr Gynecol Obstet 1993; 88:297–312.
12. Grand A. [Pregnancy and cardiovascular agents]. Ann Cardiol Angeiol (Paris) 1992; 41:549–564.
13. Farnsworth NR, Bingel AS, Cordell GA, Crane FA, Fong HH. Potential value of plants as sources of new antifertility agents II. J Pharm Sci 1975; 64:717–753.
14. McGuffin M, Hobbs C, Upton R, Goldberg A. American Herbal Products Association's Botanical Safety Handbook. Boca Raton, FL: CRC Press, 1997:231.
15. Soyka LF. Digoxin: placental transfer, effects on the fetus, and therapeutic use in the newborn. Clin Perinatol 1975; 2:23–35.
16. Brinker F. The Toxicology of Botanical Medicines. Sandy, OR: Eclectic Medical Publications, 2000:296.
17. The Review of Natural Products by Facts and Comparisons. St. Louis, MO: Wolters Kluwer Co., 1999.
18. Blumenthal M, Busse WR, Goldberg A et al. The Complete German Commission E Monographs: Therapeutic Guide to Herbal Medicines. Boston, MA: American Botanical Council, 1998.
19. Burnham TH. Drug Facts and Comparisons. Facts and Comparisons. St. Louis, MO, updated monthly.
20. Ellenhorn MJ, Schonwald S, Ordog G, Wasserberger J. Ellenhorn's Medical Toxicology: Diagnoses and Treatment of Human Poisoning. Baltimore, MD: Williams & Wilkins, 1997.

GARLIC

Allium sativum

Synonyms/common names/related substances[1]

Aged garlic extract, ail, ajo, allii aativi bulbus, allium, camphor of the poor, clove garlic, garlic clove, nectar of the gods, poor man's treacle, rust treacle, stinking rose

Indications

Garlic

*Hypercholesterolemia (mild effect):[2–14]	Evidence grade A
Mild hypertension:[3,12,13,15–17]	Evidence grade A
Cancer prevention – stomach and colorectal:[18–21]	Evidence grade A
Hypertriglyceridemia:[7–9,11,13]	Evidence grade B1
Atherosclerosis:[3,16,22–24]	Evidence grade B1
Anti-platelet aggregation:[16,23,25]	Evidence grade B1
Unstable angina pectoris:[26]	Evidence grade B2
Coronary artery disease:[11,22]	Evidence grade B2
Diabetes:[16,27]	Evidence grade B2
Tick repellant:[28]	Evidence grade B2
Upper respiratory tract infection:[29]	Evidence grade B2
Acute otitis media (with *Verbascum thapsus*, *Calendula flores*, and *Hypericum perforatum*):[30]	Evidence grade B2
Cancer prevention – thyroid, breast, endometrial:[31–33]	Evidence grade C
Rheumatoid arthritis:[34]	Evidence grade C
Anti-fungal:[35–40]	Evidence grade C
Cryptococcal meningitis:[41]	Evidence grade D
Cancer treatment:[42,43]	Evidence grade E

Anti-*Helicobacter pylori*:[44,45]	Evidence grade E

Sickle cell anemia:[46]	Evidence grade E

*A systematic review of garlic powder in the treatment of moderate hyperlipidemia concluded that garlic powder preparations significantly lowered serum triglyceride and total cholesterol compared with placebo.[4] A meta-analysis, however, concluded that garlic reduced total cholesterol by 0.65 mmol/L and was less effective in reducing total cholesterol than suggested by previous meta-analyses.[47]

Aged garlic extract

Hypercholesterolemia:[48]	Evidence grade B1

Hypertension:[48]	Evidence grade B1

Pregnancy

Minimal risk – third trimester:[49]	Evidence level 1a

A randomized controlled study was conducted where 100 primigravidae were treated with either garlic tablets (800 mg/day) or placebo during the third trimester of pregnancy to determine the effect of garlic supplementation on preeclampsia.[49] With the exception of a garlic body odor, few side effects (e.g. feeling of nausea) were reported as a result of garlic supplementation during the third trimester of pregnancy.[49] Pregnancy outcomes were comparable in both the group treated with garlic and the placebo group.[49] The authors did not report any incidence of major or minor malformations in the newborn infants nor any spontaneous abortions of the fetus.[49]

Garlic crosses into the amniotic fluid:[50]	Evidence level 1a

Amniotic fluid samples were obtained from 10 pregnant women undergoing routine amniocentesis procedure, where five of the women ingested placebo capsules while the remaining five ingested capsules containing the essential oil of garlic.[50] The odor of the amniotic fluid obtained from four of the five women who had ingested the garlic capsules was judged to be stronger or more like garlic than the samples collected from the women consuming placebo capsules.[50] Thus, it was concluded that garlic ingestion by pregnant women significantly altered the odor of their amniotic fluid.[50]

Potential abortifacient:[51]	Evidence level 4

Emmenagogue:[51]	Evidence level 4

Uterine stimulant:[51]	Evidence level 4

A review article on the potential value of plants as sources of anti-fertility agents reported that garlic was a potential abortifacient, emmenagogue and uterine stimulant.[51]

Lactation

Minimal risk:[52]	Evidence level 1

In nursing infants, maternal garlic ingestion did not significantly affect the number of times the infants fed nor the amount of milk they consumed.[52] Although benign, short-term behavioral changes were observed in the infants as nursing mothers went from placebo to garlic supplementation and vice versa.[52] The authors did not report any adverse effects in the nursing infants nor in breast milk production by the mothers.[52]

Constituents

- Sulfur-containing compounds:[9,53,54] alliin, allicin (diallyl thiosufinate), allyl propyl disulfide, diallyl disulfide, diallyl trisulfide, ajoene, vinyldithiines
- S-allymercaptocysteine[54]
- S-methylmercaptocysteine[54]
- Volatile oils[54]

Pharmacology

- Garlic has lipid-lowering effects through inhibition of the cholesterolgenic enzymes 3-hydroxy-3-methylglutaryl (HMG)-CoA reductase and acetyl-CoA synthetase, through increased loss of bile salts in feces, and through mobilization of tissue lipids into circulation.[9,55–58]
- Garlic has anti-atherogenic action in vitro and in vivo where it inhibited the proliferative activity of atherosclerotic plaques in the human aorta, reduced cholesterol accumulation in blood serum, and made low-density lipoprotein significantly more resistant to oxidation than that isolated from subjects receiving no garlic supplements.[59,60]
- Garlic inhibits platelet aggregation in healthy individuals and patients with cardiovascular disease, and inhibits platelet adhesion to collagen, fibrinogen, and von Willebrand factor.[22,61,62]
- Garlic increased fibrinolytic activity during long-term use in chronic infarction as well as during the critical acute post-infarction period.[22]
- Garlic has anti-platelet activity.[9,16,23]
- Garlic was found to reduce arterial blood pressure by causing membrane hyperpolarization and subsequent vasodilation through its action on potassium (calcium) ion channels in the membrane of vascular smooth muscle cells.
- Garlic oil reduced blood sugar levels in men and increased blood sugar levels in women.[27]
- Garlic detoxifies chemical carcinogens, prevents carcinogenesis, and directly inhibits the growth of cancer cells.[42]

- Garlic stimulates the immune system by stimulating macrophage activity, natural killer cells, and lymphokine-activated killer cells, and by increasing the production of interleukin-2, tumor necrosis factor and interferon-γ.[42]
- Garlic protects against the suppression of immunity by chemotherapy and ultraviolet radiation through the stimulation of macrophages and lymphocytes.[42]
- Garlic oil was found to reduce the activity of cytochrome P450 CYP2E1.[63]
- Garlic was shown to significantly increase maximum oxygen consumption (VO_2 max) and endurance performance time of endurance athletes.[64]
- Garlic, with *V. thapsus*, *C. flores*, and *H. perforatum*, was an effective anesthetic during acute otitis media ear pain.[31]
- Garlic has in vitro activity against *H. pylori*.[44,45]
- Garlic has anti-mycotic, anti-fungal and anti-bacterial activity.[35–40,65]

Drug interactions

Anti-coagulant/anti-platelet drugs[22,61]
Anti-glycemic drugs[16,27]
Highly active anti-retroviral therapy (HAART) drugs[66]
Oral contraceptives[1,66]
Drugs metabolized by cytochrome P450 CYP2E1 enzyme[63]

Part used[67]

Bulb

References

1. Jellin JM, Batz F, Hitchens K. Natural Medicines Comprehensive Database. Stockton, CA: Therapeutic Research Faculty, 2002:1530.
2. Ghorai M, Mandal SC, Pal M, Pal SP, Saha BP. A comparative study on hypocholesterolaemic effect of allicin, whole germinated seeds of bengal gram and guggulipid of gum guggul. Phytother Res 2000; 14:200–202.
3. Siegel G, Walter A, Engel S, Walper A, Michel F. [Pleiotropic effects of garlic]. Wien Med Wochenschr 1999; 149:217–224.
4. Silagy C, Neil A. Garlic as a lipid lowering agent – a meta-analysis. J R Coll Phys Lond 1994; 28:39–45.
5. Warshafsky S, Kamer RS, Sivak SL. Effect of garlic on total serum cholesterol. A meta-analysis. Ann Intern Med 1993; 119:599–605.
6. Jain AK, Vargas R, Gotzkowsky S, McMahon FG. Can garlic reduce levels of serum lipids? A controlled clinical study. Am J Med 1993; 94:632–635.
7. Holzgartner H, Schmidt U, Kuhn U. Comparison of the efficacy and tolerance of a garlic preparation vs. bezafibrate. Arzneimittel-Forschung 1992; 42:1473–1477.
8. Lau BHS, Lam F, Wang-Cheng R. Effect of an odor-modified garlic preparation on blood lipids. Nutr Res 1987; 7:139–149.
9. Bordia A, Verma SK, Srivastava KC. Effect of garlic (Allium sativum) on blood lipids, blood sugar, fibrinogen and fibrinolytic activity in patients with coronary artery disease. Prostaglandins Leukot Essent Fatty Acids 1998; 58:257–263.

10. Adler AJ, Holub BJ. Effect of garlic and fish-oil supplementation on serum lipid and lipoprotein concentrations in hypercholesterolemic men. Am J Clin Nutr 1997; 65:445–450.
11. Bordia A. Effect of garlic on blood lipids in patients with coronary heart disease. Am J Clin Nutr 1981; 34:2100–2103.
12. De A, Grunwald J. Effect of garlic powder tablets on blood lipids and blood pressure – a six month placebo controlled, double blind study. Br J Clin Res 1993; 4:37–44.
13. Auer W, Eiber A, Hertkorn E et al. Hypertension and hyperlipidaemia: garlic helps in mild cases. Br J Gen Pract 1990; (Suppl):3–6.
14. Kannar D, Wattanapenpaiboon N, Savige GS, Wahlqvist ML. Hypocholesterolemic effect of an enteric-coated garlic supplement. J Am Coll Nutr 2001; 20:225–231.
15. Silagy CA, Neil HA. A meta-analysis of the effect of garlic on blood pressure. J Hypertens 1994; 12:463–468.
16. Kiesewetter H, Jung F, Pindur G et al. Effect of garlic on thrombocyte aggregation, microcirculation, and other risk factors. Int J Clin Pharmacol Ther Toxicol 1991; 29:151–155.
17. Andrianova IV, Fomchenkov IV, Orekhov AN. [Hypotensive effect of long-acting garlic tablets allicor (a double-blind placebo-controlled trial)]. Terapevticheskii Arkhiv 2002; 74:76–78.
18. Fleischauer AT, Arab L. Garlic and cancer: a critical review of the epidemiologic literature. J Nutr 2001; 131:1032S–1040S.
19. Buiatti E, Palli D, Decarli A et al. A case-control study of gastric cancer and diet in Italy. Int J Cancer 1989; 44:611–616.
20. You WC, Blot WJ, Chang YS et al. Allium vegetables and reduced risk of stomach cancer. J Natl Cancer Inst 1989; 81:162–164.
21. Gao CM, Takezaki T, Ding JH, Li MS, Tajima K. Protective effect of allium vegetables against both esophageal and stomach cancer: a simultaneous case-referent study of a high-epidemic area in Jiangsu Province, China. Jpn J Cancer Res 1999; 90:614–621.
22. Bordia AK, Joshi HK, Sanadhya YK, Bhu N. Effect of essential oil of garlic on serum fibrinolytic activity in patients with coronary artery disease. Atherosclerosis 1977; 28:155–159.
23. Kiesewetter H, Jung F, Jung EM et al. Effect of garlic on platelet aggregation in patients with increased risk of juvenile ischaemic attack. Eur J Clin Pharmacol 1993; 45:333–336.
24. Koscielny J, Klussendorf D, Latza R et al. The antiatherosclerotic effect of Allium sativum. Atherosclerosis 1999; 144:237–249.
25. Kiesewetter H, Jung F, Jung EM et al. Effects of garlic coated tablets in peripheral arterial occlusive disease. Clin Investig 1993; 71:383–386.
26. Li G, Shi Z, Jia H et al. A clinical investigation on garlicin injectio for treatment of unstable angina pectoris and its actions on plasma endothelin and blood sugar levels. J Traditional Chinese Med 2000; 20:243–246.
27. Zhang XH, Lowe D, Giles P et al. Gender may affect the action of garlic oil on plasma cholesterol and glucose levels of normal subjects. J Nutr 2001; 131: 1471–1478.
28. Stjernberg L, Berglund J. Garlic as an insect repellent. JAMA 2000; 284:831.
29. Josling P. Preventing the common cold with a garlic supplement: a double-blind, placebo-controlled survey. Adv Ther 2001; 18:189–193.

30. Sarrell EM, Mandelberg A, Cohen HA. Efficacy of naturopathic extracts in the management of ear pain associated with acute otitis media. Arch Pediatr Adolesc Med 2001; 155:796–799.
31. Dorant E, van den Brandt PA, Goldbohm RA. Allium vegetable consumption, garlic supplement intake, and female breast carcinoma incidence. Breast Cancer Res Treat 1995; 33:163–170.
32. Wang ZY, Boice JDJ, Wei LX et al. Thyroid nodularity and chromosome aberrations among women in areas of high background radiation in China. J Natl Cancer Inst 1990; 82:478–485.
33. Levi F, Franceschi S, Negri E, La Vecchia C. Dietary factors and the risk of endometrial cancer. Cancer 1993; 71:3575–3581.
34. Denisov LN, Andrianova IV, Timofeeva SS. [Garlic effectiveness in rheumatoid arthritis] Effektivnost' chesnoka pri revmatoidnom artrite. Terapevticheskii Arkhiv 1999; 71:55–58.
35. Ledezma E, Lopez JC, Marin P et al. Ajoene in the topical short-term treatment of tinea cruris and tinea corporis in humans. Randomized comparative study with terbinafine. Arzneimittelforschung 1999; 49:544–547.
36. Ledezma E, Marcano K, Jorquera A et al. Efficacy of ajoene in the treatment of tinea pedis: a double-blind and comparative study with terbinafine. J Am Acad Dermatol 2000; 43:829–832.
37. Sandhu DK, Warraich MK, Singh S. Sensitivity of yeasts isolated from cases of vaginitis to aqueous extracts of garlic. Mykosen 1980; 23:691–698.
38. Naganawa R, Iwata N, Ishikawa K et al. Inhibition of microbial growth by ajoene, a sulfur-containing compound derived from garlic. Appl Environ Microbiol 1996; 62:4238–4242.
39. Pai ST, Platt MW. Antifungal effects of Allium sativum (garlic) extract against the Aspergillus species involved in otomycosis. Lett Appl Microbiol 1995; 20:14–18.
40. Davis LE, Shen J, Royer RE. In vitro synergism of concentrated allium sativum extract and amphotericin B against cryptococcus neoformans. Planta Med 1994; 60:546–549.
41. Anonymous. Garlic in cryptococcal meningitis: a preliminary report of 21 cases. Chin Med J (Engl) 1980; 93:123–126.
42. Lamm DL, Riggs DR. The potential application of Allium sativum (garlic) for the treatment of bladder cancer. Urol Clin North Am 2000; 27:157–162.
43. Hageman G, Krul C, van Herwijnen M, Schilderman P, Kleinjans J. Assessment of the anticarcinogenic potential of raw garlic in humans. Cancer Lett 1997; 114:161–162.
44. Jonkers D, van den Broek E, van Dooren I et al. Antibacterial effect of garlic and omeprazole on Helicobacter pylori. J Antimicrob Chemother 1999; 43:837–839.
45. McNulty CA, Wilson MP, Havinga W et al. A pilot study to determine the effectiveness of garlic oil capsules in the treatment of dyspeptic patients with Helicobacter pylori. Helicobacter 2001; 6:249–253.
46. Ohnishi ST, Ohnishi T, Ogunmola GB. Sickle cell anemia: a potential nutritional approach for a molecular disease. Nutrition 2000; 16:330–338.
47. Neil HA, Silagy CA, Lancaster T et al. Garlic powder in the treatment of moderate hyperlipidaemia: a controlled trial and meta-analysis. J R Coll Phys Lond 1996; 30:329–334.
48. Steiner M, Khan AH, Holbert D, Lin RI. A double-blind crossover study in moderately hypercholesterolemic men that compared the effect of aged garlic extract and placebo administration on blood lipids. Am J Clin Nutr 1996; 64:866–870.

49 Ziaei S, Hantoshzadeh S, Rezasoltani P, Lamyian M. The effect of garlic tablet on plasma lipids and platelet aggregation in nulliparous pregnants at high risk of preeclampsia. Eur J Obstet Gynec Reprod Biol 2001; 99:201–206.
50. Mennella JA, Johnson A, Beauchamp GK. Garlic ingestion by pregnant women alters the odor of amniotic fluid. Chemical Senses 1995; 20:207–209.
51. Farnsworth NR, Bingel AS, Cordell GA, Crane FA, Fong HH. Potential value of plants as sources of new antifertility agents I. J Pharm Sci 1975; 64:535–598.
52. Mennella JA, Beauchamp GK. The effects of repeated exposure to garlic-flavored milk on the nursling's behavior. Pediatr Res 1993; 34:805–808.
53. Bordia A, Bansal HC, Arora SK, Singh SV. Effect of the essential oils of garlic and onion on alimentary hyperlipemia. Atherosclerosis 1975; 21:15–19.
54. Newall CA, Anderson LA, Phillipson JD. Herbal Medicines: A Guide for Health-care Professionals. London, UK: Pharmaceutical Press, 1996:296.
55. Gupta N, Porter TD. Garlic and garlic-derived compounds inhibit human squalene monooxygenase. J Nutr 2001; 131:1662–1667.
56. Qureshi AA, Abuirmeileh N, Din ZZ, Elson CE, Burger WC. Inhibition of cholesterol and fatty acid biosynthesis in liver enzymes and chicken hepatocytes by polar fractions of garlic. Lipids 1983; 18:343–348.
57. Qureshi AA, Crenshaw TD, Abuirmeileh N, Peterson DM, Elson CE. Influence of minor plant constituents on porcine hepatic lipid metabolism. Impact on serum lipids. Atherosclerosis 1987; 64:109–115.
58. Qureshi AA, Din ZZ, Abuirmeileh N et al. Suppression of avian hepatic lipid metabolism by solvent extracts of garlic: impact on serum lipids. J Nutr 1983; 113:1746–1755.
59. Munday JS, James KA, Fray LM, Kirkwood SW, Thompson KG. Daily supplementation with aged garlic extract, but not raw garlic, protects low density lipoprotein against in vitro oxidation. Atherosclerosis 1999; 143:399–404.
60. Orekhov AN, Tertov VV, Sobenin IA, Pivovarova EM. Direct anti-atherosclerosis-related effects of garlic. Ann Med 1995; 27:63–65.
61. Steiner M, Lin RS. Changes in platelet function and susceptibility of lipoproteins to oxidation associated with administration of aged garlic extract. J Cardiovasc Pharmacol 1998; 31:904–908.
62. Steiner M, Li W. Aged garlic extract, a modulator of cardiovascular risk factors: a dose-finding study on the effects of AGE on platelet functions. J Nutr 2001; 131:980S–984S.
63. Gurley BJ, Gardner SF, Hubbard MA et al. Cytochrome P450 phenotypic ratios for predicting herb–drug interactions in humans. Clin Pharmacol Ther 2002; 72:276–287.
64. Ince DI, Sonmez GT, Ince ML. Effects garlic on aerobic performance. Turkish J Med Sci 2000; 30:557–561.
65. Rich GE. Garlic an antibiotic? Med J Aust 1982; 1:60.
66. Piscitelli SC, Burstein AH, Welden N, Gallicano KD, Falloon J. The effect of garlic supplements on the pharmacokinetics of saquinavir. Clin Infect Dis 2002; 34:234–238.
67. Brinker F. Herb Contraindications and Drug Interactions. Sandy, OR: Eclectic Medical Publications, 2001:432.

GENTIAN
Gentiana lutea

Synonyms/common names/related compounds[1]
Bitter root, bitterwort, gall weed, gentiana, *Gentianae radix*, pale gentian, stemless gentian, yellow gentian, wild gentian

Indications

Chronic and acute sinusitis (with elderberry, vervain, primrose and sorrel):[2,3]	Evidence grade B1
Digestive disorders, appetite disorders and constipation (with rhubarb, boldus and cascara):[4]	Evidence grade B1

Pregnancy

Potential mutagen:[5,6]	Evidence level 3

The gentian constituents gentisin and isogentisin were reported to have mutagenic effects on bacteria.[6]

Emmenagogue:[5]	Evidence level 4

A herbal compendium reported that gentian is an emmenagogue.[5] There are no reports in the scientific literature of gentian being either safe or contraindicated during pregnancy.

Lactation

Potential mutagen:[5,6]	Evidence level 3

The gentian constituents gentisin and isogentisin were reported to have mutagenic effects on bacteria.[6]

Unknown:	Evidence level 5

There are no reports in the scientific literature of gentian being either safe or contraindicated during lactation.

Contraindications
Acute gastrointestinal inflammation or irritation[7]
Peptic ulcer[7]

Constituents

- Iridoid monoterpenes:[7] amarogentin, gentiopicrin, swertiamarin, sweroside
- Hydroxyxanthones:[6] gentisin, isogentisin

Toxicity

100 g of gentian root was reported to yield approximately 100 mg of total mutagenic compounds, of which gentisin and isogentisin comprised 76%.[6]

Pharmacology

- The bitter constituents, gentiamarin, gentiopicrin, amarogentin and swertiamarin, appear to increase saliva and digestive secretion.[5,8]
- Gentianine may have anti-inflammatory activity.[9]
- Gentisin and isogentisin have been shown to be mutagenic in bacterial studies.[5]
- Gentiopicrin is lethal to mosquito larvae.[9]

Drug interactions[1,10]

Antacids[10]
H2 antagonists[10]
Proton pump inhibitors[10]

Part used

Root[1]

References

1. Jellin JM, Batz F, Hitchens K. Natural Medicines Comprehensive Database. Stockton, CA: Therapeutic Research Faculty, 2002:1530.
2. Marz RW, Ismail C, Popp MA. [Profile and effectiveness of a phytogenic combination preparation for treatment of sinusitis]. Wien Med Wochenschr 1999; 149:202–208.
3. Neubauer N, Marz RW. Placebo-controlled, randomized, double-blind, clincal trial with Sinupret sugar coated tablets on the basis of a therapy with antibiotics and decongestant nasal drops in acute sinusitis. Phytomedicine 1994; 1:177–181.
4. Borgia M, Camarri E, Cataldi V et al. A double-blind double-controlled multicenter study of the therapeutic efficacy of a well-known combination of medicinal herbs. Clinica Terapeutica 1985; 114:401–409.
5. Newall CA, Anderson LA, Phillipson JD. Herbal Medicines: A Guide for Health-care Professionals. London, UK: Pharmaceutical Press, 1996:296.
6. Morimoto I, Nozaka T, Watanabe F et al. Mutagenic activities of gentisin and isogentisin from Gentianae radix (Gentianaceae). Mutat Res 1983; 116:103–117.
7. Brinker F. The Toxicology of Botanical Medicines. Sandy, OR: Eclectic Medical Publications, 2000:296.
8. Blumenthal M, Busse WR, Goldberg A et al. The Complete German Commission E Monographs: Therapeutic Guide to Herbal Medicines. Boston, MA: American Botanical Council, 1998.
9. Leung AY, Foster S. Encyclopedia of Common Natural Ingredients Used in Food, Drugs and Cosmetics. New York, NY: John Wiley & Sons, 1996:649.
10. Brinker F. Herb Contraindications and Drug Interactions. Sandy, OR: Eclectic Medical Publications, 1998.

GINGER
Zingiber officinalis

Synonyms/common names/related compounds[1]

African ginger, black ginger, cochin ginger, gingembre, ginger root, imber, Jamaica ginger, jiang, race ginger, shoga, *Zingiberis rhizome*

Indications

Nausea and vomiting:[2]	Evidence grade A
Hyperemesis gravidarum – nausea and vomiting of pregnancy:[3–9]	Evidence grade B1
Hyperemesis gravidarum – nausea and vomiting of pregnancy (with vitamin B6):[3]	Evidence grade B1
Postoperative nausea and vomiting:[10–12]	Evidence grade B1
Chemotherapy-induced nausea:[13,14]	Evidence grade B2
Vomiting from motion sickness:[15,16]	Evidence grade B2
Rheumatoid arthritis:[17,18]	Evidence grade D

Pregnancy

Minimal risk (up to 1500 mg of dried ginger per day):[3–9]	Evidence level 1a

A randomized controlled trial was conducted on 120 women (<20 weeks pregnant) with symptoms of morning sickness.[4] Patients received a ginger extract, equivalent to 1500 mg of dried ginger, for 4 days.[4] After 4 days, there were significant improvements in nausea and retching.[4] Post-delivery follow-up revealed birthweights, gestational age, and APGAR scores to be within the normal ranges.[4] The frequency of congenital abnormalities in the ginger group infants was comparable to that in the general population of infants born at the time of this study.[4]

Another randomized controlled trial was conducted on 70 pregnant women where they received 1000 mg of dried ginger per day.[5] Nausea and vomiting decreased significantly and no adverse effects on pregnancy or pregnancy outcomes were reported.[5] Similar results were found in two other studies where pregnant women took 1000 mg per day.[6,9]

Another randomized controlled trial was conducted on 138 pregnant women (<16 weeks pregnant) where one group received 500 mg of ginger and the other received 10 mg of vitamin B6.[3] In both groups, symptoms of nausea and vomiting were improved, and no adverse effects during pregnancy and after delivery were reported. A similar study was conducted on ginger and vitamin B6 with 291 pregnant women and reported the same results.[8]

Unlikely cause of spontaneous abortion:[6]	Evidence level 1a

During a randomized double-blind crossover trial, one woman in the study experienced a spontaneous abortion in her twelfth week of pregnancy.[6] The authors reported that one spontaneous abortion in 27 pregnancies was not a suspiciously high rate of fetal wastage in early pregnancy.[6]

Does not increase rates of major malformations:[7]	Evidence level 1b

A prospective cohort study with matched controls was conducted on 187 pregnancies where the pregnant women had taken ginger during their pregnancy.[7] The researchers concluded that ginger does not increase the rates of major malformations above the baseline rate of 1–3%.[7]

Non-mutagenic, non-teratogenic:[19]	Evidence level 3
Mutagenic constituents:[20,21]	Evidence level 3
Anti-mutagenic constituents:[22]	Evidence level 3

Ginger extracts when administered to pregnant rats during the period of organogenesis, caused neither maternal nor developmental toxicity at daily doses of up to 1000 mg/kg body weight.[19] The constituents 6-gingerol and shogaol have been shown to be mutagenic in bacterial cultures while zingerone has been shown to be anti-mutagenic and offset the mutagenic effects of 6-gingerol and shogaol.[20–22]

Potential embryotoxicity:[23]	Evidence level 3

A study on rats reported that in utero exposure to ginger tea resulted in increased early embryo loss and in increased growth in surviving fetuses.[23] Embryonic loss in the ginger tea treatment groups was double that of the controls.[23]

Non-teratogenic:[24]	Evidence level 4

A review article on the treatments for nausea during pregnancy reported that the existing treatments, including ginger, showed no evidence of teratogenicity.[24]

Potential testosterone receptor blocker:[25]	Evidence level 4

Via inhibition of thromboxane synthetase, it has been proposed that ginger may affect testosterone receptor binding in the fetus, thereby potentially affecting sex steroid differentiation of the fetal brain.[25]

Unsafe:[26]	Evidence level 4

A literature survey of 300 non-medical sources reported that 16 sources report ginger as unsafe during pregnancy.[26]

Potential abortifacient:[27]	Evidence level 4

A review article on the potential value of plants as sources of anti-fertility agents reported that ginger is a potential abortifacient.[27]

Dose >1000 mg daily

Emmenagogue:[28]	Evidence level 4
Mutagenic:[28]	Evidence level 4
Anti-platelet:[28]	Evidence level 4

A botanical safety compendium reported that consuming more that 1000 mg of ginger per day during pregnancy was not advised due to potential emmenagogue, mutagenic, and anti-platelet effects.[28]

Lactation

Mutagenic constituents:[20,21]	Evidence level 3
Anti-mutagenic constituents:[22]	Evidence level 3

The constituents 6-gingerol and shogaol have been shown to be mutagenic while zingerone has been shown to be anti-mutagenic and offset the mutagenic effects of 6-gingerol and shogaol.[20–22]

Unknown:	Evidence level 5

There are no reports in the scientific literature of ginger being either safe or contraindicated during lactation.

Caution

Gallstones[29]
Gastric ulcers

Constituents

- Non-volatile constituents:[30] 6-gingerol, (6)-shogaol, (6)- and (10)-dehyro-gingerdione, (6)- and (10)-gingerdione, zingerone
- Oleoresins[30]
- Proteolytic enzyme:[30] zingibain (a)

Toxicity

- LD_{50} (intraperitoneal): 500 mg/kg[31]
- No evidence of teratogenicity or mutagenicity at daily doses of up to 1000 mg/kg body weight in rats[19]

Pharmacology

- The constituent 6-gingerol is believed to be responsible for ginger's anti-emetic activity.[32]
- Most of ginger's anti-emetic activity is localized to the gastrointestinal tract.[32]
- The constituent galanolactone acts primarily on 5-HT3 receptors in the ileum, which are the same receptors affected by some prescription anti-emetics.[32]
- Ginger's anti-emetic activity may also involve the central nervous system, where the constituents 6-shogaol and galanolactone act on serotonin receptors.[32]
- Ginger does not affect gastrointestinal emptying time.[33,34]
- Ginger may inhibit cyclooxygenase and lipoxygenase pathways, thereby having anti-inflammatory activity.[18]
- Ginger may inhibit platelet thromboxane, thereby having anti-platelet activity.[35]
- The constituents 6-gingerol and shogaol have been shown to be mutagenic in bacterial cultures whereas zingerone has been shown to be anti-mutagenic and to offset the mutagenic effects of 6-gingerol and shogaol.[20–22]
- A study on rats reported that in utero exposure to ginger tea resulted in increased early embryo loss and in increased growth in surviving fetuses.[23]
- Ginger may have hypoglycemic, hypotensive or hypertensive, hypocholesterolemic, anthelmintic, and gastroprotective effects.[36]
- Via inhibition of thromboxane synthetase, it has been proposed that ginger may affect testosterone receptor binding in the fetus, thereby potentially affecting sex steroid differentiation of the fetal brain.[25]

Drug interactions[1]

Acid-inhibiting drugs[37]
Anticoagulant/antiplatelet drugs[38,39]
Barbiturates[40]
Blood pressure therapy[38]
Cardiac drugs[38,41]
Diabetic drugs[38,41]

Parts used[1]

Rhizome and root

References

1. Jellin JM, Batz F, Hitchens K. Natural Medicines Comprehensive Database. Stockton, CA: Therapeutic Research Faculty, 2002:1530.
2. Ernst E, Pittler MH. Efficacy of ginger for nausea and vomiting: a systematic review of randomized clinical trials. Br J Anaesth 2000; 84:367–371.

3. Sripramote M, Lekhyananda N. A randomized comparison of ginger and vitamin B6 in the treatment of nausea and vomiting of pregnancy. J Med Assoc Thai 2003; 86:846–853.
4. Willetts KE, Ekangaki A, Eden JA. Effect of a ginger extract on pregnancy-induced nausea: a randomised controlled trial. Aust N Z J Obstet Gynaecol 2003; 43:139–144.
5. Vutyavanich T, Kraisarin T, Ruangsri R. Ginger for nausea and vomiting in pregnancy: randomized, double-masked, placebo-controlled trial. Obstet Gynecol 2001; 97:577–582.
6. Fischer-Rasmussen W, Kjaer SK, Dahl C et al. Ginger treatment of hyperemesis gravidarum. Eur J Obstet Gynecol Reprod Biol 1990; 38:19–24.
7. Portnoi G, Chng LA, Karimi-Tabesh L et al. Prospective comparative study of the safety and effectiveness of ginger for the treatment of nausea and vomiting in pregnancy. Am J Obstet Gynecol 2003; 189:1374–1377.
8. Smith C, Crowther C, Willson K, Hotham N, McMillian V. A randomized controlled trial of ginger to treat nausea and vomiting in pregnancy. Obstet Gynecol 2004; 103:639–645.
9. Keating A, Chez RA. Ginger syrup as an antiemetic in early pregnancy. Altern Ther Health Med 2002; 8:89–91.
10. Bone ME, Wilkinson DJ, Young JR, McNeil J, Charlton S. Ginger root – a new antiemetic. The effect of ginger root on postoperative nausea and vomiting after major gynaecological surgery. Anaesthesia 1990; 45:669–671.
11. Phillips S, Ruggier R, Hutchinson SE. Zingiber officinale (ginger) – an antiemetic for day case surgery. Anaesthesia 1993; 48:715–717.
12. Arfeen Z, Owen H, Plummer JL et al. A double-blind randomized controlled trial of ginger for the prevention of postoperative nausea and vomiting. Anaesth Intensive Care 1995; 23:449–452.
13. Meyer K, Schwartz J, Crater D, Keyes B. Zingiber officinale (ginger) used to prevent 8–Mop associated nausea. Dermatol Nurs 1995; 7:242–244.
14. Pace J, Conlin DS. Oral ingestion of encapsulated ginger and reported self-care actions for the relief of chemotherapy-associated nausea and vomiting. Diss Abstr Int 1987; 47:3297–3298.
15. Grontved A, Brask T, Kambskard J, Hentzer E. Ginger root against seasickness. A controlled trial on the open sea. Acta Otolaryngol 1988; 1–5:45–48.
16. Mowrey DB, Clayson DE. Motion sickness, ginger, and psychophysics. Lancet 1982; 1:655–657.
17. Srivastava KC, Mustafa T. Ginger (Zingiber officinale) in rheumatism and musculoskeletal disorders. Med Hypotheses 1992; 39:342–348.
18. Srivastava KC, Mustafa T. Ginger (Zingiber officinale) and rheumatic disorders. Med Hypotheses 1989; 29:25–28.
19. Weidner MS, Sigwart K. Investigation of the teratogenic potential of a zingiber officinale extract in the rat. Reprod Toxicol 2001; 15:75–80.
20. Nakamura H, Yamamoto T. Mutagen and anti-mutagen in ginger, Zingiber officinale. Mutat Res 1982; 103:119–126.
21. Nakamura H, Yamamoto T. The active part of the [6]-gingerol molecule in mutagenesis. Mutat Res 1983; 122:87–94.
22. Nagabhushan M, Amonkar AJ, Bhide SV. Mutagenicity of gingerol and shogaol and antimutagenicity of zingerone in Salmonella/microsome assay. Cancer Lett 1987; 36:221–233.

23. Wilkinson JM. Effect of ginger tea on the fetal development of Sprague-Dawley rats. Reprod Toxicol 2000; 14:507–512.
24. Jewell D, Young G. Interventions for nausea and vomiting in early pregnancy. Cochrane Database Syst Rev 2003:CD000145.
25. Backon J. Ginger in preventing nausea and vomiting of pregnancy: a caveat due to its thromboxane synthetase activity and effect on testosterone binding. Eur J Obstet Gynecol Reprod Biol 1991; 42:163–164.
26. Wilkinson JM. What do we know about herbal morning sickness treatments? A literature survey. Midwifery 2000; 16:224–228.
27. Farnsworth NR, Bingel AS, Cordell GA, Crane FA, Fong HH. Potential value of plants as sources of new antifertility agents I. J Pharm Sci 1975; 64:535–598.
28. McGuffin M, Hobbs C, Upton R, Goldberg A. American Herbal Products Association's Botanical Safety Handbook. Boca Raton, FL: CRC Press, 1997:231.
29. Yamahara J, Miki K, Chisaka T et al. Cholagogic effect of ginger and its active constituents. J Ethnopharmacol 1985; 13:217–225.
30. www.naturalstandard.com. Ginger (Zingiber officinale Roscoe) Natural Standard Monograph.
31. Jagetia GC, Baliga MS, Verkatesh P, Ulloor JN. Influence of ginger rhizome (Zongiber officinale Rosc) on survivla, glutathione and lipid peroxidation in mice after whole-body exposure to gamma radiation. Radiat Res 2003; 160:584–592.
32. Lumb AB. Mechanism of antiemetic effect of ginger. Anaesthesia 1993; 48:1118.
33. Phillips S, Hutchinson S, Ruggier R. Zingiber officinale does not affect gastric emptying rate. A randomised, placebo-controlled, crossover trial. Anaesthesia 1993; 48:393–395.
34. Stewart JJ, Wood MJ, Wood CD, Mims ME. Effects of ginger on motion sickness susceptibility and gastric function. Pharmacology 1991; 42:111–120.
35. Srivastava KC. Effect of onion and ginger consumption on platelet thromboxane production in humans. Leukot Essent Fatty Acids 1989; 35:183–185.
36. Leung AY, Foster S. Encyclopedia of Common Natural Ingredients Used in Food, Drugs and Cosmetics. New York, NY: John Wiley & Sons, 1996:649.
37. Brinker F. Herb Contraindications and Drug Interactions. Sandy, OR: Eclectic Medical Publications, 1998.
38. Newall CA, Anderson LA, Phillipson JD. Herbal Medicines: A Guide for Health-care Professionals. London, UK: Pharmaceutical Press, 1996:296.
39. Heck AM, DeWitt BA, Lukes AL. Potential interactions between alternative therapies and warfarin. Am J Health Syst Pharm 2000; 57:1221–1227.
40. The Review of Natural Products by Facts and Comparisons. St. Louis, MO: Wolters Kluwer Co., 1999.
41. Blumenthal M, Busse WR, Goldberg A et al. The Complete German Commission E Monographs: Therapeutic Guide to Herbal Medicines. Boston, MA: American Botanical Council, 1998.

GINKGO
Ginkgo biloba

Synonyms/common names/related substances[1]

Adiantifolia, bai guo ye, fossil tree, *Ginkgo folium*, ginkgo leaf, ginkyo, Japanese silver apricot, kew tree, maidenhair tree, salisburia, *Salisburia adiantifolia*, yinhsing, baiguo

Indications

Leaf

Intermittent claudication – peripheral vascular disease:[2–4]	Evidence grade A
Dementia (Alzheimer disease and other):[5–7]	Evidence grade A
Cerebrovascular insufficiency:[8–10]	Evidence grade A
Tinnitus:[11,12]	Evidence grade A
Age-associated memory impairment:[13–15]	Evidence grade B1
Memory enhancement in healthy individuals:[16–18]	Evidence grade B1
Altitude sickness:[19]	Evidence grade B1
Vertigo:[9]	Evidence grade B1
Premenstrual syndrome:[20]	Evidence grade B1
Macular degeneration:[21]	Evidence grade B2
Erectile dysfunction:[22–25]	Evidence grade C
Antidepressant-induced sexual dysfunction:[26]	Evidence grade C
Chemotherapy adjunct:[27,28]	Evidence grade C
Multiple sclerosis:[29]	Evidence grade D
Light-induced retinal damage:[30]	Evidence grade E

Seed

Cough, expectorant, asthma, bronchitis:[1]	Evidence grade E

Skin sores and scabies (topical):[1]	Evidence grade E

Pregnancy

Leaf

Unsafe when adultered with colchicine:[31]	Evidence level 1c

A case series in the literature reported the presence of colchicine in the placental blood of pregnant women having taken ginkgo.[31] The source of colchicine was traced back to the consumption of commercially available *Ginkgo biloba* products that contained colchicine.[31] Given that colchicine is not a common constituent of ginkgo, the observed finding is most likely due to an adulteration of a ginkgo product by a herb containing colchicine.

Antiplatelet:[30,32,33]	Evidence level 3

The antiplatelet properties of ginkgo leaf may prolong bleeding during delivery.[30,32,33]

Emmenagogue:[34]	Evidence level 4

Hormonal changes:[34]	Evidence level 4

A herb toxicology and drug interaction compendium reported that ginkgo leaf is an emmenagogue and can cause hormonal changes.[34] Ginkgo leaf was not reported in the medical literature as being an emmenagogue or causing hormonal changes, nor was it reported as being contraindicated in pregnancy.

Roasted seed

Possibly safe if taken as food:[35]	Evidence level 4

A toxicology compendium reported that roasted ginkgo seeds may be potentially safe if eaten as a food during pregnancy.[35] Roasted ginkgo seed was not reported in the literature as being either safe or contraindicated in pregnancy.

Raw Seed

Possibly unsafe:[36]	Evidence level 4

A toxicology compendium reported that raw ginkgo seeds (nonroasted) may be a concern in pregnancy if they are used medicinally.[36] Raw ginkgo seeds were not reported in the literature as being either safe or contraindicated in pregnancy.

Lactation

Leaf

Unknown:	Evidence level 5

Ginkgo leaf was not reported in the literature as being either safe or contraindicated in lactation.

Roasted seed

Possibly safe if taken as food[35]:	Evidence level 4

A toxicology compendium reported that roasted ginkgo seeds may be potentially safe if eaten as a food during lactation.[35] Roasted ginkgo seed was not reported in the literature as being either safe or contraindicated in lactation.

Raw seed

Possibly unsafe:[36]	Evidence level 4

A toxicology compendium reported that raw ginkgo seeds (nonroasted) may be a concern in lactation if they are used medicinally.[36] Raw ginkgo seeds were not reported in the literature as being either safe or contraindicated in lactation.

Constituents

Leaf

Flavonoids:[37] rutin, isorhamnetine, quercetin, kaempferol, proanthocyanidins
Terpenoids:[5] ginkgolides A, B, C, M and J, bilobalide
Organic acids[1]

Seed

Cyanogenic glycosides[36]
Ginkgotoxin[35,36]

Toxicity

Leaf

- LD_{50} in mice: 7725 mg[38]
- Crude extracts of ginkgo leaf may contain ginkgolic acids, which are suspected to have cytotoxic, allergenic, mutagenic, and carcinogenic properties.[39,40]

Seed

- Ginkgotoxin, found in ginkgo seed, may cause seizures, loss of consciousness and death.[35,36]

Pharmacology

Leaf

- Ginkgo increases cerebral and peripheral blood circulation.[41,42]
- Ginkgo reduces vascular permeability, causes vascular contraction, improves venous tone, inhibits phosphodiesterase type 4 (PDE4), relaxes vascular smooth muscle via a nitric oxide pathway and improves blood flow to the corpus cavernosum of the penis.[22,41–43]
- Ginkgo reduces platelet aggregation by competitively binding platelet activating factor (PAF) and by inhibiting the formation of platelet thromboxane A2.[30,32,33,44]
- The ginkgo flavonoids have antioxidant and free radical scavenging properties.[5,7,30,32,45]
- Partially due to its antioxidant activity, ginkgo inhibits the toxicity and cell death induced by beta-amyloid plaques in Alzheimer disease.[46]
- Ginkgo decreases systolic and diastolic blood pressure, increases fasting plasma insulin and C-peptide, decreases cortisol secretion and decreases the secretion of corticotropic releasing hormone (CRH).[32,47,48]
- Ginkgo may have cholinergic effects and may or may not have a monoamine oxidase inhibitor (MAOI) effect in the central nervous system.[7,49–51]
- Ginkgo may reverse the decline in brain alpha-adrenoceptor activity that occurs with aging.[45]
- Ginkgo decreases phagocyte chemotaxis, decreases smooth muscle contraction, prevents degranulation of neutrophils, decreases free radical production, decreases damaging glycine production after brain injury and reduces excitatory amino acid receptor function.[5,45,52]
- Ginkgo may inhibit cytochrome P450 3A4, induce cytochrome P450 3A5 and mildly inhibit cytochrome P450 1A2 and 2D6.[1,53,54]

Seed

Cyanogenic glycosides may have antibacterial and antifungal effects.[1,36]

Drug interactions

Leaf

Anti-coagulant/anti-platelet drugs[30,32,33]
Fluoxetine[55]
Buspirone[55]
St John's wort[55]
Melatonin[55]
Insulin[32]
Monoamine oxidase inhibitors[46–48]
Seizure threshold lowering drugs[56,57]

Thiazide diuretics[58]
Trazodone[54]
Warfarin[59]
Drugs metabolized by cytochrome P450 3A4, P450 3A5, P450 1A2 and P450 2D6 enzymes[1,53,54]

Parts used

Leaf, seed[1]

References

1. Jellin JM, Batz F, Hitchens K. Natural Medicines Comprehensive Database, 3rd ed. Stockton, CA: Therapeutic Research Faculty, 2002:1530.
2. Schweizer J, HC. Comparison of two dosages of ginkgo biloba extract EGb 761 in patients with peripheral arterial occlusive disease Fontaine's stage IIb. A randomised, double-blind, multicentric clinical trial. Arzneimittelforschung 1999; 49:900–904.
3. Pittler MH, Ernst E. Ginkgo biloba extract for the treatment of intermittent claudication: a meta-analysis of randomized trials. Am J Med 2000; 108:276–281.
4. Ernst E. [Ginkgo biloba in treatment of intermittent claudication. A systematic research based on controlled studies in the literature]. Fortschr Med 1996; 114:85–87.
5. Oken BS, Storzbach DM, Kaye JA. The efficacy of Ginkgo biloba on cognitive function in Alzheimer disease. Arch Neurol 1998; 55:1409–1415.
6. Kanowski S, Herrmann WM, Stephan K, Wierich W, Horr R. Proof of efficacy of the ginkgo biloba special extract EGb 761 in outpatients suffering from mild to moderate primary degenerative dementia of the Alzheimer type or multi-infarct dementia. Pharmacopsychiatry 1996; 29:47–56.
7. Le Bars PL, Katz M, Berman N et al. A placebo-controlled, double-blind, randomized trial of an extract of Ginkgo biloba for dementia. North American EGb Study Group. JAMA 1997; 278:1327–1332.
8. Kleijnen J, Knipschild P. Ginkgo biloba for cerebral insufficiency. Br J Clin Pharmacol 1992; 34:352–358.
9. Haguenauer JP, Cantenot F, Koskas H, Pierart H. [Treatment of equilibrium disorders with Ginkgo biloba extract. A multicenter double-blind drug vs. placebo study]. Presse Med 1986; 15:1569–1572.
10. Hopfenmuller W. [Evidence for a therapeutic effect of Ginkgo biloba special extract. Meta-analysis of 11 clinical studies in patients with cerebrovascular insufficiency in old age]. Arzneimittelforschung 1994; 44:1005–1013.
11. Meyer B. [Multicenter randomized double-blind drug vs. placebo study of the treatment of tinnitus with Ginkgo biloba extract]. Presse Med 1986; 15:1562–1564.
12. Holstein N. [Ginkgo special extract EGb 761 in tinnitus therapy. An overview of results of completed clinical trials]. Fortschr Med Orig 2001; 118:157–164.
13. Allain H, Raoul P, Lieury A et al. Effect of two doses of Gingko biloba extract (EGb 761) on the dual-coding test in elderly subjects. Clin Ther 1993; 15:549–558.
14. Semlitsch HV, Anderer P, Saletu B, Binder GA, Decker KA. Cognitive psychophysiology in nootropic drug research: effects of Ginkgo biloba on event-related potentials (P300) in age-associated memory impairment. Pharmacopsychiatry 1995; 28:134–142.

15 Brautigam MR, B F, Verleye G et al. Treatment of age-related memory complaints with Ginkgo biloba extract: a randomized double blind placebo-controlled study. Phytomedicine 1998;5:425–434.
16. Rigney U, Kimber S, Hindmarch I. The effects of acute doses of standardized Ginkgo biloba extract on memory and psychomotor performance in volunteers. Phytother Res 1999; 13:408–415.
17. Mix JA, Crews WD Jr. An examination of the efficacy of Ginkgo biloba extract EGb761 on the neuropsychologic functioning of cognitively intact older adults. J Altern Complement Med 2000; 6:219–229.
18. Kennedy DO, Scholey A, Wesnes KA. The dose-dependent cognitive effects of acute administration of Ginkgo biloba to healthy young volunteers. Psychopharmacology (Berl) 2000; 151:416–423.
19. Roncin JP, Schwartz F, D'Arbigny P. EGb 761 in control of acute mountain sickness and vascular reactivity to cold exposure. Aviat Space Environ Med 1996; 67:445–452.
20. Tamborini A, Taurelle R. [Value of standardized Ginkgo biloba extract (EGb 761) in the management of congestive symptoms of premenstrual syndrome]. Rev Fr Gynecol Obstet 1993; 88(7–9):447–457.
21. Lebuisson DA, Leroy L, Rigal G. [Treatment of senile macular degeneration with Ginkgo biloba extract. A preliminary double-blind drug vs. placebo study]. Presse Med 1986; 15:1556–1558.
22. Paick JS, Lee JH. An experimental study of the effect of ginkgo biloba extract on the human and rabbit corpus cavernosum tissue. J Urol 1996; 156:1876–1880.
23. Sohn M, Sikora R. Ginkgo biloba extract in the therapy of erectile dysfunction. J Sex Educ Ther 1991;17:53–61.
24. Sikora R, Sohn M, Engelke B et al. Randomized placebo-controlled study on the effects of oral treatment with Gingko biloba extract in patients with erectile dysfunction. J Urol 1998; 159(Suppl 5):240.
25. Sikora R, Sohn M, Deutz FJ et al. Ginkgo biloba extract in the therapy of erectile dysfunction. J Urol 1989; 141:188A.
26. Cohen AJ, Bartlik B. Ginkgo biloba for antidepressant-induced sexual dysfunction. J Sex Marital Ther 1998; 24:139–143.
27. Hauns B, Haring B, Kohler S et al. Phase II study with 5-fluorouracil and ginkgo biloba extract (GBE 761 ONC) in patients with pancreatic cancer. Arzneimittelforschung 1999; 49:1030–1034.
28. Hauns B, Haring B, Kohler S, Mross K, Unger C. Phase II study of combined 5-fluorouracil/Ginkgo biloba extract (GBE 761 ONC) therapy in 5-fluorouracil pretreated patients with advanced colorectal cancer. Phytother Res 2001; 15:34–38.
29. Brochet B, Orgogozo J, Guinot P, Dartigues JF, Henry P, Loiseau P. [Pilot study of Ginkgolide B, a PAF-acether specific inhibitor in the treatment of acute outbreaks of multiple sclerosis]. Rev Neurol (Paris) 1992; 148:299–301.
30. Ranchon I, Gorrand J, Cluzel J, Droy-Lefaix MT, Doly M. Functional protection of photoreceptors from light-induced damage by dimethylthiourea and Ginkgo biloba extrac. Invest Ophthalmol Vis Sci 1999; 40:1191–1199.
31. Petty HR, Fernando M, Kindzelskii AL et al. Identification of colchicine in placental blood from patients using herbal medicines. Chem Res Toxicol 2001; 14:1254–1258.
32. Kudolo GB. The effect of 3-month ingestion of Ginkgo biloba extract on pancreatic beta-cell function in response to glucose loading in normal glucose tolerant individuals. J Clin Pharmacol 2000; 40:647–654.

33. Kudolo GB, Dorsey S, Blodgett J. Effect of the ingestion of Ginkgo biloba extract on platelet aggregation and urinary prostanoid excretion in healthy and Type 2 diabetic subjects. Thromb Res 2002; 108:151–160.
34. Brinker F. The Toxicology of Botanical Medicines. Sandy, OR: Eclectic Medical Publications, 2000:296.
35. Leung AY, Foster S. Encyclopedia of Common Natural Ingredients Used in Food, Drugs and Cosmetics, 2nd ed. New York, NY: John Wiley & Sons, 1996:649.
36. Newall CA, Anderson LA, Phillipson JD. Herbal Medicines: A Guide for Health-care Professionals. London, UK: Pharmaceutical Press, 1996:296.
37. Jan GS, Tong WN, Chan AM, Hui TW, Lo JW. Recovery from mivacurium block with or without anticholinesterase following continuous infusion in obstetric patients. Anaesth Intensive Care 1996; 24:585–589.
38. www.naturalstandard.com.
39. Kressmann S, Muller W, Blume HH. Pharmaceutical quality of different Ginkgo biloba brands. J Pharm Pharmacol 2002; 54:661–669.
40. Hecker H, Johannisson R, Koch E, Siegers CP. In vitro evaluation of the cytotoxic potential of alkylphenols from Ginkgo biloba L. Toxicology 2002; 177:167–177.
41. Campos-Toimil M, Lugnier C, Droy-Lefaix MT, Takeda K. Inhibition of type 4 phosphodiesterase by rolipram and Ginkgo biloba extract (EGb 761) decreases agonist-induced rises in internal calcium in human endothelial cells. Arterioscler Thromb Vasc Biol 2000; 20:E34–E40.
42. Diamond BJ, Shiflett S, Feiwel N et al. Ginkgo biloba extract: mechanisms and clinical indications. Arch Phys Med Rehabil 2000; 81:668–678.
43. Chen X, SS, Lee TJ. Extracts of Ginkgo biloba and ginsenosides exert cerebral vasorelaxation via a nitric oxide pathway. Clin Exp Pharmacol Physiol 1997; 24:958–959.
44. Logani S, Chen M, Tran T, Le T, Raffa RB. Actions of Ginkgo Biloba related to potential utility for the treatment of conditions involving cerebral hypoxia. Life Sci 2000; 67:1389–1396.
45. Bastianetto S, Ramassamy C, Dore S et al. The Ginkgo biloba extract (EGb 761) protects hippocampal neurons against cell death induced by beta-amyloid. Eur J Neurosci 2000; 12:1882–1890.
46. Fowler JS, Wang GJ, Volkow ND et al. Evidence that gingko biloba extract does not inhibit M, AO, A and B in living human brain. Life Sci 2000; 66:PL 141–146.
47. Porsolt RD, Roux S, Drieu K. Evaluation of a ginkgo biloba extract (EGb 761) in functional tests for monoamine oxidase inhibition. Arzneimittelforschung 2000; 50:232–235.
48. White HL, Scates P, Cooper BR. Extracts of Ginkgo biloba leaves inhibit monoamine oxidase. Life Sci 1996; 58:1315–1321.
49. Marcilhac A, Dakine N, Bourhim N et al. Effect of chronic administration of Ginkgo biloba extract or Ginkgolide on the hypothalamic-pituitary-adrenal axis in the rat. Life Sci 1998; 62:2329–2340.
50. Amri H, OS, Boujrad N, Drieu K, Papadopoulos V. In vivo regulation of peripheral-type benzodiazepine receptor and glucocorticoid synthesis by Ginkgo biloba extract EGb 761 and isolated ginkgolides. Endocrinology 1996; 137:5707–5718.
51. Kudolo G. Ingestion of Ginkgo biloba extract significantly inhibits collagen-induced platelet aggregation and thromboxane A2 synthesis. Alt Ther 2001; 7:105.
52. Gardiner P, Wornham W. Recent review of complementary and alternative medicine used by adolescents. Curr Opin Pediatr 2000; 12:298–302.

53. Budzinski JW, Foster BC, Vandenhoek S, Arnason JT. An in vitro evaluation of human cytochrome P450 3A4 inhibition by selected commercial herbal extracts and tinctures. Phytomedicine 2000; 7:273–282.
54. Galluzzi S, Zanetti O, Binetti G, Trabucchi M, Frisoni GB. Coma in a patient with Alzheimer's disease taking low dose trazodone and gingko biloba. J Neurol Neurosurg Psychiatry 2000; 68:679–680.
55. Spinella M, Eaton L. Hypomania induced by herbal and pharmaceutical psychotropic medicines following mild traumatic brain injury. Brain Inj 2002; 16:359–367.
56. Granger AS. Ginkgo biloba precipitating epileptic seizures. Age Ageing 2001; 30:523–525. Links 2001.
57. Gregory PJ. Seizure associated with Ginkgo biloba? Ann Intern Med 2001; 134:344.
58. Shaw D, LC, Kolev S, Murray V. Traditional remedies and food supplements. A 5-year toxicological study (1991–1995). Drug Saf 1997; 17:342–356.
59. Matthews MJ. Association of Ginkgo biloba with intracerebral hemorrhage. Neurology 1998; 50:1933–1934.

GOLDENSEAL
Hydrastis canadensis

Synonyms/common names/related substances[1]

Eye balm, eye root, goldenroot, goldsiegel, ground raspberry, *Hydrastis*, Indian dye, Indian plant, Indian tumeric, jaundice root, orange root, sceau d'or, warnera, wild curcuma, yellow Indian paint, yellow paint, yellow puccoon, yellow root

Indications

Chloroquine-resistant malaria (with pyrimethamine):[2]	Evidence grade B1
Infectious diarrhea:[3,4]	Evidence grade B1
Trachoma (*Chlamydia trachomatis* eye infection):[5,6]	Evidence grade B2
Congestive heart failure:[7]	Evidence grade C
Anti-*Helicobacter pylori*:[8]	Evidence grade E
Anti-tubercular:[9]	Evidence grade E
Narcotic concealment:[10,11]	Evidence grade E
Upper respiratory tract infections:[12,13]	Evidence grade E
Cancer prevention:[14–16]	Evidence grade E

Pregnancy

May cause newborn jaundice (kernicterus):[17]	Evidence level 3

In rats, berberine displaces bilirubin bound to albumin.[17] Berberine (10–20 μg/g) was administered intraperitoneally to adult rats on a daily basis for 1 week.[17] After 1 week, a significant decrease in mean bilirubin serum protein binding was observed due to an in vivo displacement effect by berberine.[17] A persistent elevation in serum concentrations of unbound and total bilirubin was also observed.[17]

Uterine stimulant:[18–20]	Evidence level 4

A review article on the potential value of plants as sources of anti-fertility agents reported that goldenseal contains the uterine stimulant berberine.[18,19] A herbal and drug interaction compendium reported that goldenseal also contains the uterine stimulant components hydrastine, canadine, and hydrastinine.[20]

Oxytoxic effects:[18,21]	Evidence level 4

Two herbal toxicology compendia reported that goldenseal has oxytocic effects during pregnancy.[18,21] Goldenseal, however, was not reported in the evidence-based medical literature as having oxytocic properties.

Lactation

May cause or aggravate newborn jaundice (kernicterus):[17] Evidence level 3

In rats, berberine displaces bilirubin bound to albumin.[17] Berberine (10–20 μg/g) was administered intraperitoneally to adult rats on a daily basis for 1 week.[17] After 1 week, a significant decrease in mean bilirubin serum protein binding was observed due to an in vivo displacement effect by berberine.[17] A persistent elevation in serum concentrations of unbound and total bilirubin was also observed.[17]

Contraindication

Newborn jaundice (kernicterus)[17]

Constituents

Isoquinoline alkaloids:[8,20,22] hydrastine, berberine, tetrahydroberberastine, berberastine, canadaline, canadine, hydrastinine, β-hydrastine

Toxicity

LD_{50} of berberine in humans:[18] 27.5 mg/kg

Pharmacology

- Berberine was found to displace bilirubin bound to albumin in vitro.[17] Berberine was found to be about 10 times superior to phenylbutazone, a known potent displacer of bilirubin, and about 100 times superior to papaverine, a berberine-type alkaloid.[17]
- Hydrastine and berberine have been shown to have antibacterial activity.[12,13,23–26]
- Hydrastine and berberine have been shown to have amebicidal, anti-parasitic (trypanocidal) and anti-fungal activity.[23,27–30]
- Berberine and beta-hydrastine were shown to have anti-*Helicobacter pylori* activity in vitro.[8]
- Berberine derived from goldenseal has been shown to have anti-tubercular activity in vitro.[9]
- At low doses hydrastine may have a hypotensive effect and at higher doses hydrastine constricts peripheral blood vessels and may potentially cause a hypertensive effect.[21]
- In low doses, berberine may act as a cardiac and respiratory stimulant and in high doses it may act as a cardiac and respiratory depressant.[18,23,31]
- Berberine was shown to have anti-platelet activity.[32]
- Goldenseal was shown to increase immune function and berberine was shown to have anti-inflammatory effects.[33–37]
- Berberine was found to have antidiarrheal effects.[38]

- Berberine was found to inhibit parathyroid hormone-stimulated bone resorption, inhibit osteoclastic bone resorption, and prevent a decrease in bone mineral density of the lumbar vertebra.[39]
- Goldenseal may interfere with cytochrome P450 3A4 (CYP3A4) enzyme.[40]

Drug interactions

Acid-inhibiting drugs[1,41]
Anti-hypertensive agents[21]
Barbiturates[21]
Anticoagulant drugs[32]
Highly protein-bound drugs[17]
Sedative drugs[21]
Drugs metabolized by cytochrome P450 3A4 (CYP3A4) enzyme[40]

Parts used[20]

Root, rhizome

References

1. Jellin JM, Batz F, Hitchens K. Natural Medicines Comprehensive Database, 3rd ed. Stockton, CA: Therapeutic Research Faculty, 2002:1530.
2. Sheng WD, Jiddawi MS, Hong XQ, Abdulla SM. Treatment of chloroquine-resistant malaria using pyrimethamine in combination with berberine, tetracycline or cotrimoxazole. East Afr Med J 1997; 74:283–284.
3. Rabbani GH, Butler T, Knight J, Sanyal SC, Alam K. Randomized controlled trial of berberine sulfate therapy for diarrhea due to enterotoxigenic Escherichia coli and Vibrio cholerae. J Infect Dis 1987; 155:979–984.
4. Swabb EA, Tai YH, Jordan L. Reversal of cholera toxin-induced secretion in rat ileum by luminal berberine. Am J Physiol 1981; 241:G248–G252.
5. Khosla PK, Neeraj VI, Gupta SK, Satpathy G. Berberine, a potential drug for trachoma. Rev Int Trach Pathol Ocul Trop Subtrop Sante Publique 1992; 69:147–165.
6. Mohan M, Pant CR, Angra SK, Mahajan VM. Berberine in trachoma. (A clinical trial). Indian J Ophthalmol 1982; 30:69–75.
7. Zeng X, Zeng X. Relationship between the clinical effects of berberine on severe congestive heart failure and its concentration in plasma studied by HPLC. Biomed Chromatogr 1999; 13:442–444.
8. Mahady GB, Pendland SL, Stoia A, Chadwick LR. In vitro susceptibility of Helicobacter pylori to isoquinoline alkaloids from Sanguinaria canadensis and Hydrastis canadensis. Phytother Res 2003; 17:217–221.
9. Gentry EJ, Jampani HB, Keshavarz-Shokri A et al. Antitubercular natural products: berberine from the roots of commercial Hydrastis canadensis powder. Isolation of inactive 8-oxotetrahydrothalifendine, canadine, beta-hydrastine, and two new quinic acid esters, hycandinic acid esters-1 and -2. J Nat Prod 1998; 61:1187–1193.
10. Wu AH, Forte E, Casella G et al. CEDIA for screening drugs of abuse in urine and the effect of adulterants. J Forensic Sci 1995; 40:614–618.
11. Mikkelsen SL, Ash KO. Adulterants causing false negatives in illicit drug testing. Clin Chem 1988; 34:2333–2336.

12. Stermitz FR, Lorenz P, Tawara JN, Zenewicz LA, Lewis K. Synergy in a medicinal plant: antimicrobial action of berberine potentiated by 5′-methoxyhydnocarpin, a multidrug pump inhibitor. Proc Natl Acad Sci USA 2000; 97:1433–1437.
13. Stermitz FR, Tawara-Matsuda J, Lorenz P et al. 5′-Methoxyhydnocarpin-D and pheophorbide A: Berberis species components that potentiate berberine growth inhibition of resistant Staphylococcus aureus. J Nat Prod 2000; 63:1146–1149.
14. Anis KV, Rajeshkumar NV, Kuttan R. Inhibition of chemical carcinogenesis by berberine in rats and mice. J Pharm Pharmacol 2001; 53:763–768.
15. Chung JG, Chen GW, Hung CF et al. Effects of berberine on arylamine N-acetyltransferase activity and 2-aminofluorene-DNA adduct formation in human leukemia cells. Am J Chin Med 2000; 28:227–238.
16. Fukuda K, Hibiya Y, Mutoh M et al. Inhibition by berberine of cyclooxygenase-2 transcriptional activity in human colon cancer cells. J Ethnopharmacol 1999; 66:227–233.
17. Chan E. Displacement of bilirubin from albumin by berberine. Biol Neonate 1993; 63:201–208.
18. McGuffin M, Hobbs C, Upton R, Goldberg A. American Herbal Products Association's Botanical Safety Handbook. Boca Raton, FL: CRC Press, 1997:231.
19. Farnsworth NR, Bingel AS, Cordell G, Crane FA, Fong HH. Potential value of plants as sources of new antifertility agents I. J Pharm Sci 1975; 64:535–598.
20. Brinker F. The Toxicology of Botanical Medicines. Sandy, OR: Eclectic Medical Publications, 2000:296.
21. Newall CA, Anderson LA, Phillipson JD. Herbal Medicines: A Guide for Health-care Professionals. London, UK: Pharmaceutical Press, 1996:296.
22. Weber HA, Zart MK, Hodges AE et al. Method validation for determination of alkaloid content in goldenseal root powder. J AOAC Int 2003; 86:476–483.
23. Leung AY, Foster S. Encyclopedia of Common Natural Ingredients Used in Food, Drugs and Cosmetics, 2nd ed. New York, NY: John Wiley & Sons, 1996:649.
24. Abel G. [Chromosome-damaging effect of beta-asaron on human lymphocytes]. Planta Med 1987; 53:251–253.
25. Hwang BY, Roberts SK, Chadwick LR, Wu CD, Kinghorn AD. Antimicrobial constituents from Goldenseal (the Rhizomes of Hydrastis canadensis) against selected oral pathogens. Planta Med 2003; 69:623–627.
26. Scazzocchio F, Cometa MF, Tomassini L, Palmery M. Antibacterial activity of Hydrastis canadensis extract and its major isolated alkaloids. Planta Med 2001; 67:561–564.
27. Ghosh AK, Bhattacharyya FK, Ghosh DK. Leishmania donovani: amastigote inhibition and mode of action of berberine. Exp Parasitol 1985; 60:404–413.
28. Ghosh AK, Rakshit MM, Ghosh DK. Effect of berberine chloride on Leishmania donovani. Indian J Med Res 1983; 78:407–416.
29. Mahajan VM, Sharma A, Rattan A. Antimycotic activity of berberine sulphate: an alkaloid from an Indian medicinal herb. Sabouraudia 1982; 20:79–81.
30. Goel M, Singh UP, Jha RN, Pandey VB, Pandey MB. Individual and combined effect of (+/−)-alpha-hydrastine and (+/−)-beta-hydrastine on spore germination of some fungi. Folia Microbiol (Praha) 2003; 48:363–368.
31. Foster S, Tyler VE. Tyler's Honest Herbal. Binghamton, NY: Haworth Herbal Press, 1999.

32. Huang CG, Chu ZL, Wei SJ, Jiang H, Jiao BH. Effect of berberine on arachidonic acid metabolism in rabbit platelets and endothelial cells. Thromb Res 2002; 106:223–227.
33. Rehman J, Dillow JM, Carter SM et al. Increased production of antigen-specific immunoglobulins G and M following in vivo treatment with the medicinal plants Echinacea angustifolia and Hydrastis canadensis. Immunol Lett 1999; 68:391–395.
34. Ivanovska N, Philipov S. Study on the anti-inflammatory action of Berberis vulgaris root extract, alkaloid fractions and pure alkaloids. Int J Immunopharmacol 1996; 18:553–561.
35. Ivanovska N, Philipov S, Hristova M. Influence of berberine on T-cell mediated immunity. Immunopharmacol Immunotoxicol 1999; 21:771–786.
36. Kupeli E, Kosar M, Yesilada E, Husnu K, Baser C. A comparative study on the anti-inflammatory, antinociceptive and antipyretic effects of isoquinoline alkaloids from the roots of Turkish Berberis species. Life Sci 2002; 72:645–657.
37. Yesilada E, Kupeli E. Berberis crataegina DC. root exhibits potent anti-inflammatory, analgesic and febrifuge effects in mice and rats. J Ethnopharmacol 2002; 79:237–248.
38. Zhang MF, Shen YQ. [Antidiarrheal and anti-inflammatory effects of berberine]. Zhongguo Yao Li Xue Bao 1989; 10:174–176.
39. Li H, Miyahara T, Tezuka Y et al. The effect of kampo formulae on bone resorption in vitro and in vivo. II. Detailed study of berberine. Biol Pharm Bull 1999; 22:391–396.
40. Budzinski JW, Foster BC, Vandenhoek S, Arnason JT. An in vitro evaluation of human cytochrome P450 3A4 inhibition by selected commercial herbal extracts and tinctures. Phytomedicine 2000; 7:273–282.
41. Brinker F. Herb Contraindications and Drug Interactions, 2nd ed. Sandy, OR: Eclectic Medical Publications, 1998.

GREEN TEA
Camellia sinensis

Synonyms/common names/related substances[1]

C. thea, *C. theifera*, Chinese tea, EGCG, Japanese tea, tea, tea green, *Thea sinensis*, *T. boeha*, *T. viridis*

Indications

Cancer prevention:[2–8]	Evidence grade A
Oral leukoplakia:[9]	Evidence grade B1
Improves cognitive performance:[10]	Evidence grade C
Elevated cholesterol and triglycerides:[11]	Evidence grade C
Cardiovascular disease prevention:[11]	Evidence grade C
Liver disease prevention:[11]	Evidence grade C
Parkinsonism prevention:[12]	Evidence grade C

Pregnancy

Minimal risk:[13]	Evidence level 1b

A comparison study on the effects of green tea consumption on iron absorption during pregnancy was conducted.[13] Pregnant women were given sodium ferrous citrate along with green tea in one group and water in another.[13] The authors reported that green tea did not interfere with iron absorption nor did they report any serious side effects in the pregnant women.[13]

Spontaneous abortion:[14,15]	Evidence level 1b

A case–control study of 3149 pregnant women reported that serum paraxanthine concentration, a caffeine metabolite, was higher in women who had spontaneous abortions than in controls.[14] A case–control study of 1498 pregnant women reported that the consumption of 375 mg or more caffeine per day during pregnancy may increase the risk of spontaneous abortion.[15]

Increased risk of stillbirth:[16]	Evidence level 1b

A prospective follow-up study of 18 478 singleton pregnancies in women with valid information about coffee consumption during pregnancy reported that pregnant women who drink eight or more cups of coffee per day have double the risk of stillbirth when compared with women who do not drink coffee during pregnancy.[16] Although this study was related to coffee, there could also be an increased risk of stillbirth with proportional intake of green tea.

Low birthweight infants:[17,18]	Evidence level 1b

A large prospective study on 2291 mothers reported that women consuming more than 600 mg of caffeine per day are at greater risk for having low birthweight infants.[18] A prospective study on 63 women reported that pregnant nonsmokers consuming caffeine more than 300 mg/day had statistically significant lower weights of newborns and placentas ($p<0.05$).[17]

Teratogenic compounds:[19–22]	Evidence level 3

Elevated caffeine intake causes histopathologically teratogenic effects on newborn rat cornea.[19] A review study, however, reported that when caffeine is administered in fractioned quantities during the day, as is the case with human caffeine intake, caffeine is no longer a teratogen in animals.[23]

Harmful to the fetus:[24]	Evidence level 4

A compendium on the safety of drugs in pregnancy and lactation reported that over 300 mg of caffeine a day may be harmful to the fetus.[24]

300 mg of caffeine throughout the day – possibly safe:[25,26]	Evidence level 4

A drug compendium and a review study reported that approximately 300 mg of caffeine consumed throughout the day seems safe during pregnancy.[25,26]

Lactation

Teratogenic compounds:[19–22]	Evidence level 3

Elevated caffeine intake causes histopathologically teratogenic effects on newborn rat cornea.[19] Since caffeine appears in breast milk at half the concentration as in the mother's plasma, newborns may be exposed to teratogenic compounds.[27] A review study, however, reported that when caffeine is administered in fractioned quantities during the day, as it is the case with human caffeine intake, caffeine is no longer a teratogen in animals.[23]

May cause sleeping disorders:[28]	Evidence level 4

A compendium on herbal medicine reported that nursing mothers who consume caffeine may have infants with sleeping disorders.[28]

Constituents

- Polyphenols:[29,30] gallic acid
- Catechins:[29,30] epigallocatechin gallate (EGCG), epigallocatechin (EGC), epicatechin gallate (ECG), epicatechin (EC)
- Caffeine 2–4% or 10–80 mg caffeine per cup.[31–33]

Toxicity

Caffeine in doses greater than 1 g/(body surface in m^2) taken three times daily is associated with a higher incidence of side effects.[34]

Pharmacology

- ECG appears to induce apoptosis in cancer cells by reactive oxygen species formation and mitochondrial depolarization.[30]
- EGCG may have anti-angiogenic activity by preventing new blood vessel growth in tumors and may inhibit tumor cell proliferation.[34–37]
- The catechins may reduce lipoprotein oxidation and proliferation of vascular smooth muscle that occurs with high concentrations of low-density lipoproteins.[38–41]
- Topically, EGCG and epicatechin-3-gallate may protect against UVA and UVB sunburn.[1]
- EGCG may prevent oxidation and apoptosis of neurons, which may protect people from developing Alzheimer disease.[42]
- Green tea is an antioxidant, thereby reduces oxidative DNA damage, lipid peroxidation and free radical generation.[43]
- Green tea may reduce mutagenic activity in smokers.[44]
- The tannins may have anti-diarrheal properties.[45]
- The polyphenols increase levels of lactobacilli and bifidobacteria, and reduce levels of Enterobacteriaceae.[46]
- Through caffeine preventing adenosine's inhibition of dopaminergic transmission, green tea may reduce the clinical expression of parkinsonism.[47]
- Green tea may have antiplatelet activity.[3,48,49]

Caffeine

- Caffeine is a central nervous system stimulant.[28,29,50]
- Caffeine increases blood pressure, heart rate and heart contractility.[39,50,51]
- Caffeine improves cognitive performance.[10]
- Caffeine stimulates gastric acid secretion.[50]
- Caffeine is a diuretic.[50]

Drug interactions

Adenosine (Adenocard)[52]
Anti-coagulant, anti-platelet agents[3,48,49]
Anti-psychotic drugs[53,54]
Aspirin, acetaminophen (Tylenol)[55]
Barbiturates[56]
Benzodiazepines[52]
β-Adrenergic agonists[50]
Chlorpromazine (Thorazine)[52]
Cimetidine (Tagamet)[57]
Clozapine (Clozaril)[52,56,58]
Disulfiram (Antabuse)[50]

Ephedrine[52]
Ergotamine (Ergomar)[50]
Lithium (Eskalith, Lithobid)[59,60]
Monoamine oxidase inhibitors[52]
Mexiletine (Mexitil)[61]
Oral contraceptives[57]
Phenylpropanolamine (Propagest, Rhindecon)[52]
Phenytoin (Dilantin)[52]
Quinolones[61–64]
Theophylline (Theo-Dur)[56]
Verapamil (Calan, Isoptin)[57]
Warfarin (Coumadin)[48,65–68]

Parts used

Leaf bud, leaf, and stem[1]

References

1. Jellin JM, Batz F, Hitchens K. Natural Medicines Comprehensive Database, 3rd ed. Stockton, CA: Therapeutic Research Faculty, 2002:1530.
2. Mitscher LA, Jung M, Shankel D et al. Chemoprotection: a review of the potential therapeutic antioxidant properties of green tea (Camellia sinensis) and certain of its constituents. Med Res Rev 1997; 17:327–365.
3. Bushman JL. Green tea and cancer in humans: a review of the literature. Nutr Cancer 1998; 31:151–159.
4. Ohno Y, Aoki K, Obata K, Morrison AS. Case-control study of urinary bladder cancer in metropolitan Nagoya. Natl Cancer Inst Monogr 1985; 69:229–234.
5. Inoue M, Tajima K, Mizutani M et al. Regular consumption of green tea and the risk of breast cancer recurrence: follow-up study from the Hospital-based Epidemiologic Research Program at Aichi Cancer Center (HERPACC), Japan. Cancer Lett 2001; 167:175–182.
6. Zhang M, Binns CW, Lee A. Tea consumption and ovarian cancer risk: a case–control study in China. Cancer Epidemiol Biomarkers Prev 2002; 11:713–718.
7. Kaegi E. Unconventional therapies for cancer: 2. Green tea. The Task Force on Alternative Therapies of the Canadian Breast Cancer Research Initiative. CMAJ 1998; 158:1033–1035.
8. Setiawan VW, Zhang ZF, Yu G et al. Protective effect of green tea on the risks of chronic gastritis and stomach cancer. Int J Cancer 2001; 92:600–604.
9. Li N, Sun Z, Han C, Chen J. The chemopreventive effects of tea on human oral precancerous mucosa lesions. Proc Soc Exp Biol Med 1999; 220:218–224.
10. Durlach PJ. The effects of a low dose of caffeine on cognitive performance. Psychopharmacoloy 1998; 140:116–119.
11. Imai K, Nakachi K. Cross sectional study of effects of drinking green tea on cardiovascular and liver diseases. BMJ 1995; 310:693–696.
12. Ross GW, Abbott RD, Petrovitch H et al. Association of coffee and caffeine intake with the risk of parkinson disease. JAMA 2000; 283:2674–2679.
13. Mitamura T, Kitazono M, Yoshimura O, Yakushiji M. [The influence of green tea upon the improvement of iron deficiency anemia with pregnancy treated by sodium ferrous citrate]. Nippon Sanka Fujinka Gakkai Zasshi 1989; 41:688–694.

14. Klebanoff MA, Levine RJ, DerSimonian R, Clemens JD, Wilkins DG. Maternal serum paraxanthine, a caffeine metabolite, and the risk of spontaneous abortion. N Engl J Med 1999; 341:1639–1644.
15. Rasch V. Cigarette, alcohol, and caffeine consumption: risk factors for spontaneous abortion. Acta Obstet Gynecol Scand 2003; 82:182–188.
16. Wisborg K, Kesmodel U, Bech B, Hedegaard M, Henriksen TB. Maternal consumption of coffee during pregnancy and stillbirth and infant death in first year of life: prospective study. BMJ 2003; 326:420.
17. Balat O, Balat A, Ugur M, Pence S. The effect of smoking and caffeine on the fetus and placenta in pregnancy. Clin Exp Obstet Gynecol 2003; 30:57–59.
18. Bracken MB, Triche EW, Belanger K, Hellenbrand K, Leaderer BP. Association of maternal caffeine consumption with decrements in fetal growth. Am J Epidemiol 2003; 157:456–466.
19. Evereklioglu C, Sari I, Alasehirli B et al. High dose of caffeine administered to pregnant rats causes histopathological changes in the cornea of newborn pups. Med Sci Monit 2003; 9:BR168–173.
20. Ajarem JS, Ahmad M. Teratopharmacological and behavioral effects of coffee in mice. Acta Physiol Pharmacol Bulg 1996; 22:51–61.
21. Brinker F. The Toxicology of Botanical Medicines. Sandy, OR: Eclectic Medical Publications, 2000:296.
22. Palm PE, Arnold EP, Nick M, Valentine JR, Doerfler TE. Two-year toxicity/carcinogenicity study of fresh-brewed coffee in rats initially exposed in utero. Toxicol Appl Pharmacol 1984; 74:364–382.
23. Nehlig A, Debry G. Consequences on the newborn of chronic maternal consumption of coffee during gestation and lactation: a review. J Am Coll Nutr 1994; 13:6–21.
24. Briggs GB, Freeman RK, Yaffe SJ. Drugs in Pregnancy and Lactation. 5th ed. Philadelphia: Lippincott Williams & Wilkins, 1998.
25. McKevoy GK. Drug Information. Bethesda, MD: American Society of Health-System Pharmacists, 1998.
26. Nehlig A, Debry G. [Effects of coffee and caffeine on fertility, reproduction, lactation, and development. Review of human and animal data]. J Gynecol Obstet Biol Reprod (Paris) 1994; 23:241–256.
27. Boyd JR. Facts and Comparisons. St Louis, MO: J.B. Lippincott Co., 1985.
28. Gruenwald J, Brendler T, Jaenicke C. PDR for Herbal Medicines. Montvale, NJ: Medical Economics Company, 1998.
29. Nemecz G. Green tea. US Pharmacist 2000:67–70.
30. Chung LY, Cheung TC, Kong SK et al. Induction of apoptosis by green tea catechins in human prostate cancer DU145 cells. Life Sci 2001; 68:1207–1214.
31. Robbers JE, Tyler VE. Tyler's Herbs of Choice: The Therapeutic Use of Phytomedicinals. New York, NY: The Haworth Herbal Press, 1999.
32. Foster S, Duke JA. Eastern/Central Medicinal Plants. New York, NY: Houghton Mifflin Co., 1990.
33. Kaegi E. Unconventional therapies for cancer: Green tea. The Task Force on Alternative Therapies of the Canadian Breast Cancer Research Initiative. CMAJ 1998; 158:1033–1035.
34. Pisters KM, Newman RA, Coldman B et al. Phase I trial of oral green tea extract in adult patients with solid tumors. J Clin Oncol 2001; 19:1830–1838.
35. Garbisa S, Biggin S, Cavallarin N et al. Tumor invasion: molecular shears blunted by green tea. Nat Med 1999; 5:1216.

36. Cao Y, Cao R. Angiogenesis inhibited by drinking tea. Nature 1999; 398:381.
37. L'Allemain G. [Multiple actions of EGCG, the main component of green tea]. Bull Cancer 1999; 86:721–724.
38. Leenen R, Roodenburg AJ, Tijburg LB et al. A single dose of tea with or without milk increases plasma antioxidant activity in humans. Eur J Clin Nutr 2000; 54:87–92.
39. Hodgson JM, Puddey IB, Burke V et al. Effects on blood pressure of drinking green and black tea. J Hypertens 1999; 17:457–463.
40. Leung LK, Su Y, Chen R et al. Theaflavins in black tea and catechins in green tea are equally effective antioxidants. J Nutr 2001; 131:2248–2251.
41. Locher R, Emmanuele L, Suter PM et al. Green tea polyphenols inhibit human vascular smooth muscle cell proliferation stimulated by native low-density lipoprotein. Eur J Pharmacol 2002; 434:1–7.
42. Choi YT, Jung CH, Lee SR et al. The green tea polyphenol (−)-epigallocatechin gallate attenuates beta-amyloid-induced neurotoxicity in cultured hippocampal neurons. Life Sci 2001; 70:603–614.
43. Klaunig JE, Xu Y, Han C et al. The effect of tea consumption on oxidative stress in smokers and nonsmokers. Proc Soc Exp Biol Med 1999; 220:249–254.
44. Lee IP, Kim YH, Kang MH et al. Chemopreventive effect of green tea (Camellia sinensis) against cigarette smoke induced mutations in humans. J Cell Biochem Suppl 1997; 27:68–75.
45. Schulz V, Hansel R, Tyler VE, Terry C. Rational Phytotherapy: A Physician's Guide to Herbal Medicine, 3rd ed. Berlin: Springer, 1998.
46. Weisburger JH. Tea and health: the underlying mechanisms. Proc Soc Exp Biol Med 1999; 220:271–275.
47. Ross GW, Abbott RD, Petrovitch H et al. Association of coffee and caffeine intake with the risk of parkinson disease. JAMA 2000; 283:2674–9.
48. Ali M, Afzal M. A potent inhibitor of thrombin stimulated platelet thromboxane formation from unprocessed tea. Prostaglandins Leukot Med 1987; 27:9–13.
49. Ardlie NG, Glew G, Schultz BG, Schwartz CJ. Inhibition and reversal of platelet aggregation by methyl xanthines. Thromb Diath Haemorrh 1967; 18:670–673.
50. McKevoy GK. AHFS Drug Information. Bethesda, MD: American Society of Health-System Pharmacists, 1998.
51. Nurminen ML, Niittynen L, Korpela R, Vapaatalo H. Coffee, caffeine and blood pressure: a critical review. Eur J Clin Nutr 2000; 54:234–238.
52. Brinker F. Herb Contraindications and Drug Interactions, 2nd ed. Sandy, OR: Eclectic Medical Publications, 1998.
53. Lasswell WLJ, Weber SS, Wilkins JM. In vitro interaction of neuroleptics and tricylic antidepressants with coffee, tea, and gallotannic acid. J Pharm Sci 1984; 73:1056–1058.
54. Kulhanek F, Linde OK, Meisenberg G. Precipitation of antipsychotic drugs in interaction with coffee or tea. Lancet 1979; ii:1130.
55. Tyler VE. Herbs of Choice. Binghamton, NY: Pharmaceutical Products Press, 1994.
56. Sklar S et al. Drug therapy screening system. Indianapolis, IN: First Data Bank:99.
57. MICROMEDEX. Micromedex Healthcare Series. Englewood, CO: MICROMED EX.
58. Hagg S, Spigset O, Mjorndal T, Dahlqvist R. Effect of caffeine on clozapine pharmacokinetics in healthy volunteers. Br J Clin Pharmacol 2000; 49:59–63.

59. Mester R, Toren P, Mizrachi I et al. Caffeine withdrawal increases lithium blood levels. Biol Psychiatry 1995; 37:348–350.
60. Jefferson JW. Lithium tremor and caffeine intake: two cases of drinking less and shaking more. J Clin Psychiatry 1988; 49:72–73.
61. Joeres R, Klinker H, Heusler H et al. Influence of mexiletine on caffeine elimination. Pharmacol Ther 1987; 33:163–169.
62. Harder S, Fuhr U, Staib AH, Wolff T. Ciprofloxacin-caffeine: a drug interaction established using in vivo and in vitro investigations. Am J Med 1989; 87:89S–91S.
63. Carbo M, Segura J, De la Torre R et al. Effect of quinolones on caffeine disposition. Clin Pharmacol Ther 1989; 45:234–240.
64. Healy DP, Polk RE, Kanawati L et al. Interaction between oral ciprofloxacin and caffeine in normal volunteers. Antimicrob Agents Chemother 1989; 33:474–478.
65. Booth SL, Madabushi HT, Davidson KW et al. Tea and coffee brews are not dietary sources of vitamin K-1 (phylloquinone). J Am Diet Assoc 1995; 95:82–83.
66. Taylor JR, Wilt VM. Probable antagonism of warfarin by green tea. Ann Pharmacother 1999; 33:426–428.
67. Lou FQ, Zhang MF, Zhang XG et al. A study on tea-pigment in prevention of atherosclerosis. Chin Med J (Engl) 1989; 102:579–583.
68. Graham HN. Green tea composition, consumption, and polyphenol chemistry. Prev Med 1992; 21:334–350.

GUGGUL
Commiphora mukul

Synonyms/common names/related compounds[1]

Guggal, guggul gum resin, guggulipid, guggulipids, guggulu, guggulsterone, guggulsterones, gum guggal, gum gugglu, gum guggulu, Indian bdellium-tree, mukul myrrh, mukul myrrh tree

Indications

*Conflicting evidence – hyperlipidemia:[2–8]	Evidence grade B1
Nodulocystic acne:[9]	Evidence grade C
Obesity:[10,11]	Evidence grade C
Rheumatoid arthritis:[12,13]	Evidence grade D
Osteoarthritis (with gold):[14,15]	Evidence grade D
Osteoarthritis:[16]	Evidence grade E

*A number of studies, including randomized controlled trials, reported that guggul has lipid-lowering effects.[2–8] A 2003 randomized controlled trial on guggul, however, reported that guggulipid did not appear to improve levels of serum cholesterol in adults with hypercholesterolemia, and might in fact raise levels of low-density lipoprotein-C.[17] Given that this contradicts a number of previously published trials, further investigation is required.

Pregnancy

Potential abortifacient:[18]	Evidence level 4
Emmenagogue:[18]	Evidence level 4
Uterine stimulant:[19,20]	Evidence level 4

A review article on the potential value of plants as sources of anti-fertility agents reported that guggul was a potential abortifacient and an emmenagogue.[18] A herbal toxicology and drug interaction compendium and a herb safety compendium reported that guggul was a uterine stimulant.[19,20]

Lactation

Unknown:	Evidence level 5

There are no reports in the literature of guggul being either safe or contraindicated during lactation.

Constituents

- Ketonic steroids:[1] Z-guggulsterone and E-guggulsterone
- Essential oils:[22] curzerenone, furanodiene-6-one and furanoeudesma-1,3-diene
- Resin

Toxicity

LD_{50}: 1.6 g/kg[21]

Pharmacology

- Guggul extract, also known as guggulipid (usually standardized to 2.5% guggulsterones), is an ethyl acetate extract of the gum resin that contains both Z- and E-guggulsterones.[17,23]
- Guggulsterones inhibit the synthesis of cholesterol in the liver and appear to have an antioxidant effect on lipids.[23,24]
- Guggul may lower lipoprotein (a) and C-reactive protein.[17]
- Guggul is an antagonist ligand for farnesoid X receptor (FXR) where it decreases expression of bile acid-activated genes.[25]
- Guggulsterones may have thyroid-stimulating activity where they increase the conversion of T4 to T3.[24,26,27]
- Guggul may have a protective effect against drug-induced myocardial necrosis.[28]
- In acne, guggulipid may reduce secretion of sebum and inhibit bacterial metabolism of triglycerides.[9]
- Guggul may have anti-inflammatory activity.[16]
- Guggul may have anti-platelet and anti-coagulant activity.[23,29]

Drug interactions[1]

Anti-coagulant/anti-platelet drugs[23,29]
Diltiazem[30]
Propranolol[30]
Thyroid drugs[26,27]

Parts used[1]

Gum resin

References

1. Jellin JM, Batz F, Hitchens K. Natural Medicines Comprehensive Database, 3rd ed. Stockton, CA: Therapeutic Research Faculty, 2002:1530.
2. Nityanand S, Srivastava JS, Asthana O. Clinical trials with gugulipid. A new hypolipidaemic agent. J Assoc Physicians India 1989; 37:323–328.
3. Gaur SP, Garg RK, Kar AM, et al. Guggulipid, a new hypolipidaemic agent, in patients of acute ischaemic stroke: effect on clinical outcome, platelet function and serum lipids. Asia Pacif J Pharm 1997; 12:65–69.
4. Verma SK, Bordia A. Effect of Commiphora mukul (gum guggulu) in patients of hyperlipidemia with special reference to HDL-cholesterol. Indian J Med Res 1988; 87:356–360.

5. Kotiyal JP, Singh DS, Bisht DB. Gum guggulu (Commiphora mukul) fraction 'A' in obesity – a double-blind clinical trial. J Res Ayur Siddha 1985; 6:20–35.
6. Kuppurajan K, Rajagopalan SS, Rao T, Sitaraman R. Effect of guggulu (Commiphora mukul-Engl.) on serum lipids in obese, hypercholesterolemic and hyperlipemic cases. J Assoc Physicians India 1978; 26:367–373.
7. Ghorai M, Mandal SC, Pal M, Pal SP, Saha BP. A comparative study on hypocholesterolaemic effect of allicin, whole germinated seeds of bengal gram and guggulipid of gum gugglu. Phytother Res 2000; 14:200–202.
8. Thompson Coon JS, Ernst E. Herbs for serum cholesterol reduction: a systematic view. J Fam Pract 2003; 52:468–478.
9. Thappa DM, Dogra J. Nodulocystic acne: oral gugulipid versus tetracycline. J Dermatol 1994; 21:729–731.
10. Bhatt AD, Dalal DG, Shah S et al. Conceptual and methodologic challenges of assessing the short-term efficacy of Guggulu in obesity: data emergent from a naturalistic clinical trial. J Postgrad Med 1995; 41:5–7.
11. Sidhu LS, Sharma K, Puri AS et al. Effect of gum guggul on body weight and subcutaneous tissue folds. J Res Indian Med Yoga Hom 1976; 11:16–22.
12. Kishore P, Devi Das KV, Banarjee S. Clinical studies on the treatment of Amavata-Rheumatoid arthritis with Sunthi-Guggulu. J Res Ayur Siddha 1982; 3(3–4):133–146.
13. Mahesh S, Pandit M, Hakala C. A study of Shuddha Guggulu on rheumatoid arthritis. Rheumatism 1981; 16:54–67.
14. Majumdar KA. A clinical study of R-Arthritis with A-Compound – a herbal formulation. Rheumatism 1984; 19:66–74.
15. Majumdar KA. Role of gum guggulu with gold in rheumatic and other allied disorders. Rheumatism 1984; 20:9–15.
16. Singh BB, Mishra L, Aquilina N, Kohlbeck F. Usefulness of guggul (Commiphora mukul) for osteoarthritis of the knee: an experimental case study. Altern Ther Health Med 2001; 7:112–114.
17. Szapary PO, Wolfe ML, Bloedon LT et al. Guggulipid for treatment of hypercholesterolemia: a randomized controlled trial. JAMA 2003; 290:765–772.
18. Farnsworth NR, Bingel AS, Cordell G, Crane FA, Fong HH. Potential value of plants as sources of new antifertility agents I. J Pharm Sci 1975; 64:535–598.
19. Brinker F. The Toxicology of Botanical Medicines. Sandy, OR: Eclectic Medical Publications, 2000:296.
20. McGuffin M, Hobbs C, Upton R, Goldberg A. American Herbal Products Association's Botanical Safety Handbook. Boca Raton, FL: CRC Press, 1997:231.
21. Bradshaw C, Nguyen A, Surles J. Gugulipid (Gum Guggul, Guggulu). Vol. 2004: http://www.dotek.de/ebooks/documents/html/gugulipid_.html
22. Saeed MA, Sabir AW. Irritant potential of some constituents from oleo-gum-resin of Commiphora myrrha. Fitoterapia 2004; 75:81–84.
23. Singh RB, Niaz MA, Ghosh S. Hypolipidemic and antioxidant effects of Commiphora mukul as an adjunct to dietary therapy in patients with hypercholesterolemia. Cardiovasc Drugs Ther 1994; 8:659–664.
24. Panda S, Kar A. Gugulu (Commiphora mukul) induces triiodothyronine production: possible involvement of lipid peroxidation. Life Sci 1999; 65:PL137–141.
25. Cui J, Huang L, Zhao A et al. Guggulsterone is a farnesoid × receptor antagonist in coactivator association assays but acts to enhance transcription of bile salt export pump. J Biol Chem 2003; 278:10214–10220. Epub 2003 Jan 13.

26. Antonio J, Colker CM, Torina GC et al. Effects of a standardized guggulsterone phosphate supplement on body composition in overweight adults: a pilot study. Curr Ther Res 1999; 60:220–227.
27. Tripathi YB, Tripathi P, Malhotra OP, Tripathi SN. Thyroid stimulatory action of (Z)-guggulsterone: mechanism of action. Planta Med 1988; 54:271–277.
28. Kaul S, Kapoor NK. Cardiac sarcolemma enzymes and liver microsomal cytochrome P450 in isoproterenol treated rats. Indian J Med Res 1989; 90:62–68.
29. Mester L, Mester M, Nityanand S. Inhibition of platelet aggregation by 'guggulu' steroids. Planta Med 1979; 37:367–369.
30. Dalvi SS, Nayak VK, Pohujani SM et al. Effect of gugulipid on bioavailability of diltiazem and propranolol. J Assoc Physicians India 1994; 42:454–455.

HAWTHORN

Crataegus oxycantha, C. cuneata, C. laevigata

Synonyms/common names/related substances[1]

Aubepine, blanca spino, crataegi flos, crataegi folium, crataegi folium cum flore, crataegi fructus, English hawthorn, epine blanche, epine de mai, haagdorn, hagedorn, harthorne, haw, hawthorn extract, hawthorn flower, hawthorne fruit, hawthorn leaf, hawthorne, hedgethorn, may, maybush, maythorn, mehlbeebaum, meidorn, nan shanzha, oneseed hawthorn, shazha, weissdorn

Indications

Congestive heart failure:[2]	Evidence grade A
Coronary artery disease (angina):[3]	Evidence grade B1
Functional cardiovascular disorders (with camphor):[4]	Evidence grade B1

Pregnancy

Uterine activity:[5]	Evidence level 4

A herbal medicine compendium reported that hawthorn has uterine activity and is unsafe during pregnancy.[5] There are no reports in the medical literature of hawthorn being safe or contraindicated during pregnancy.

Lactation

Unknown:	Evidence level 5

There are no reports in the literature of hawthorn being safe or contraindicated during lactation.

Constituents

Flavonoids[6]
Procyanidins[6]
Vtexin[6]
Rutin[6]
Hyperoside[6]

Toxicity

- LD_{50}: 18–24 mL/kg (intravenous) and 18.5–33.8 mL/kg (oral)[7–9]
- Acute toxicity (LD_{50}) of isolated flavonoid constituents: 50–2600 mg/kg (intravenous) and 6 g/kg (oral)[7–9]

Pharmacology

- Hawthorn acts on the myocardium by increasing the force of contraction and by lengthening the refractory period.[6,10]
- Hawthorn has antiarrhythmic activity by prolonging refractory period of the action potential.[11]
- Hawthorn reduces peripheral vascular resistance and oxygen consumption, and increases nerve conductivity.[6,12]
- Hawthorn increases coronary blood flow, vasodilation, and has a positive inotropic effects by increasing calcium membrane permeability and inhibiting phosphodiesterase (which increases intracellular cyclic AMP).[12,13]
- Hawthorn reduces lipid levels.[1]
- Hawthorn has antibacterial properties.[14]
- Hawthorn has spasmolytic and analgesic effects.[14]
- Hawthorn may decrease uterine tone and motility.[1]

Drug interactions

Cardiovascular drugs[5,15]
Central nervous system depressants[5,6]
Coronary vasodilators[6]
Digoxin[6,15]

Parts used[1]

Leaf, fruit, and flower

References

1. Jellin JM, Batz F, Hitchens K. Natural Medicines Comprehensive Database, 3rd ed. Stockton, CA: Therapeutic Research Faculty, 2002:1530.
2. Weihmayr T, Ernst E. [Therapeutic effectiveness of Crataegus]. Fortschr Med 1996; 114:27–29.
3. Weng WL, Zhang WQ, Liu F et al. Therapeutic effect of Crataegus pinnatifida on 46 cases of angina pectoris – a double blind study. J Tradit Chin Med 1984; 4:293–294.
4. Schmidt U, Albrecht M, Schmidt S. [Effects of an herbal crataegus-camphor combination on the symptoms of cardiovascular diseases]. Arzneimittelforschung 2000; 50:613–619.
5. Newall CA, Anderson LA, Phillipson JD. Herbal Medicines: A Guide for Health-care Professionals. London, UK: Pharmaceutical Press, 1996:296.
6. Upton R. Hawthorn leaf with flower: analytical, quality control, and therapeutic monograph. Santa Cruz, CA American Herbal Pharmacopoeia: 1999:1–29.
7. Ammon HP, Handel M. [Crataegus, toxicology and pharmacology. Part III: Pharmacodynamics and pharmacokinetics (author's transl)]. Planta Med 1981; 43:313–322.
8. Ammon HP, Handel M. [Crataegus, toxicology and pharmacology. Part II: Pharmacodynamics (author's transl)]. Planta Med 1981; 43:209–239.
9. Ammon HP, Handel M. [Crataegus, toxicology and pharmacology, Part I: Toxicity (author's transl)]. Planta Med 1981; 43:105–120.

10. Pittler MH, Schmidt K, Ernst E. Hawthorn extract for treating chronic heart failure: meta-analysis of randomized trials. Am J Med 2003; 114:665–674.
11. Zbinden S, Seiler C. [Phytotherapy in cardiovascular medicine]. Ther Umsch 2002; 59:301–306.
12. Gruenwald J, Brendler T, Jaenicke C. PDR for Herbal Medicines. Montvale, NJ: Medical Economics Company, 1998.
13. Johnson JA, Lalonde RL. Congestive heart failure. In: DiPiro JT, ed. Pharmacotherapy, 3rd ed. Stamford: Appleton and Lange, 1997.
14. Leung AY, Foster S. Encyclopedia of Common Natural Ingredients Used in Food, Drugs and Cosmetics, 2nd ed. New York, NY: John Wiley & Sons, 1996:649.
15. McGuffin M, Hobbs C, Upton R, Goldberg A. American Herbal Products Association's Botanical Safety Handbook. Boca Raton, FL: CRC Press, 1997:231.

HORSECHESTNUT

Aesculus hippocastanum

Synonyms/common names/related substances[1]

Buckeye, chestnut, escine, Hippocastani cortex, Hippocastani flos, Hippocastani folium, Hippocastani semen, horse chestnut, marron europeen, Spanish chestnut, venastat, venostat, venostasin retard

Indications

Horse chestnut seed extract (HCSE)

Chronic venous insufficiency:[2–21]	Evidence grade A

Escin gel (2%) – topical

Hematoma:[22]	Evidence grade B2

Escin

Postoperative edema and thrombosis:[23,24]	Evidence grade B2

Esculin

Hemorrhoids:[25]	Evidence grade C

Pregnancy

HCSE

Minimal risk:[26]	Evidence level 1a

A randomized placebo-controlled trial of 52 women with leg edema attributed to pregnancy-induced venous insufficiency failed to observe any serious adverse effects after 2 weeks.[26] Subjects received 300 mg twice daily of Venostasin[reg] retard (240–290 mg of horse chestnut seed extract, standardized to 50 mg escin).[26]

Unprocessed (raw) horsechestnut preparations

Toxic – contraindicated in pregnancy and lactation:[27,28]	Evidence level 4

Unprocessed (raw) horsechestnut preparations (seed, bark, flower, leaf) can be lethal when ingested.[28] In adults, a few chestnuts can cause severe symptoms, whereas in children, a few chestnuts can be lethal.[27] It has been reported that roasting horsechestnut appears to destroy its toxins.[27] Unprocessed horsechestnut was not reported in the literature as being either contraindicated or safe for use during pregnancy.

Lactation

HCSE

Unknown:	Evidence level 5

There are no reports in the literature of horse chestnut seed extract being either safe or contraindicated during lactation.

Unprocessed (raw) horsechestnut preparations

Toxic – contraindicated in pregnancy and lactation:[27,28]	Evidence level 4

Unprocessed (raw) horsechestnut preparations (seed, bark, flower, leaf) can be lethal when ingested.[28] In adults, a few chestnuts can cause severe symptoms, whereas in children, a few chestnuts can be lethal.[27] It has been reported that roasting horsechestnut appears to destroy its toxins.[27] Unprocessed horsechestnut was not reported in the literature as being either contraindicated or safe for use during lactation.

Caution

Diabetes or glucose intolerance[29]

Constituents

- Triterpene saponins:[1,29–32] triterpene oligoglycosides (escins Ia, Ib, IIa, IIb, IIIa), acylated polyhydroxyoleanene triterpene oligoglycosides (escins IIIb, IV, V, VI), isoescins (Ia, Ib, V)
- Sapogenols:[1,29–32] hippocaesculin, barringtogenol-C
- Hydroxycoumarin lactone glycoside:[27] esculin
- Sterols:[1,29–32] stigmasterol, α-spinasterol, β-sitosterol
- Fatty acids:[1,29–32] linolenic, palmitic, stearic acids
- Flavonoids[1,29–32]
- Tannins[1,29–32]
- Quinines[1,29–32]

Toxicity

- The constituent esculin is associated with significant toxicity.[28]
- HCSE which is standardized to escin content should not contain clinically relevant levels of esculin, and thus most toxicities will not be of concern.[28]

Pharmacology

Unprocessed (raw) horsechestnut preparations

- Esculin causes neural stimulation and increases antithrombin activity, thereby leading to increased bleeding time.[27]
- Esculin is a mucous membrane irritant.[27]

HCSE

- Escin, the active ingredient in horse chestnut seed extract has anti-exudative and vascular-tightening effects.[31]
- HCSE reduces vascular permeability, reduces the activity of lysosomal enzymes and inhibits the breakdown of glycoacalyx in the capillary walls.[31]
- HCSE contracts canine and human isolated saphenous veins in vitro, possibly due to preferential formation of the vasoconstrictive eicosanoid PGF2-α.[33–35]
- HCSE increases femoral venous pressure and flow, decreases the formation of edema, and suppresses plasma extravasation and leucocyte emigration into the pleural cavity.[34,36]
- HCSE has antioxidant effects.[34]

Drug interactions

Hypoglycemic agents[29]
Anti-coagulant/anti-platelet therapy[27]

Parts containing toxins[27]

Seeds, bark, leaves, pericarp of fruit twigs, and non-medicinal flowers

References

1 Jellin JM, Batz F, Hitchens K. Natural Medicines Comprehensive Database, 3rd ed. Stockton, CA: Therapeutic Research Faculty, 2002:1530.
2. Bielanski TE, Piotrowski ZH. Horse-chestnut seed extract for chronic venous insufficiency. J Fam Pract 1999; 48:171–172.
3. Bisler H, Pfeifer R, Kluken N et al. [Effects of horse-chestnut seed extract on transcapillary filtration in chronic venous insufficiency]. Dtsch Med Wochenschr 1986; 111:1321–1329.
4. Diehm C, Trampisch HJ, Lange S, Schmidt C. Comparison of leg compression stocking and oral horse-chestnut seed extract therapy in patients with chronic venous insufficiency. Lancet 1996; 347:292–294.
5. Diehm C, Vollbrecht D, Amendt K et al. [Medical edema protection – clinical benefit in patients with chronic deep vein incompetence. A placebo controlled double blind study]. Vasa 1992; 21:188–192.
6. Dworschak E, Antal M, Biro L et al. Medical activities of Aesculus hippocastaneum (horse-chestnut) saponins. Adv Exp Med Biol 1996; 404:471–474.
7. Ehringer H. [On the vein tonicising principle of horse chestnut extract. Effect of pure horse chestnut extract and aescin on the venous capacity, venous tonus and circulation of the extremities]. Med Welt 1968; 33:1781–1785.

8. Gerova Z, Stvrtinova V, Sefranek V, Illek B. [Beta-aescin in the treatment of chronic venous insufficiency]. Cas Lek Cesk 1991; 130:15–19.
9. Greeske K, Pohlmann BK. [Horse chestnut seed extract – an effective therapy principle in general practice. Drug therapy of chronic venous insufficiency]. Fortschr Med 1996; 114:196–200.
10. Hirsch J. [Leg disorders – disorders of blood supply. The effect of Essaven ultra in chronic venous insufficiency]. Fortschr Med 1982; 100:436–438.
11. Hitzenberger G. [The therapeutic effectiveness of chestnut extract]. Wien Med Wochenschr 1989; 139:385–389.
12. Klemm J. [Flow velocity of blood in varicose veins of the lower extremities. The effect of a venous therapeutic agent (venostasin) (author's transl)]. MMW Munch Med Wochenschr 1982; 124:579–582.
13. Kronberger L, Golles J. [On the prevention of thrombosis with aesculus extract]. Med Klin 1969; 64:1207–1209.
14. Montagnani A. [Treatment of chronic venous insufficiency with phlebotropic drugs]. Clin Ter 1984; 108:91–98.
15. Nehring U. [On the demonstration of efficacy of horse chestnut extract on venous tonus following its oral administration]. Med Welt 1966; 32:1662–1665.
16. Neumann-Mangoldt P. [Experiences in the use of Essaven capsules in the treatment of venous leg diseases. Results of a double-blind study]. Fortschr Med 1979; 97:2117–2119.
17. Nill HJ, Fischer H. [Comparative investigations concerning the effect of extract of horse chestnut upon the pressure-volume-diagramm of patients with venous disorders]. Arztl Forsch 1970; 24:141–143.
18. Pittler MH, Ernst E. Horse-chestnut seed extract for chronic venous insufficiency. A criteria-based systematic review. Arch Dermatol 1998; 134:1356–1360.
19. Rehn D, Unkauf M, Klein P et al. [Comparative clinical efficacy and tolerability of oxerutins and horse chestnut extract in patients with chronic venous insufficiency]. Arzneimittelforschung 1996; 46:483–487.
20. Saenko VF, Sukharev II, Viktorov AP, Goloopykho LI. [Experience with the clinical use of Essaven gel in treating venous diseases]. Klin Khir 1996; 7:13–14.
21. Steiner M. [Conservative therapy of chronic venous insufficiency. The extent of the edema-preventive effect of horse chestnut seed extract]. Vasa Suppl 1991; 33:217.
22. Calabrese C, Preston P. Report of the results of a double-blind, randomized, single-dose trial of a topical 2% escin gel versus placebo in the acute treatment of experimentally-induced hematoma in volunteers. Planta Med 1993; 59:394–397.
23. Prexl HJ, Suppan G, Kronberger D, Fueger GF. [A prospective study on the occurrence of postoperative thrombosis of leg-veins and the possible influence of aescin in its prevention (author's transl)]. Wien Klin Wochenschr 1976; 88:326–329.
24. Wilhelm K, Feldmeier C. [Thermometric investigations about the efficacy of beta-escin to reduce postoperative edema (author's transl)]. Med Klin 1977; 72:128–134.
25. Damianov L, Katsarova M. [Our experience in using the preparation Proctosedyl from the Roussel firm in pregnant women with hemorrhoids]. Akush Ginekol (Sofiia) 1993; 32:71.
26. Steiner M. Untersuchungen zur odemvermindernden und odemportektiven wirking von ro kastaniensamenextrakt. Phlebol Prokto 1990; 19:239–242.
27. Brinker F. The Toxicology of Botanical Medicines. Sandy, OR: Eclectic Medical Publications, 2000:296.

28. Ellenhorn MJ, Schonwald S, Ordog G, Wasserberger J. Ellenhorn's Medical Toxicology: Diagnoses and Treatment of Human Poisoning, 2nd ed. Baltimore, MD: Williams & Wilkins, 1997.
29. Yoshikawa M, Murakami T, Yamahara J, Matsuda H. Bioactive saponins and glycosides. XII. Horse chestnut. Structures of escins IIIb, IV, V, and VI and isoescins Ia, Ib, and V, acylated polyhydroxyoleanene triterpene oligoglycosides, from the seeds of horse chestnut tree (Aesculus hippocastanum L., Hippocastanaceae). Chem Pharm Bull (Tokyo) 1998; 46:1764–1769.
30. Blumenthal M, Busse WR, Goldberg A et al. The Complete German Commission E Monographs: Therapeutic Guide to Herbal Medicines. Boston, MA: American Botanical Council, 1998.
31. Leung AY, Foster S. Encyclopedia of Common Natural Ingredients Used in Food, Drugs and Cosmetics, 2nd ed. New York, NY: John Wiley & Sons, 1996:649.
32. Yoshikawa M, Murakami T, Otuki K, Yamahara J, Matsuda H. [Bioactive saponins and glycosides. XIII. Horse chestnut. Quantitative analysis of escins Ia, Ib, IIa, and IIb by means of high performance liquid chromatography]. Yakugaku Zasshi 1999; 119:81–87.
33. Brunner F, Hoffmann C, Schuller-Petrovic S. Responsiveness of human varicose saphenous veins to vasoactive agents. Br J Clin Pharmacol 2001; 51:219–224.
34. Guillaume M, Padioleau F. [Veinotonic effect, vascular protection, antiinflammatory and free radical scavenging properties of horse chestnut extract]. Arzneimittelforschung 1994; 44:25–35.
35. Longiave D, Omini C, Nicosia S et al. The mode of action of aescin on isolated veins: relationship with PGF2 alpha. T Pharmacol Res Commun 1978; 10:145–152.
36. Masaki H, Sakaki S, Atsumi T et al. Active-oxygen scavenging activity of plant extracts. Biol Pharm Bull 1995; 18:162–166.

JUNIPER
Juniperus communis

Synonyms/common names/related compounds[1]

Common juniper berry, enebro, geniévre, ginepro, *Juniperi fructus*, wacholderbeeren, zimbro

Indications

Common cold (with peppermint oil, cajeput oil, eucalyptus oil and methylquinolinium oil):[2]	Evidence grade C
Renoprotective:[3]	Evidence grade E
Anti-mycobacterial activity:[4]	Evidence grade E
Hypoglycemic:[5]	Evidence grade E
Antibacterial and antifungal:[6]	Evidence grade E
Diuretic and aquaretic:[7,8]	Evidence grade F
Cystitis:[7]	Evidence grade F

Pregnancy

Abortifacient:[9–13]	Evidence level 3
Blocks progesterone production:[14]	Evidence level 3

Juniper was reported to cause abortions in pregnant cattle.[9] Isocupressic acid is believed to be the primary abortifacient compound in juniper.[9] Cows fed juniper needles subsequently aborted after 3–4 days.[10] Other studies on isocupressic acid have also shown that it has an abortive effect in pregnant cattle.[11,12] A review article on the potential value of plants as sources of anti-fertility agents reported that juniper was an abortifacient.[13]

Isocupressic acid was reported to block progesterone production in bovine luteal cells.[14] It was concluded that isocupressic acid can induce pregnant cows to abort partly through blocking luteal function.[14]

Anti-implantation activity and interferes with fertility:[15–18]	Evidence level 3

A study on the anti-implantation activity in female albino rats of a number of herbs found that juniper had 60–70% anti-implantation activity.[16] An editorial review of contraceptive products reported that the Drug Research Institute in Lucknow, India, US National Institutes of Health, the World Health Organization, and the Indian Council of Medical Research confirm that juniper has anti-implantation effects.[15]

Emmenagogue:[13]	Evidence level 4

Uterine stimulant:[17,18]	Evidence level 4

A review article on the potential value of plants as sources of anti-fertility agents reported that juniper was an emmenagogue.[13] A herbal toxicology and drug interaction compendium and a herbal medicine compendium reported that juniper is a uterine stimulant.[17,18]

Lactation

May cross into breast milk:[19]	Evidence level 3

Supplementing the diet of rabbit does with aromatic juniper berries before and after pregnancy led offspring to have a preference for juniper berries in their diet.[19] The authors theorized that this may imply a transfer of the preference from mother to offspring through breast-feeding.[19]

Contraindications

Nephritis[17]
Pyelitis[17]

Caution

- Avoid use for more than 4 weeks without medical advice.[17]
- Topical use over large skin wounds or in individuals with acute skin conditions.[20]
- Some authors report that long-term use of juniper may cause convulsions or kidney damage,[21,22] others report that it is non-toxic.[23]

Constituents

- Volatile monoterpenes:[7,17] α-pinene, β-pinene, β-myrcene
- Volatile alcohol:[17,18] terpinen-4-ol
- Isocupressic acid[9]

Toxicity

- LD_{50} of juniper extract in mice (intraperitoneal injection): 3 g/kg[24]
- LD_{50} of juniper oil in rats (oral): 6.28 g/kg[17]
- LD_{50} of terpinen-4-ol in mice and rats (intramuscular): 0.78 mL/kg and 1.5 mL/kg, respectively[17]

Pharmacology

- Animal studies have found that juniper oil did not induce changes in function or morphology of the kidneys and was reported as non-toxic.[23]

- The diuretic action of juniper is attributed to the terpinen-4-ol portion which is purported to stimulate glomerular filtration.[18,25]
- The volatile monoterpenes are irritants to the urinary mucosa.[17]
- Studies have identified isocupressic acid as the primary abortifacient compound in juniper.[9] In vitro and in vivo studies have shown isocupressic acid is rapidly metabolized to agathic acid, dihydroagathic acid, and tetrahydroagathic acid.[9]
- Juniper demonstrated hypoglycemic activity in both rats and mice.[26,27]
- Juniper was shown to have antifungal, antiviral (against herpes simplex virus 1) and anti-inflammatory properties.[6,18]
- Oral administration of an extract of juniper berries was seen to decrease experimentally induced foot edema in rats.[28]
- Juniper oil was found to inhibit the growth of *Mycobacterium tuberculosis* and *M. avium*.[4]

Drug interactions[1]

Anti-diabetic drugs[18]
Diuretics[8,18]

Parts used[1,17]

Berries and oil

References

1. Jellin JM, Batz F, Hitchens K. Natural Medicines Comprehensive Database, 3rd ed. Stockton, CA: Therapeutic Research Faculty, 2002:1530.
2. Hansen B, Babiak G, Schilling M et al. A mixture of volatile oils in treatment of common cold. Therapiewoche 1984; 34:2015–2019.
3. Butani L, Afshinnik A, Johnson J et al. Amelioration of tacrolimus-induced nephrotoxicity in rats using juniper oil. Transplantation 2003; 76:306–311.
4. Jimenez-Arellanes A, Meckes M, Ramirez R, Torres J, Luna-Herrera J. Activity against multidrug-resistant Mycobacterium tuberculosis in Mexican plants used to treat respiratory diseases. Phytother Res 2003; 17:903–908.
5. Sanchez de Medina F, Gamez MJ, Jiminez I et al. Hypoglycemic activity of juniper 'berries'. Planta Med 1994; 60:197–200.
6. Filipowicz N, Kaminski M, Kurlenda J, Asztemborska M, Ochocka JR. Antibacterial and antifungal activity of juniper berry oil and its selected components. Phytother Res 2003; 17:227–231.
7. Mitchell W. Botanical Applications – Botanical Remedies in Naturopathic Medicine. Seattle, WA: Aush, 1982.
8. Robbers JE, Tyler VE. Tyler's Herbs of Choice: The Therapeutic Use of Phytomedicinals. New York, NY: The Haworth Herbal Press, 1999.
9. Lee ST, Gardner DR, Garrosian M et al. Development of enzyme-linked immunosorbent assays for isocupressic acid and serum metabolites of isocupressic acid. J Agric Food Chem 2003; 51:3228–3233.
10. Gardner DR, Panter KE, James L, Stegelmeier BL. Abortifacient effects of lodgepole pine (Pinus contorta) and common juniper (Juniperus communis) on cattle. Vet Hum Toxicol 1998; 40:260–263.

11. Garrossian M, Gardner DR, Panter K, James LF. Preparation of tetrahydroagathic acid: a serum metabolite of isocupressic acid, a cattle abortifacient in ponderosa pine. J Agric Food Chem 2002; 50:2235–2240.
12. Gardner DR, Panter KE, James L. Pine needle abortion in cattle: metabolism of isocupressic acid. J Agric Food Chem 1999; 47:2891–2897.
13. Farnsworth NR, Bingel AS, Cordell G, Crane FA, Fong HH. Potential value of plants as sources of new antifertility agents I. J Pharm Sci 1975; 64:535–598.
14. Wu LS, Chen JC, Sheu S et al. Isocupressic acid blocks progesterone production from bovine luteal cells. Am J Chin Med 2002; 30:533–541.
15. Chaudhury RR. The quest for a herbal contraceptive. Natl Med J India 1993; 6:199–201.
16. Prakash AO, Saxena V, Shukla S et al. Anti-implantation activity of some indigenous plants in rats. Acta Eur Fertil 1985; 16:441–448.
17. Brinker F. The Toxicology of Botanical Medicines. Sandy, OR: Eclectic Medical Publications, 2000:296.
18. Newall CA, Anderson LA, Phillipson JD. Herbal Medicines: A Guide for Health-care Professionals. London, UK: Pharmaceutical Press, 1996:296.
19. Bilko A, Altbacker V, Hudson R. Transmission of food preference in the rabbit: the means of information transfer. Physiol Behav 1994; 56:907–912.
20. Gruenwald J, Brendler T, Jaenicke C. PDR for Herbal Medicines. Montvale, NJ: Medical Economics Company, 1998.
21. Brinker F. Herb Contraindications and Drug Interactions, 2nd ed. Sandy, OR: Eclectic Medical Publications, 1998.
22. Wichtl M, Czygan FC, Frohne D et al. Herbal Drugs and Phytopharmaceuticals. Stuttgart, DE: Medpharm-CRC Press, 1994:566.
23. Schilcher H, Leuschner F. [The potential nephrotoxic effects of essential juniper oil]. Arzneimittelforschung 1997; 47:855–858.
24. Fenaroli's handbook for flavor ingredients, 2nd ed. Boca Raton: CRC Press, 1975.
25. Tyler VE. Herbs of choice. Binghamton, NY: Pharmaceutical Products Press, 1994.
26. Sanchez de Medina F, Gamez M, Jimenez I et al. Hypoglycemic activity of juniper 'berries'. Planta Medica 1994; 60:197–200.
27. Swanston-Flatt S, Day C, Bailey C, Flatt P. Traditional plant treatments for diabetes. Studies in normal and streptozotocin mice. Diabetologia 1990; 33:462–464.
28. Mascolo N, Autore G, Capasso G et al. Biological screening of Italian medicinal plants for anti-inflammatory activity. Phytother Res 1987; 1:28–31.

SAFETY SCALE

Pregnancy safety scale	Lactation safety scale
Safe	Safe
Caution	Caution
Unsafe	Unsafe
Unknown	Unknown

HERBAL MEDICINES

Herb	Pregnancy	Lactation
Aconite	Caution	Caution
Alfalfa	Caution	Caution
Aloe	Caution	Caution
Ashwaghanda	Caution	Unknown
Astragalus	Unknown	Unknown
Barberry	Unsafe	Unsafe
Black Cohosh	Caution	Caution
Blazing Star	Caution	Caution
Blue Cohosh	Unsafe	Caution
Borage	Unsafe	Safe
Calamus	Unsafe	Unsafe
Calendula	Caution	Unknown
Chastetree	Caution	Caution
Coffee	Caution	Caution
Cranberry	Safe	Unknown
Damiana	Caution	Unknown
Dandelion	Unknown	Unknown
Deadly nightshade	Unsafe	Caution
Dong quai	Caution	Unknown
Echinacea	Safe	Safe
Ephedra	Unsafe	Unsafe

Evening primrose	Evening primrose
False unicorn	False unicorn
Fennel	Fennel
Fenugreek	Fenugreek
Feverfew	Feverfew
Flax	Flax
Foxglove	Foxglove
Garlic	Garlic
Gentian	Gentian
Ginger	Ginger
Ginkgo	Ginkgo
Goldenseal	Goldenseal
Green tea	Green tea
Guggul	Guggul
Hawthorn	Hawthorn
Horsechestnut	Horsechestnut
Juniper	Juniper
Kava	Kava
Korean ginseng	Korean ginseng
Lemon balm	Lemon balm
Licorice	Licorice
Milk thistle	Milk thistle
Nettle	Nettle
Oregon grape	Oregon grape
Parsley	Parsley
Passionflower	Passionflower
Pennyroyal	Pennyroyal
Peppermint	Peppermint
Raspberry	Raspberry
Red clover	Red clover

SAFETY SCALE

Pregnancy safety scale	Lactation safety scale
Safe	Safe
Caution	Caution
Unsafe	Unsafe
Unknown	Unknown

HERBAL MEDICINES cont.

Rye ergot	Rye ergot
Senna	Senna
Siberian ginseng	Siberian ginseng
Squaw vine	Squaw vine
St John's wort	St John's wort
Turmeric	Turmeric
Valerian	Valerian
Wild yam	Wild yam
Yarrow	Yarrow

Contraindications

Existing liver disease[12]
Parkinson disease[12]
Existing pulmonary disease[12]

Caution

Avoid long-term use[12]
Avoid daily doses above 300 mg[12]
Operating heavy machinery[12]
Endogenous depression[10,13]

Constituents

Kavalactones (also called kavapyrones):[14,15] methysticin, dihydromethysticin (DMH), yangonin, dihydrokavain (DHK), kawain (kavalin)

Toxicity

- LD_{50} of kavalactones: approximately 300–400 mg/kg[16]
- LD_{50} (oral) of dihydrokavain: 920 mg/kg[16]
- LD_{50} (oral) of dihydromethysticin: 1050 mg/kg[16]
- LD_{50} of standardized kava extract (containing 70% kava lactones): 16 g/kg (oral, rats), 1.8 g/kg (oral, mice), 370 mg/kg (intraperitoneal, rats) and 380 mg/kg (intraperitoneal, mice)[17]
- Doses of 50 mg/kg of dihydrokavain three times a week for 3 months to rats produced no evidence of chronic toxicity[18]

Pharmacology

- People consuming kava have reported feeling more sociable, tranquil, and generally happy.[19]
- Kava's sedative effects may result from an increase in the number of γ-aminobutyric acid binding sites.[15,20,21]
- Kava's sedative effects may also result from dopamine antagonism, particularly by the vangonin constituent.[22–25]
- The kavapyrones methycystine and kavain may inhibit the uptake of noradrenaline, thereby contributing to the psychotropic actions of kava.[22]
- Kava has not been shown to affect benzodiazepine receptors.[26,27]
- Kava may affect the limbic system.[28]
- Kava appears to produce motor sedation without affecting respiratory processes.[29]
- Kava may cause muscle paralysis and numb the mouth through a mechanism similar to local anesthetics such as cocaine.[19,30]
- The kavapyrones desmethoxyyangonin and methysticin appear to competitively inhibit monoamine oxidase B.[31]
- Kava may inhibit enzymes in the cyclooxygenase-1 and -2 pathways.[32]
- The kavapyrone kavain inhibits cyclooxygenase and decreases the synthesis of thromboxane A2, thereby decreasing platelet aggregation.[33]

- Kava may affect the following cytochrome P450 enzymes: P450 2C19 (CYP2C19), P450 1A2 (CYP1A2), P450 2C9 (CYP2C9), P450 2D6 (CYP2D6), and P450 3A4 (CYP3A4)[34]

Drug interactions[1]

Alprazolam[35]
Anti-coagulant/anti-platelet drugs[33]
Central nervous system depressants[4,36]
Drugs metabolized by cytochrome P450 2C19 (CYP2C19), P450 1A2 (CYP1A2), P450 2C9 (CYP2C9), P450 2D6 (CYP2D6) and P450 3A4 (CYP3A4)[34]
Hepatotoxic drugs[5,37]
Levodopa (Larodopa, Dopar)[38]
Monoamine oxidase inhibitors[31]

Parts used[1]

Rhizome, root, and stem

References

1. Jellin JM, Batz F, Hitchens K. Natural Medicines Comprehensive Database, 3rd ed. Stockton, CA: Therapeutic Research Faculty, 2002:1530.
2. Pittler MH, Ernst E. Kava extract for treating anxiety. Cochrane Database Syst Rev 2002; CD003383.
3. Pittler MH, Ernst E. Kava extract for treating anxiety. Cochrane Database Syst Rev 2003; CD003383.
4. Pittler MH, Ernst E. Efficacy of kava extract for treating anxiety: systematic review and meta-analysis. J Clin Psychopharmacol 2000; 20:84–89.
5. Escher M, Desmeules J, Giostra E, Mentha G. Drug points: hepatitis associated with kava, a herbal remedy for anxiety. BMJ 2001; 322:139.
6. Teschke R, Gaus W, Loew D. Kava extracts: safety and risks including rare hepatotoxicity. Phytomedicine 2003; 10:440–446.
7. Schulze J, Raasch W, Siegers C. Toxicity of kava pyrones, drug safety and precautions – a case study. Phytomedicine 2003; 10(Suppl 4):68–73.
8. Russmann S, Lauterberg BH, Helbling A. Kava hepatotoxicity [letter]. Ann Intern Med 2001; 135:68.
9. Shaver K. Liver toxicity with kava. Pharmacist's Letter/Prescriber's Letter 2001; 18:180115.
10. Singh YN. Kava: an overview. J Ethnopharmacol 1992; 37:13–45.
11. Brinker F. The Toxicology of Botanical Medicines. Sandy, OR: Eclectic Medical Publications, 2000:296.
12. www.naturalstandard.com. Kava (Piper methysticum) Natural Standard Monograph, 2004.
13. Jamieson DD, Duffield PH, Cheng D, Duffield AM. Comparison of the central nervous system activity of the aqueous and lipid extract of kava (Piper methysticum). Arch Int Pharmacodyn Ther 1989; 301:66–80.
14. Garner LF, Klinger JD. Some visual effects caused by the beverage kava. J Ethnopharmacol 1985; 13:307–311.

15. Baum SS, Hill R, Rommelspacher H. Effect of kava extract and individual kavapyrones on neurotransmitter levels in the nucleus accumbens of rats. Prog Neuropsychopharmacol Biol Psychiatry 1998; 22:1105–1120.
16. Meyer HJ. [Pharmacology of the active priciples of kavaroot (Piper methysticum Forst)]. Arch Int Pharmacodyn Ther 1962; 138:505–536.
17. Hansel R, Woelk H. Spektrum Kava-kava. Arzneimitteltherapie heute: Phytopharmaka; Bd. 6. Aesopus Verlag: Basel, 1994:40.
18. Meyer HJ. Postdoctoral thesis: Pharmakologie der Kawa-Droge. Freiburg: Pharmakologie Institut der Albert-Ludwig Universitat, 1966.
19. Pierce A. The American Pharmaceutical Association Practical Guide to Natural Medicines. New York, NY: The Stonesong Press, 1999:19.
20. Jussofie A, Schmiz A, Hiemke C. Kavapyrone enriched extract from Piper methysticum as modulator of the GABA binding site in different regions of rat brain. Psychopharmacology 1994; 116:469–474.
21. Boonen G, Pramanik A, Rigler R, Haberlein H. Evidence for specific interactions between kavain and human cortical neurons monitored by fluorescence correlation spectroscopy. Planta Med 2000; 66:7–10.
22. Seitz U, Schule A, Gleitz J. [3H]-monoamine uptake inhibititon properties of kava pyrones. Planta Med 1997; 63:548–549.
23. Schelosky L, Raffaup C, Jendroska K, Poewe W. Kava and dopamine antagonism. J Neurol Neurosurg Psychiatry 1995; 58:639–640.
24. Meseguer E, Taboada R, Sanchez V et al. Life-threatening parkinsonism induced by kava-kava. Mov Disord 2002; 17:195–196.
25. Bilia AR, Gallori S, Vincieri FF. Kava-kava and anxiety: growing knowledge about the efficacy and safety. Life Sci 2002; 70:2581–2597.
26. Pizzorno JE, Murray MT. Textbook of Natural Medicine, 2nd ed. Edinburgh: Churchill Livingstone, 1999.
27. Davies LP, Drew CA, Duffield P et al. Kava pyrones and resin: studies on GABA-A, GABA-B, and benzodiazepine binding sites in rodent brain. Pharmacol Toxicol 1992; 71:120–126.
28. Fetrow CW, Avala JR. Professional's Handbook of Complementary and Alternative Medicines: Springhouse Corporation, 1999.
29. Lehmann E, Kinzler E, Friedemann J. Efficacy of a special Kava extract (Piper methysticum) in patients with states of anxiety, tension and excitedness of non-mental origin: a double-blind placebo-controlled study of four weeks treatment. Phytomedicine 1996; 3:113–119.
30. Singh YN. Effects of kava on neuromuscular transmission and muscle contractility. J Ethnopharmacol 1983; 7:267–276.
31. Uebelhack R, Franke L, Schewe HJ. Inhibition of platelet MAO-B by kava pyrone-enriched extract from Piper methysticum Forster (kava-kava). Pharmacopsychiatry 1998; 31:187–192.
32. Wu D, Yu L, Nair MG et al. Cyclooxygenase enzyme inhibitory compounds with antioxidant activities from Piper methysticum (kava kava) roots. Phytomedicine 2002; 9:41–47.
33. Gleitz J, Beile A, Wilkens P et al. Antithrombotic action of the kava pyrone (+)-kavain prepared from Piper methysticum on human platelets. Planta Med 1997; 63:27–30.

34. Mathews JM, Etheridge AS, Black SR. Inhibition of human cytochrome P450 activities by kava extract and kavalactones. Drug Metab Dispos 2002; 30:1153–1157.
35. Almeida JC, Grimsley EW. Coma from the health food store: interaction between kava and alprazolam. Ann Intern Med 1996; 125:940–941.
36. Munte TF, Heinze HJ, Matzke M, Steitz J. Effects of oxazepam and an extract of kava roots (Piper methysticum) on event-related potentials in a word recognition task. Neuropsychobiology 1993; 27:46–53.
37. Russmann S, Lauterberg BH, Hebling A. Kava hepatotoxicity [letter]. Ann Intern Med 2001; 135:68.
38. Brinker F. Herb Contraindications and Drug Interactions, 2nd ed. Sandy, OR: Eclectic Medical Publications, 1998.

KOREAN GINSENG

Panax ginseng, P. schinseng

Synonyms/common names/related substances[1]

Asian ginseng, Asiatic ginseng, Chinese ginseng, ginseng, ginseng asiatique, *Ginseng radix*, ginseng root, guigai, hong shen, Japanese ginseng, jen-shen, jinsao, jintsam, insam, Korean ginseng, Korean panax ginseng, Korean red ginseng, ninjin, Oriental ginseng, *Panax ginseng*, *Radix ginseng rubra*, red ginseng, ren shen, renshen, renxian, sang, seng, sheng shai shen, white ginseng

Indications

Erectile dysfunction:[2]	Evidence grade B1
Premature ejaculation:[3]	Evidence grade B1
Type 2 diabetes:[4]	Evidence grade B1
Improves memory (with *Ginkgo biloba*):[5,6]	Evidence grade B1
Potentiates against influenza and the common cold (with influenza vaccine):[7]	Evidence grade B1
Improves cognitive function:[8]	Evidence grade B2
Chronic bronchitis (with antibiotics):[9]	Evidence grade C
Cancer prevention:[10,11]	Evidence grade C

Pregnancy

Conflicting evidence

Non-estrogenic:[12]	Evidence level 1a
Estrogenic:[13]	Evidence level 2

A randomized controlled trial of 384 women receiving either ginseng extract or placebo for 16 weeks showed that the beneficial effects in the treatment of menopause are most likely not mediated by hormone replacement-like effects, as physiologic parameters such as follicle-stimulating hormone and estradiol levels, endometrial thickness, maturity index, and vaginal pH were not affected by the treatment.[12]

On the other hand, there are case reports and animal studies of estrogenic activity, postmenopausal vaginal bleeding, and increased serum ceruloplasmin oxidase activity and that ginsenoside Rb1 acts as a phytoestrogen.[14–20] A review article on the potential value of plants as sources of anti-fertility agents also reported that Korean ginseng has estrogenic activity.[13]

Minimal risk:[21]	Evidence level 1b

Treatment of intrauterine growth retardation:[21]	Evidence level 1b

A comparison study on pregnant women with intrauterine growth retardation was conducted where one group of women received Korean ginseng while the other group acted as controls.[21] The height of fundus, fetal diparietal diameter, urinary estrogens/creatinine, serum human placental lactogen, and neonatal weights approached normal pregnancy values.[21] The authors did not report any adverse effects associated with ginseng supplementation.[21]

No evidence to support androgenization:[22,23]	Evidence level 2

A case was reported of a 30-year-old woman who gave birth to a full-term baby boy with signs of androgenization following ingestion of 'ginseng' during her pregnancy.[23] After further investigation, the herbal preparation used by the mother appeared to be adultered by the herb silk vine (*Periploca sepium*) and not Siberian ginseng (*Eleutherococcus senticosus*).[22]

Protects neonatal brain against ethanol damage:[24]	Evidence level 3

A study reported that ginseng extract prevented ethanol-induced reduction of neonatal brain weight in rats.[24] The ginseng saponins, including ginsenosides Rg1, Rb2, Rd, Rf, and Re, were shown to stimulate a potent recovery of cerebellum growth.[24]

Teratogenic:[25]	Evidence level 3

A study on organogenesis found that ginsenosides exert direct teratogenic effects on rat embryos.[25]

Activates DNA polymerase delta in placenta:[26]	Evidence level 3

Ginsenosides from *P. ginseng* were found to activate DNA polymerase delta in bovine placenta.[26]

May cause neonatal death:[27]	Evidence level 4

An evidence-based natural product compendium reported that there is one report of neonatal death following use of *P. ginseng*.[27] There were no reports in the scientific literature of *P. ginseng* causing neonatal death.

Traditionally used during pregnancy:[28]	Evidence level 4

Researchers conducted a review of the herbs used during pregnancy in Singapore.[28] Korean ginseng was used in various combinations and in various amounts in herbal prescriptions during pregnancy.[28] The researchers could not confirm that the claims made by Chinese herbalists on the efficacy of Korean ginseng in pregnancy were substantiated.[28] They concluded that there is no specific effect on the pregnant woman, but that it does not exclude the possibility of a beneficial psychosomatic effect.[28] The researchers also noted that the active principles can cross the placenta and reach the fetus.[28] The authors did not discuss if Korean ginseng was safe or contraindicated during pregnancy.[28]

Lactation

Minimal risk:[29–31]	Evidence level 3

Cows with subclinical mastitis caused by *Staphylococcus aureus* were subjected to subcutaneous injections with an extract from the root of Korean ginseng.[29] Based on blood leukocyte measurements, ginseng treatment was found to activate the innate immunity of cows and contribute to the cow's recovery from mastitis.[29] The authors did not report any adverse effects associated with the use of Korean ginseng during lactation.[29] Two other studies by the same authors conducted in lactating cows found similar results where Korean ginseng increased leukocyte activity and no adverse effects were reported.[30,31]

Constituents

Triterpenoid saponins:[32] ginsenosides (Rg1, Rb1)
Polyacetylenic constituents:[32] panaxynol, panaxydol, panaxytriol
Panaxagin[33]
Essential oil[34]
Phytosterol[34]
Pectin[35]
B vitamins[35]
Flavonoids[35]

Toxicity

Very low incidence of toxicity has been observed in ginseng clinical trials using well-characterized preparations.[36]

Pharmacology

- Ginseng is frequently used as a general tonic, adaptogen and restorative due to its anti-fatigue, immunologic, and hormonal qualities.[23]
- Ginsenosides increase serum cortisol levels, stimulate adrenal function, and, in women, increase dehydroepiandrosterone sulfate.[37–40]
- Ginsenoside Rb1 lowers blood pressure and acts as a central nervous system depressant.[35]
- Ginsenosides interfere with platelet aggregation and coagulation.[41]

- Ginsenosides have analgesic and anti-inflammatory effects.[42]
- Ginsenosides potentiate nerve growth factor and may have a neuroprotective effect through nicotinic activity.[35,43]
- Ginsenosides have anti-asthmatic effects through the relaxation of human bronchial smooth muscle by stimulating the release of nitrous oxide from airway epithelium.[44]
- *P. ginseng* has anti-tumor activity.[11,32,45] The polyacetylenic constituent panaxydol seems to have anti-proliferative effects on various types of cancer cell.[32]
- *P. ginseng* has shown inhibitory activity on *Helicobacter pylori*.[46]
- *P. ginseng* promotes the growth of normal intestinal flora while inhibiting clostridial species.[47]
- *P. ginseng* may lower cholesterol and triglycerides.[42]
- *P. ginseng* may prevent insulin resistance and change gene expression in type 2 diabetes.[48]
- There is conflicting evidence on whether or not *P. ginseng* has estrogenic activity.[12,14–20]
- The protein isolate panaxagin may have anti-viral and anti-fungal activity where it appears to inhibit human immunodeficiency virus reverse transcriptase and ribosomal activity of some fungi.[33]
- *P. ginseng* may mildly inhibit cytochrome P450.[49]
- *P. ginseng* increases penile vibratory threshold and reduces the amplitude of penile somatosensory evoked potentials.

Drug interactions

Anti-coagulant/anti-platelet agents[50,51]
Anti-diabetic drugs[4]
Anti-psychotic drugs[52]
Caffeine[53]
Furosemide[54]
Immunosuppressants[11]
Insulin[53]
Monoamine oxidase inhibitors[55,56]
Stimulant drugs[57]
Warfarin (Coumadin)[50,51,58]
Drugs metabolized by cytochrome P450 enzymes[49]

Part used

Root[1]

References

1. Jellin JM, Batz F, Hitchens K. Natural Medicines Comprehensive Database, 3rd ed. Stockton, CA: Therapeutic Research Faculty, 2002:1530.
2. Hong B, Ji YH, Hong J, Nam KY, Ahn TY. A double-blind crossover study evaluating the efficacy of korean red ginseng in patients with erectile dysfunction: a preliminary report. J Urol 2002; 168:2070–2073.
3. Choi HK, Jung GW, Moon KH et al. Clinical study of SS-Cream in patients with lifelong premature ejaculation. Urology 2000; 55:257–261.
4. Sotaniemi EA, Haapakoski E, Rautio A. Ginseng therapy in non-insulin dependent diabetic patients. Diabetes Care 1993; 16:8–15 1995; 18:1373–1375.
5. Wesnes KA, Ward T, McGinty A, Petrini O. The memory enhancing effects of a Ginkgo biloba/Panax ginseng combination in healthy middle-aged volunteers. Psychopharmacology (Berl) 2000; 152:353–361.
6. Scholey AB, Kennedy DO. Acute, dose-dependent cognitive effects of Ginkgo biloba, Panax ginseng and their combination in healthy young volunteers: differential interactions with cognitive demand. Hum Psychopharmacol 2002; 17:35–44.
7. Scaglione F, Cattaneo G, Alessandria M, Cogo R. Efficacy and safety of the standardised Ginseng extract G115 for potentiating vaccination against the influenza syndrome and protection against the common cold [corrected]. Drugs Exp Clin Res 1996; 22:65–72.
8. Sorensen H, Sonne JA. A double-masked study of the effects of ginseng on cognitive functions. Curr Ther Res Clin Exp 1996; 57:959–968.
9. Scaglione F, Weiser K, Alessandria M. Effects of the standardized ginseng extract G115 (Reg.) in patients with chronic bronchitis: a nonblinded, randomized, comparative pilot study. Clin Drug Invest 2001; 21:41–45.
10. Yun TK, Soi Y. Non-organ specific cancer prevention of ginseng: a prospective study in Korea. Int J Epidemiol 1998; 27:359–364.
11. Shin HR, Kim JY, Yun TK et al. The cancer-preventive potential of Panax ginseng: a review of human and experimental evidence. Cancer Causes Control 2000; 11:565–576.
12. Wiklund IK, Mattsson LA, Lindgren R et al. Effects of a standardized ginseng extract on quality of life and physiological parameters in symptomatic postmenopausal women: a double-blind, placebo-controlled trial. Int J Clin Pharmacol Res 1999; 19:89–99.
13. Farnsworth NR, Bingel AS, Cordell GA, Crane FA, Fong HH. Potential value of plants as sources of new antifertility agents II. J Pharm Sci 1975; 64:717–753.
14. Palmer BV, Montgomery AC, Monteiro JC et al. Gin Seng and mastalgia [letter]. BMJ 1978; 1:1284.
15. Hopkins MP, Androff L, Benninghoff AS. Ginseng face cream and unexplained vaginal bleeding. Am J Obstet Gynecol 1988; 159:1121–1122.
16. Greenspan EM. Ginseng and vaginal bleeding [letter]. JAMA 1983; 249:2018.
17. Hammond TG, Whitworth JA. Adverse reactions to ginseng [letter]. Med J Aust 1981; 1:492.
18. Punnonen R, Lukola A. Oestrogen-like effect of ginseng. Br Med J 1980; 281:1110.
19. Eagon PK, Elm MS, Hunter DS et al. Medicinal herbs: modulation of estrogen action, Era of Hope Mtg, Dept Defense, Atlanta, GA, Jun 8–11, 2000. Breast Cancer Res Prog.
20. Lee YJ, Jin YR, Lim WC et al. Ginsenoside-Rb1 acts as a weak phytoestrogen in MCF-7 human breast cancer cells. Arch Pharm Res 2003; 26:58–63.

21. Zhang WY, Teng H, Zheng Y. [Ginseng saponin treatment for intrauterine growth retardation]. Zhonghua Yi Xue Za Zhi 1994; 74:608–610, 646.
22. Awang DV. Maternal use of ginseng and neonatal androgenization. JAMA 1991; 266:363.
23. Koren G, Randor S, Martin S, Danneman D. Maternal ginseng use associated with neonatal androgenization. JAMA 1990; 264:2866.
24. Okamura N, Kobayashi K, Akaike A, Yagi A. Protective effect of ginseng saponins against impaired brain growth in neonatal rats exposed to ethanol. Biol Pharm Bull 1994; 17: 270–274.
25. Chan LY, Chiu PY, Lau T. An in-vitro study of ginsenoside Rb1-induced teratogenicity using a whole rat embryo culture model. Hum Reprod 2003; 18:2166–2168.
26. Cho SW, Cho EH, Choi S. Ginsenosides activate DNA polymerase delta from bovine placenta. Life Sci 1995; 57:1359–1365.
27. www.naturalstandard.com. Panax Ginseng, 2004.
28. Wong HB. Effects of herbs and drugs during pregnancy and lactation. J Singapore Paediatr Soc 1979; 21(3–4):169–178.
29. Hu S, Concha C, Johannisson A, Meglia G, Waller KP. Effect of subcutaneous injection of ginseng on cows with subclinical Staphylococcus aureus mastitis. J Vet Med B Infect Dis Vet Public Health 2001; 48:519–528.
30. Concha C, Hu S, Holmberg O. The proliferative responses of cow stripping milk and blood lymphocytes to pokeweed mitogen and ginseng in vitro. Vet Res 1996; 27:107–115.
31. Hu S, Concha C, Cooray R, Holmberg O. Ginseng-enhanced oxidative and phagocytic activities of polymorphonuclear leucocytes from bovine peripheral blood and stripping milk. Vet Res 1995; 26:155–161.
32. Moon J, Yu SJ, Kim HS, Sohn J. Induction of G cell cycle arrest and p27(KIP1) increase by panaxydol isolated from Panax ginseng. Biochem Pharmacol 2000; 59:1109–1116.
33. Ng TB, Wang H. Panaxagin, a new protein from Chinese ginseng possesses antifungal, anti-viral, translation-inhibiting and ribonuclease activities. Life Sci 2001; 68:739–749.
34. Foster S. Panax ginseng. American Botanical Council, 1996.
35. Leung AY, Foster S. Encyclopedia of Common Natural Ingredients Used in Food, Drugs and Cosmetics, 2nd ed. New York, NY: John Wiley & Sons, 1996:649.
36. Chang YS, Seo EK, Gyllenhaal C, Block KI. Panax ginseng: a role in cancer therapy? Integr Cancer Ther 2003; 2:13–33.
37. Tode T, Kikuchi Y, Hirata J et al. Effect of Korean red ginseng on psychological functions in patients with severe climacteric syndromes. Int J Gynaecol Obstet 1999; 67:169–174.
38. Hiai S, Yokoyama H, Oura H et al. Stimulation of pituitary-adrenocortical system by ginseng saponin. Endocrinol Jpn 1979; 26:661–665.
39. Kase Y, Saitoh K, Ishige A et al. Mechanisms by which Hange-shashin-to reduces prostaglandin E2 levels. Biol Pharm Bull 1998; 21:1277–1281.
40. Robbers JE, Speedie MK, Tyler VE. Pharmacognosy and Pharmacobiotechnology. Baltimore, MD: Williams & Wilkins, 1996.
41. Park HJ, Lee JH, Song YB, Park KH. Effects of dietary supplementation of lipophilic fraction from Panax ginseng on cGMP and cAMP in rat platelets and on blood coagulation. Biol Pharm Bull 1996; 19:1434–1439.

42. The Review of Natural Products by Facts and Comparisons. St. Louis, MO: Wolters Kluwer Co., 1999.
43. Lewis R, Wake G, Court G et al. Non-ginsenoside nicotinic activity in ginseng species. Phytother Res 1999; 13:59–64.
44. Tamaoki J, Nakata J, Kawatani K. Ginsenoside-induced relaxation of human bronchial smooth muscle via release of nitric oxide. Br J Pharmacol 2000; 130:1859–1864.
45. Keum YS, Park KK, Lee JM et al. Antioxidant and anti-tumor promoting activities of the methanol extract of heat-processed ginseng. Cancer Lett 2000; 150:41–48.
46. Belogortseva NI, Yoon JY, Kim KH. Inhibition of Helicobacter pylori hemagglutination by polysaccharide fractions from roots of Panax ginseng. Planta Med 2000; 66:217–220.
47. Schulz V, Hansel R, Tyler VE, Terry C. Rational Phytotherapy: A Physician's Guide to Herbal Medicine, 3rd ed. Berlin: Springer, 1998.
48. Pan SJ, Ding Z, Ivy JL. Ginseng's effects on glucose tolerance and mRNA profiles in a animal model of Type II diabetes. Alt Ther 2001; 7:S26.
49. Gurley BJ, Gardner SF, Hubbard MA. Clinical assessment of potential cytochrome P450-mediated herb-drug interactions. AAPS Annual Meeting & Expo, Indianapolis, IN, 29 Oct–2 Nov, 2000.
50. Janetzky K, Morreale AP. Probable interaction between warfarin and ginseng. Am J Health Syst Pharm 1997; 54:692–693.
51. Cheng TO. Ginseng-warfarin interaction. ACC Curr J Rev 2000; 9:84.
52. Newall CA, Anderson LA, Phillipson JD. Herbal Medicines: A Guide for Health-care Professionals. London, UK: Pharmaceutical Press, 1996:296.
53. Brinker F. Herb Contraindications and Drug Interactions, 2nd ed. Sandy, OR: Eclectic Medical Publications, 1998.
54. Becker BN. Ginseng-induced diuretic resistance. JAMA 1996; 276:606–607.
55. Shader RI, Greenblatt DJ. Phenylzine and the dream machine-ramblings and reflections. J Clin Psychopharmacol 1985; 5:65.
56. Jones BD, Runikis AM. Interaction of ginseng with phenelzine. J Clin Psychopharmacol 1987; 7:201–202.
57. McGuffin M, Hobbs C, Upton R, Goldberg A. American Herbal Products Association's Botanical Safety Handbook. Boca Raton, FL: CRC Press, 1997:231.
58. Zhu M, Chan KW, Ng LS et al. Possible influences of ginseng on the pharmacodynamics of warfarin in rats. J Pharm Pharmacol 1999; 51:175–180.

LEMON BALM
Melissa officinalis

Synonyms/common names/related compounds[1]

Balm, cure-all, dropsy plant, honey plant, melissa, *Melissae folium*, melissenblatt, sweet balm, sweet mary

Indications

Lemon balm extract

Mild to moderate Alzheimer disease:[2–4]	Evidence grade B1
Cold sores (herpes labialis):[5,6]	Evidence grade B2
Sleep quality and quantity:[7]	Evidence grade B2
Dyspepsia (with bitter candy tuft, chamomile flower, peppermint leaves, caraway fruit, licorice root, angelica root, celandine herbs, and milk thistle fruit):[8]	Evidence grade B2
Chronic colitis (with *Taraxacum officinale*, *Hypericum perforatum*, *Calendula officinalis*, and *Foeniculum vulgare*):[9]	Evidence grade C
Anti-ulcerogenic:[10]	Evidence grade E

Oil

Severe dementia:[11]	Evidence grade B1

Pregnancy

Emmenagogue:[12]	Evidence level 4
Hormonal changes:[13]	Evidence level 4

A review article on the potential value of plants as sources of anti-fertility agents reported that lemon balm was an emmenagogue.[12] A herbal toxicology and drug interaction compendium reported that lemon balm causes hormonal changes.[13]

Anti-gonadotrophic activity:[12]	Evidence level 4

A review article on the potential value of plants as sources of anti-fertility agents reported that lemon balm had anti-gonadotrophic activity in rats.[12]

Lactation

Hormonal changes:[13]	Evidence level 4

A herbal toxicology and drug interaction compendium reported that lemon balm causes hormonal changes.[13] There are no reports in the scientific literature of lemon balm being either safe or contraindicated during lactation.

Constituents

- Monoterpenoid aldehydes:[1] citronellal, neral, and geranial
- Polyphenolic compounds:[14] rosmarinic acid
- Flavonoids:[15] luteolin 3′-O-β-D-glucuronide

Pharmacology

- Lemon balm induces a calming effect and reduces alertness.[16]
- In vitro lemon balm extracts have cholinergic binding properties and may effectively ameliorate the cognitive deficits associated with Alzheimer disease.[16]
- Lemon balm may have nicotinic and muscarinic binding properties.[16]
- The terpenes in the essential oil of lemon balm are rapidly absorbed through the lungs and cross the blood–brain barrier, and may have cholinergic activity or act on γ-aminobutyric acid receptor.[17]
- Lemon balm was shown to have anti-herpes simplex 1 activity and antiviral effects.[18–20]
- Lemon balm was shown to have anti-human immunodeficiency virus-1 activity.[21]
- Rosmarinic acid may have anti-thyroid effects.[22]
- Rosmarinic acid may have anti-inflammatory activity through its inhibitory effects on complement C3-convertase.[14]
- Lemon balm was shown to have protective effects against enzyme-dependent and -independent lipid peroxidation.[23]

Drug interactions[1]

Barbiturates[16]
Sedative drugs[16]
Thyroid hormone[22]

Parts used[1]

Leaf oil

References

1. Jellin JM, Batz F, Hitchens K. Natural Medicines Comprehensive Database, 3rd ed. Stockton, CA: Therapeutic Research Faculty, 2002:1530.
2. Akhondzadeh S, Noroozian M, Mohammadi M et al. Melissa officinalis extract in the treatment of patients with mild to moderate Alzheimer's disease: a double blind, randomised, placebo controlled trial. J Neurol Neurosurg Psychiatry 2003; 74:863–866.

3. Kennedy DO, Scholey AB, Tildesley N, Perry EK, Wesnes KA. Modulation of mood and cognitive performance following acute administration of Melissa officinalis (lemon balm). Pharmacol Biochem Behav 2002; 72:953–964.
4. Kennedy DO, Wake G, Saveley S et al. Modulation of mood and cognitive performance following acute administration of single doses of Melissa officinalis (Lemon balm) with human CNS nicotinic and muscarinic receptor-binding properties. Neuropsychopharmacology 2003; 28:1871–1881.
5. Wolbling RH, Leonhardt K. Local therapy of herpes simplex with dried extract from Melissa officinalis. Phytomedicine 1994;1:25–31.
6. Koytchev R, Alken RG, Dundarov S. Balm mint extract (Lo-701) for topical treatment of recurring herpes labialis. Phytomedicine 1999; 6:225–230.
7. Cerny A, Schmid K. Tolerability and efficacy of valerian/lemon balm in healthy volunteers (a double blind, placebo-controlled, multicentre study). Fitoterapia 1999; 70:221–228.
8. Madisch A, Melderis H, Mayr G, Sassin I, Hotz J. [A plant extract and its modified preparation in functional dyspepsia. Results of a double-blind placebo controlled comparative study]. Z Gastroenterol 2001; 39:511–517.
9. Chakurski I, Matev M, Koichev A, Angelova I, Stefanov G. [Treatment of chronic colitis with an herbal combination of Taraxacum officinale, Hipericum perforatum, Melissa officinaliss, Calendula officinalis and Foeniculum vulgare]. Vutr Boles 1981; 20:51–54.
10. Khayyal MT, el-Ghazaly MA, Kenawy S et al. Antiulcerogenic effect of some gastrointestinally acting plant extracts and their combination. Arzneimittelforschung 2001; 51:545–553.
11. Ballard CG, O'Brien JT, Reichelt K, Perry EK. Aromatherapy as a safe and effective treatment for the management of agitation in severe dementia: the results of a double-blind, placebo-controlled trial with Melissa. J Clin Psychiatry 2002; 63:553–558.
12. Farnsworth NR, Bingel AS, Cordell G, Crane FA, Fong HH. Potential value of plants as sources of new antifertility agents I. J Pharm Sci 1975; 64:535–598.
13. Brinker F. Herb Contraindications and Drug Interactions. Sandy, OR: Eclectic Institute, 1997:146.
14. Englberger W, Hadding U, Etschenberg E et al. Rosmarinic acid: a new inhibitor of complement C3-convertase with anti-inflammatory activity. Int J Immunopharmacol 1988; 10:729–737.
15. Heitz A, Carnat A, Fraisse D, Carnat AP, Lamaison JL. Luteolin 3′-glucuronide, the major flavonoid from Melissa officinalis subsp. officinalis. Fitoterapia 2000; 71:201–202.
16. Kennedy DO, Scholey AB, Tildesley NT et al. Modulation of mood and cognitive performance following acute administration of Melissa officinalis (lemon balm). Pharmacol Biochem Behav 2002; 72:953–964.
17. Burns A, Byrne J, Ballard C, Holmes C. Sensory stimulation in dementia. BMJ 2002; 325:1312–1313.
18. Dimitrova Z, Dimov B, Manolova N et al. Antiherpes effect of Melissa officinalis L. extracts. Acta Microbiol Bulg 1993; 29:65–72.
19. Kucera LS, Herrmann E Jr. Antiviral substances in plants of the mint family (labiatae). I. Tannin of Melissa officinalis. Proc Soc Exp Biol Med 1967; 124:865–869.
20. May G, Willuhn G. [Antiviral effect of aqueous plant extracts in tissue culture]. Arzneimittelforschung 1978; 28:1–7.

21. Yamasaki K, Nakano M, Kawahata T et al. Anti-HIV-1 activity of herbs in Labiatae. Biol Pharm Bull 1998; 21:829–833.
22. Dr. Duke's Phytochemical and Ethnobotanical Databases. www.ars-grin.gov/cgi-bin/duke/farmacy.2pl
23. Hohmann J, Zupko I, Redei D et al. Protective effects of the aerial parts of Salvia officinalis, Melissa officinalis and Lavandula angustifolia and their constituents against enzyme-dependent and enzyme-independent lipid peroxidation. Planta Med 1999; 65:576–578.

LICORICE
Glycyrrhiza glabra

Synonyms/common names/related compounds[1]

Alcacuz, alcazuz, Chinese licorice, gan cao, gan zao, glycyrrhiza, *G. glabra typica*, *G. glabra violacea*, isoflavone, isoflavones, jethi-madh, mulhathi, lakritze, licorice root, *Liquiritiae radix*, liquirizia, liquorice, orozuz, phytoestrogen, reglisse, regliz, Russian licorice, Spanish licorice, subholz, sweet root, yashti-madhu, yashti-madhu, yashti-madhuka

Indications

Indigestion (with bitter candy, chamomile, peppermint, caraway, lemon balm, angelica, celandine, milk thistle):[2]	Evidence grade B2
Idiopathic thrombocytopenic purpura (with corticosteroids):[3]	Evidence grade B2
Hepatitis C:[4–6]	Evidence grade B2
Familial Mediterranean fever (with andrographis, Siberian ginseng, schizandra):[7]	Evidence grade B2
Hemophiliacs with HIV-1:[8]	Evidence grade C
Viral hepatitis:[9–12]	Evidence grade C
Viral hepatitis (with interferon):[13,14]	Evidence grade C
Oral lichen planus:[15]	Evidence grade C
Dental plaque:[16]	Evidence grade C
Hyperkalemia:[17]	Evidence grade C
Herpes zoster:[18]	Evidence grade D
Psoriasis (with *Tripterygium wilfordii* and erythromycia):[19]	Evidence grade D

Deglycyrrhizinated licorice (DGL)

Aphthous ulcers:[20]	Evidence grade C
Gastric and duodenal ulcers:[21–23]	Evidence grade E

Gastric mucosal damage by acetyl salicylic acid (aspirin):[24]	Evidence grade E

Pregnancy

Likely to be born before 38 weeks' gestation:[25]	Evidence level 1b
Risk of pre-term pregnancy (before 37 weeks):[26]	Evidence level 1b
Does not affect birthweight:[25]	Evidence level 1b
Does not affect maternal blood pressure:[25]	Evidence level 1b

A study of 1049 Finnish women found babies with heavy exposure to glycyrrhizin were significantly more likely to be born earlier.[25] The odds ratio for being born before 38 weeks' gestation was 2.[5,25] It was also reported that heavy glycyrrhizin exposure during pregnancy did not significantly affect birthweight or maternal blood pressure.[25] Another study of 95 women found that heavy consumption of glycyrrhizin was associated with a more than twofold increased risk of pre-term (<37 weeks) delivery.[26]

Minimal risk:[27]	Evidence level 1c

A study published 110 case reports on the use of glycyrrhizin injections for the treatment of viral hepatitis during pregnancy.[27] No adverse effects were reported.[27]

Estrogenic:[28,29]	Evidence level 3

The constituent glabridin was shown to have varying degrees of estrogen receptor agonism in different tests and demonstrated growth-inhibitory actions on human breast cancer cells.[28] A review article on the potential value of plants as sources of anti-fertility agents reported that licorice has estrogenic activity.[29]

Potential abortifacient:[30]	Evidence level 4
Emmenagogue:[30]	Evidence level 4
Uterine stimulant:[30]	Evidence level 4

A review article on the potential value of plants as sources of anti-fertility agents reported that licorice was a potential abortifacient, emmenagogue, and uterine stimulant.[31]

Causes high prolactin and estrogen levels:[31,32]	Evidence level 4

An evidence-based herbal monograph reported that licorice causes high prolactin levels and high estrogen levels in women.[31,32]

DGL

Unknown:	Evidence level 5

It is unknown if the removal of the glycyrrhizin constituent in licorice makes DGL safe during pregnancy. There are no reports in the literature of DGL being either safe or contraindicated during pregnancy.

Lactation

Hormonal effects:[31,32]	Evidence level 4

An evidence-based herbal monograph reported that licorice causes high prolactin levels and high estrogen levels in women.[31,32] There are no reports in the scientific literature of licorice being either safe or contraindicated during lactation.

DGL

Unknown:	Evidence level 5

It is unknown if the removal of the glycyrrhizin constituent in licorice makes DGL safe during lactation. There are no reports in the scientific literature of DGL being either safe or contraindicated during lactation.

Contraindications

Long-term use[32]
Hypertension[32]
Hypokalemia[32]
Cardiovascular disease[32]
Diabetes[32]
Liver disorders (cholestasis, chronic hepatitis, cirrhosis)[32]
Severe kidney insufficiency[32]

Constituents[33]

- Triterpenoid saponins:[34–40] glycyrrhizin (glycyrrhizic acid), glycyrrhetinic acid (18-β-glycyrrhetinic acid)
- Flavonoids:[34,41] liquiritin, chalcones, and isoflavonoids
- Sterols[36]

Toxicity

No significant changes were observed in rats fed 100–1000 mg/kg per day for 1 year (intragastric route).[42]

Glycyrrhizin

Long-term administration of glycyrrhizin did not induce tumors in mice.[43]

Glycyrrhetinic acid

- In rats, oral consumption of glycyrrhetinic acid caused an increase in right atrial pressure and thickening of the pulmonary vessels, suggesting pulmonary hypertension.[44]
- Patients with previous breast cancer given doses of 0.02–0.03 mmol/kg of glycyrrhetinic acid experienced hypertension or hypokalemia, which required dose reduction or discontinuance.[45]

Pharmacology

- Glycyrrhizin contributes to the mineralocorticoid effects of licorice, such as hypertension and hypokalemia, by binding directly to mineralocorticoid receptors and by decreasing the conversion of active cortisol to inactive cortisone.[46–50]
- The constituents glycyrrhizin and glycyrrhetinic acid inhibit the enzyme 11-β-hydroxysteroid dehydrogenase, which is located in the aldosterone receptor cells of the cortical collecting duct.[46,51]
- Licorice blocks the metabolism of prostaglandins E and F2 α, which may have a preventive effect on nonsteroidal anti-inflammatory drug-induced damage to the gastrointestinal mucosa.[52]
- Licorice appears to have anti-estrogenic and estrogenic activity, where the constituent glabridin has estrogenic activity at low concentrations and anti-estrogenic activity at high concentrations.[28]
- Licorice does not appear to stimulate the growth of estrogen-dependent breast cancer cells.[53]
- Intravenous preparations of glycyrrhizin and glycyrrhizic acid were shown to have activity against hepatitis B and C in humans.[13,14,54]
- Licorice may decrease testosterone production in young healthy men.[55]
- Licorice may reduce body fat but the accompanying fluid retention offsets any change in body weight.[56]

DGL

DGL may accelerate the healing of gastric and duodenal ulcer disease.[21–23]

Drug interactions[1]

Anti-hypertensive drugs[57]
Corticosteroids[52,58]
Drugs metabolized by cytochrome P450 3A4 and P450 2B6[59,60]
Digoxin[52]
Potassium-depleting diuretic drugs[58]
Estrogens[51]
Ethacrynic acid[61]
Furosemide[61]
Insulin[52]

Part used

Root

References

1. Jellin JM, Batz F, Hitchens K. Natural Medicines Comprehensive Database, 3rd ed. Stockton, CA: Therapeutic Research Faculty, 2002:1530.
2. Madisch A, Melderis H, Mayr G, Sassin I, Hotz J. [A plant extract and its modified preparation in functional dyspepsia. Results of a double-blind placebo controlled comparative study]. Z Gastroenterol 2001; 39:511–517.
3. Luo YG, Liu YQ, Hu J. Clinical study on effect of recombinant roasted licorice decoction combined with low-dose glucocorticoids in treating idiopathic thrombocytopenic purpura. Zhongguo Zhong Xi Yi Jie He Za Zhi Zhongguo Zhongxiyi Jiehe Zazhi 2001; Jul 21:501–503.
4. Van Rossum TGJ, De Jong FH, Hop W, Boomsma F, Schalm SW. 'Pseudo-aldosteronism' induced by intravenous glycyrrhizin treatment of chronic hepatitis C patients. J Gastroenterol Hepatol 2001; 16:789–795.
5. Tsubota A, Kumada H, Arase Y et al. Combined ursodeoxycholic acid and glycyrrhizin therapy for chronic hepatitis C virus infection: a randomized controlled trial in 170 patients. Eur J Gastroenterol Hepatol 1999; 11:1077–1083.
6. van Rossum TG, Vulto AG, Hop W et al. Intravenous glycyrrhizin for the treatment of chronic hepatitis C: a double-blind, randomized, placebo-controlled phase I/II trial. J Gastroenterol Hepatol 1999; 14:1093–1099.
7. Amaryan G, Astvatsatryan V, Gabrielyan E et al. Double-blind, placebo-controlled, randomized, pilot clinical trial of ImmunoGuard – a standardized fixed combination of Andrographis paniculata Nees, with Eleutherococcus senticosus Maxim, Schizandra chinensis Bail. and Glycyrrhiza glabra L. extracts in patients with Familial Mediterranean Fever. Phytomedicine 2003; 10:271–285.
8. Mori K, Sakai H, Suzuki S et al. Effects of glycyrrhizin (SNMC: Stronger Neo-Minophagen C) in hemophilia patients with HIV-1 infection. Tohoku J Exp Med 1990; 162:183–193.
9. Eisenburg J. [Treatment of chronic hepatitis B. Part 2: Effect of glycyrrhizic acid on the course of illness]. Fortschritte der Medizin 1992; 110:395–398.
10. Zhang LC, Wang WL, Xie, X. Effect of glycyrrhizin on hepato-pathology in chronic hepatitis B.Chinese J Integr Trad Western Med Liver Dis 1998; 8:54
11. Miyake K, Tango T, Ota Y et al. Efficacy of Stronger Neo-Minophagen C compared between two doses administered three times a week on patients with chronic viral hepatitis. J Gastroenterol Hepatol 2002; Nov 17:1198–1204.
12. Jiang XS, Liao YQ. Glycyrrhizin for treatment of 50 cases of chronic hepatitis B. Chinese J Integr Trad Western Med Liver Dis 1999; 9:24.
13. Abe Y, Ueda T, Kato T, Kohli Y. [Effectiveness of interferon, glycyrrhizin combination therapy in patients with chronic hepatitis C]. Nippon Rinsho 1994; 52: 1817–1822.
14. Acharya SK, Dasarathy S, Tandon A, Joshi YK, Tandon BN. A preliminary open trial on interferon stimulator (SNMC) derived from Glycyrrhiza glabra in the treatment of subacute hepatic failure. Indian J Med Res 1993; 98:69–74.
15. Da Nagao Y, Sata M, Suzuki H et al. Effectiveness of glycyrrhizin for oral lichen planus in patients with chronic HCV infection. J Gastroenterol 1996; 691–695.
16. Steinberg D, Sgan-Cohen HD, Stabholz A et al. The anticariogenic activity of glycyrrhizin: preliminary clinical trials. Isr J Dent Sci 1989; 2:153–157.
17. Serra A, Uehlinger DE, Ferrarri P et al. Glycyrrhetinic acid decreases plasma potassium concentrations in patients with anuria. J Am Soc Nephrol 2002; 13:191–196.

18. Wang YY. [Effective observation of glycyrrhizin treating 38 cases of herpes zoster] (Chinese). Chinese J Leprosy Skin Dis 2001; 17:226.
19. Yang XY, Liu XQ, Li HZ, Lin L, Chen K. [Cases evaluations of curative effect of Tripterygium wilfordii, Erythromycia and Glycyrrhizin in treating psoriasis vulgaris together]. Chinese J Dermatovenereol 2000; 14:168–169.
20. Das SK, Das V, Gulati A, Singh VP. Deglycyrrhizinated liquorice in aphthous ulcers. J Assoc Physicians India 1989; 37:647.
21. Tewari SN, Wilson AK. Deglycyrrhizinated liquorice in duodenal ulcer. Practitioner 1973; 210:820–823.
22. Turpie AG, Runcie J, Thomson TJ. Clinical trial of deglydyrrhizinized liquorice in gastric ulcer. Gut 1969; 10:299–302.
23. van Marle J, Aarsen PN, Lind A, van Weeren-Kramer J. Deglycyrrhizinised liquorice (DGL) and the renewal of rat stomach epithelium. Eur J Pharmacol 1981; 72:219–225.
24. Rees WD, Rhodes J, Wright J, Stamford LF, Bennett A. Effect of deglycyrrhizinated liquorice on gastric mucosal damage by aspirin. Scand J Gastroenterol 1979; 14:605–607.
25. Strandberg TE, Jarvenpaa AL, Vanhanen H, McKeigue PM. Birth outcome in relation to licorice consumption during pregnancy. Am J Epidemiol 2001; 153:1085–1088.
26. Strandberg TE, Andersson S, Jarvenpaa A, McKeigue PM. Preterm birth and licorice consumption during pregnancy. Am J Epidemiol 2002; 156:803–805.
27. Han GR, Su PM, Guo C. Glycyrrhizin injection for treatment of 110 cases of pregnancy with viral hepatitis. Chinese J Integr Trad Western Med Liver Dis 1999; 9:49.
28. Tamir S, Eizenberg M, Somjen D et al. Estrogenic and antiproliferative properties of glabridin from licorice in human breast cancer cells. Cancer Res 2000; 60:5704–5709.
29. Farnsworth NR, Bingel AS, Cordell GA, Crane FA, Fong HH. Potential value of plants as sources of new antifertility agents II. J Pharm Sci 1975; 64:717–753.
30. Farnsworth NR, Bingel AS, Cordell G, Crane FA, Fong HH. Potential value of plants as sources of new antifertility agents I. J Pharm Sci 1975; 64:535–598.
31. www.naturalstandard.com. Licorice (Glycyrrhyza glabra) Natural standard Monograph.
32. Brinker F. The Toxicology of Botanical Medicines. Sandy, OR: Eclectic Medical Publications, 2000:296.
33. Mills S, Bone K. Principles and Practice of Phytotherapy: Modern Herbal Medicine. London: Churchill Livingstone, 2000.
34. Wagner H, Bladt S. Plant drug analysis: a think layer chromatography atlas. Berlin: Springer-Verlag, 1996:308.
35. Hostettmann K, Marston A. Chemistry and Pharmacology of Natural Products: Saponins. Cambridge: Cambridge University Press, 1995:312–318.
36. Bisset NG. Herbal drugs and phytopharmaceuticals. Stuttgart: Medpharm Scientific Publishers, 1994:302.
37. Sticher O, Soldati F. [Glycyrrhizic acid determination in Radix liquiritiae with high pressure liquid chromatography (HPLC)]. Pharm Acta Helv 1978; 53:46–52.
38. Takino Y, Koshioka M, Shiokawa M et al. Quantitative determination of glycyrrhizic acid in liquorice roots and extracts by TLC-densitometry. Planta Med 1979; 36:74–78.
39. De Smet PAGM, Keller K, Hänsel R, Chandler RF, eds. Adverse Effects of Herbal Drugs, vol 3. Berlin: Springer-Verlag, 1997:67.

40. Killacky J, Ross MS, Turner TD et al. The determination of beta-glycyrrhetinic acid in liquorice by high pressure liquid chromatography. Planta Med 1976; 30:310–316.
41. British Herbal Medicine Association. British herbal compendium, vol 1. Bournemouth: BHMA, 1992.
42. Kelloff GJ, Crowell JA, Boone CW et al. Clinical development plan: 18beta-glycyrrhetinic acid. J Cell Biochem Suppl 1994; 20:166–175.
43. Kobuke K, Inai K, Nambu S et al. Tumorigenicity study of disodium glycyrrhizinate administered orally to mice. Food Chem Toxicol 1985; 23:979–983.
44. Rusymah BH, Nabishah BM, Aminuddin S et al. Effects of glycyrrhizic acid on right atrial pressure and pulmonary vasculature in rats. Clin Exp Hypertens 1995; 17:575–591.
45. Vogel VG, Newman RZ, Ainslie N et al. Phase I pharmacology and toxicity study of glycyrrhetinic acid as a chemopreventive drug. Proc Annu Meet Am Assoc Cancer Res 1992; 33:A1245.
46. Hussain RM. The sweet cake that reaches parts other cakes can't! Postgrad Med J 2003; 79:115–116.
47. Sigurjonsdottir HA, Franzson L, Manhem K et al. Liquorice-induced rise in blood pressure: a linear dose-response relationship. J Hum Hypertens 2001; 15:549–552.
48. Sigurjonsdottir HA, Manhem K, Wallerstedt S. Liquorice-induced hypertension – a linear, dose-response relationship. 82nd Annual Meeting of the Endocrine Society, Toronto, 21–24 June 2000.
49. Armanini D, Lewicka S, Pratesi C et al. Further studies on the mechanism of the mineralocorticoid action of licorice in humans. J Endocrinol Invest 1996; 19:624–629.
50. Krahenbuhl S, Hasler F, Frey BM et al. Kinetics and dynamics of orally administered 18 beta-glycyrrhetinic acid in humans. J Clin Endocrinol Metab 1994; 78:581–585.
51. Newall CA, Anderson LA, Phillipson JD. Herbal Medicines: A Guide for Health-care Professionals. London, UK: Pharmaceutical Press, 1996:296.
52. Brinker F. Herb Contraindications and Drug Interactions, 2nd ed. Sandy, OR: Eclectic Medical Publications, 1998.
53. Amato P, Christophe S, Mellon PL. Estrogenic activity of herbs commonly used as remedies for menopausal symptoms. Menopause 2002; 9:145–150.
54. Zhang XH, Lowe D, Giles P et al. Gender may affect the action of garlic oil on plasma cholesterol and glucose levels of normal subjects. J Nutr 2001; 131:1471–1478.
55. Armanini D, Bonanni G, Palermo M et al. Reduction of serum testosterone in men by licorice. N Engl J Med 1999; 341:1158.
56. Armanini D, De Palo CB, Mattarello MJ et al. Effect of licorice on reduction of body fat mass in healthy subjects. J Endocrinol Invest 2003; 26:646–650.
57. Foster S, Tyler VE. Tyler's Honest Herbal. Binghamton, NY: Haworth Herbal Press, 1999.
58. Yoshida S, Takayama Y. Licorice-induced hypokalemia as a treatable cause of dropped head syndrome. Clin Neurol Neurosurg 2003; 105:286–287.
59. Budzinski JW, Foster BC, Vandenhoek S, Arnason JT. An in vitro evaluation of human cytochrome P450 3A4 inhibition by selected commercial herbal extracts and tinctures. Phytomedicine 2000; 7:273–282.
60. Kent UM, Aviram M, Rosenblat M, Hollenberg PF. The licorice root derived isoflavan glabridin inhibits the activities of human cytochrome P450S 3A4, 2B6, and 2C9. Drug Metab Dispos 2002; 30:709–715.
61. Zhang YD, Lorenzo B, Reidenberg MM. Inhibition of 11 beta hydroxysteroid dehydrogenase obtained from guinea pig kidney by furosemide, naringenin and some other compounds. J Steroid Biochem Mol Biol 1994; 49:81–85.

MILK THISTLE
Silybum marianum

Synonyms/common names/related substances[1]

Holy thistle, Lady's thistle, legalon, *Cardui mariae fructus*, *Cardui mariae herba*, marian thistle, mariendistel, Mary thistle, Our Lady's thistle, St Mary thistle, silybin, Silybum, silymarin

Indications

Alcoholic liver cirrhosis:[2–6]	Evidence grade A
Liver cirrhosis mortality:[2,4]	Evidence grade A
Non-alcoholic liver cirrhosis:[4,7]	Evidence grade B1
Chronic viral hepatitis C:[8,9]	Evidence grade B1
Acute viral hepatitis:[10]	Evidence grade B1
Diabetes mellitus-related cirrhosis:[2,11,12]	Evidence grade B1
Drug-induced liver toxicity:[13]	Evidence grade B2
Dyspepsia (with bitter candy tuft, chamomile flower, peppermint leaves, caraway fruit, licorice root, angelica root, celandine herbs, and lemon balm):[8]	Evidence grade B2
Toxicity-induced liver disease:[14,15]	Evidence grade C
Type 2 diabetes mellitus:[16]	Evidence grade C
Amanita phalloides mushroom poisoning:[2,17,18]	Evidence grade D
Primarily fatty degeneration of the liver:[19]	Evidence grade D
Hepatocellular carcinoma:[20]	Evidence grade E
Cancer prevention:[21,22]	Evidence grade E

Pregnancy

Minimal risk:[23–25]	Evidence level 1a

A 60-day trial of silymarin 400 mg daily was conducted in pregnant women and adults with 'minor liver insufficiencies'.[23] No adverse effects were reported in the mothers and offspring.[23]

Intrahepatic cholestasis of pregnancy:[24–26]	Evidence level 1c

When administered to a small group of patients over 15 days, milk thistle was shown to attenuate pruritus in pregnant women with intrahepatic cholestasis of pregnancy.[24–26] No adverse effects were reported with the use of milk thistle.[24–26]

Emmenagogue:[27]	Evidence level 4

Uterine stimulant constituent:[27]	Evidence level 4

A review article on the potential value of plants as sources of anti-fertility agents reported that milk thistle was an emmenagogue and that it contains the uterine stimulant constituent tyramine.[27]

Lactation

Unknown:	Evidence level 5

Milk thistle was not reported in the scientific literature as being contraindicated or safe during lactation.

Constituents

Flavonolignans:[28,29] silybin A and B, silydistin, silydianin, silymarin, silibinin tyramine[27]

Pharmacology

- Silybin, a milk thistle constituent, was shown to stimulate RNA polymerase A and DNA synthesis.[31] This stimulation increases the synthesis of ribosome proteins, stimulates cell development and thereby increases the regenerative capacity of the liver.[31]
- Regular consumption of standardized preparations of milk thistle were shown to control the liver enzymes aspartate aminotransferase (AST) and alanine aminotransferase (ALT).[8,32]
- Silymarin, the active constituent in milk thistle, may competitively bind some toxins and act as a free radical scavenger.[33,34]
- Silymarin may increase the hepatic contents of gluthathione (both oxidized and reduced).[35]
- Silymarin may increase the enzyme superoxidase dismutase (SOD).[36]
- Silymarin may regulate cell membrane permeability, inhibit the 5-lipoxygenase pathway, scavenge for reactive oxygen species (ROS) of the R-OH type and effect DNA-expression.[2]
- Silibinin, a constituent of milk thistle, was shown to significantly inhibit cell growth and DNA synthesis of different prostate, breast and cervical human carcinoma cells.[22]
- Silibinin treatment significantly decreased both intracellular and secreted forms of prostate specific antigen (PSA) and inhibited cell growth via a G1 arrest in cell cycle progression.[23]

- Milk thistle may affect cytochrome P450 2C9 (CYP2C9) and P450 3A4 (CYP3A4).[40,41]

Drug interactions

Estrogens[36]

Glucuronidated drugs[37,38]

Drugs metabolized by cytochrome P450 2C9 (CYP2C9) and P450 3A4 (CYP3A4)[39,40]

Part used[28]

Seeds

References

1. Jellin JM, Batz F, Hitchens K. Natural Medicines Comprehensive Database, 3rd ed. Stockton, CA: Therapeutic Research Faculty, 2002:1530.
2. Saller R, Meier R, Brignoli R. The use of silymarin in the treatment of liver diseases. Drugs 2001; 61:2035–2063.
3. Pares A, Planas R, Torres M et al. Effects of silymarin in alcoholic patients with cirrhosis of the liver: results of a controlled, double-blind, randomized and multicenter trial. J Hepatol 1998; 28:615–621.
4. Ferenci P, Dragosics B, Dittrich H et al. Randomized controlled trial of silymarin treatment in patients with cirrhosis of the liver. J Hepatol 1989; 9:105–113.
5. Feher J, Deak G, Muzes G et al. Liver-protective action of silymarin therapy in chronic alcoholic liver diseases. Orvosi Hetilap 1989; 130:2723–2727.
6. Salmi HA, Sarna S. Effect of silymarin on chemical, functional, and morphological alterations of the liver. A double-blind controlled study. Scand J Gastroenterol 1982; 17:517–521.
7. Benda L, Dittrich H, Ferenzi P. The influence of therapy with silymarin on the survival rate of patients with liver cirrhosis. Wien Klin Wochenschr 1980; 92: 678–683.
8. Buzzelli G, Moscarella S, Giusti A et al. A pilot study on the liver protective effect of silybin-phosphatidylcholine complex (IdB1016) in chronic active hepatitis. Int J Clin Pharmacol Ther Toxicol 1993; 31:456–460.
9. Kiesewetter E, Leodolter I, Thaler H. [Results of two double-blind studies on the effect of silymarine in chronic hepatitis]. Leber, Magen, Darm 1977; 7:318–323.
10. Magliulo E, Gagliardi B, Fiori GP. [Results of a double blind study on the effect of silymarin in the treatment of acute viral hepatitis, carried out at two medical centres]. Medizinische Klinik 1978; 73:1060–1065.
11. Velussi M, Cernigoi AM, De Monte A et al. Long-term (12 months) treatment with an anti-oxidant drug (silymarin) is effective on hyperinsulinemia, exogenous insulin need and malondialdehyde levels in cirrhotic diabetic patients. J Hepatol 1997; 26:871–879.
12. Velussi M, Cernigoi AM, Viezzoli L et al. Silymarin reduces hyperinsulinemia, malondialdehyde levels, and daily insulin need in cirrhotic diabetic patients. Curr Ther Res Clin Exp 1993; 53:533–545.
13. Allain H, Schuck S, Lebreton S et al. Aminotransferase levels and silymarin in de novo tacrine-treated patients with Alzheimer's disease. Dement Geriatr Cogn Disord 1999; 10:181–185.

14. Szilard S, Szentgyorgyi D, Demeter I. Protective effect of Legalon in workers exposed to organic solvents. Acta Med Hung 1988; 45:249–256.
15. Boari C, Montanari FM, Galletti GP et al. [Toxic occupational liver diseases. Therapeutic effects of silymarin]. Minerva Med 1981; 72:2679–2688.
16. Zhang JQ, Mao XM, Zhou YP. [Effects of silybin on red blood cell sorbitol and nerve conduction velocity in diabetic patients]. Zhongguo Zhong Xi Yi Jie He Za Zhi 1993; 13:725–726, 708.
17. Floersheim GL, Weber O, Tschumi P, Ulbrich M. [Clinical death-cap (Amanita phalloides) poisoning: prognostic factors and therapeutic measures. Analysis of 205 cases]. Schweiz Med Wochenschr 1982; 112:1164–1177.
18. Carducci R, Armellino MF, Volpe C et al. [Silibinin and acute poisoning with Amanita phalloides]. Minerva Anestesiol 1996; 62:187–193.
19. Poser G. [Experience in the treatment of chronic hepatopathies with silymarin]. Arzneimittelforschung 1971; 21:1209–1212.
20. Grossmann M, Hoermann R, Weiss M et al. Spontaneous regression of hepatocellular carcinoma. Am J Gastroenterol 1995; 90:1500–1503.
21. Bhatia N, Zhao J, Wolf DM, Agarwal R. Inhibition of human carcinoma cell growth and DNA synthesis by silibinin, an active constituent of milk thistle: comparison with silymarin. Cancer Lett 1999; 147:77–84.
22. Zi X, Agarwal R. Silibinin decreases prostate-specific antigen with cell growth inhibition via G1 arrest, leading to differentiation of prostate carcinoma cells: implications for prostate cancer intervention. Proc Natl Acad Sci USA 1999; 96:7490–7495.
23. Giannola C, Buogo F, Forestiere G et al. [A two-center study on the effects of silymarin in pregnant women and adult patients with so-called minor hepatic insufficiency]. Clin Ther 1985; 114:129–135.
24. Reyes H, Simon FR. Intrahepatic cholestasis of pregnancy: an estrogen-related disease. Semin Liver Dis 1993; 13:289–301.
25. Reyes H. The spectrum of liver and gastrointestinal disease seen in cholestasis of pregnancy. Gastroenterol Clin North Am 1992; 21:905–921.
26. Gonzalez MC, Reyes H, Ribalta J et al. Effect of sylimarin on pruritis of cholestasis [abstract]. Hepatology 1988; 8:1356.
27. Farnsworth NR, Bingel AS, Cordell G, Crane FA, Fong HH. Potential value of plants as sources of new antifertility agents I. J Pharm Sci 1975; 64:535–598.
28. Boon H, Smith M. The botanical pharmacy: the pharmacology of 47 common herbs. Kingston, ON: Quarry Health Books/CCNM, 1999:320.
29. Blumenthal M, Busse WR, Goldberg A et al. The Complete German Commission E Monographs: Therapeutic Guide to Herbal Medicines. Boston, MA: American Botanical Council, 1998.
30. Wellington K, Jarvis B. Silymarin: a review of its clinical properties in the management of hepatic disorders. BioDrugs 2001; 15:465–489.
31. Lang I, Nekam K, Deak G et al. Immunomodulatory and hepatoprotective effects of in vivo treatment with free radical scavengers. Ital J Gastroenterol 1990; 22:283–287.
32. Dvorak Z, Kosina P, Walterova D et al. Primary cultures of human hepatocytes as a tool in cytotoxicity studies: cell protection against model toxins by flavonolignans obtained from Silybum marianum. Toxicol Lett 2003; 137:201–212.
33. Okawa M, Kinjo J, Nohara T, Ono M. DPPH (1,1-diphenyl-2-picrylhydrazyl) radical scavenging activity of flavonoids obtained from some medicinal plants. Biol Pharm Bull 2001; 24:1202–1205.

34. Ramadan LA, Roushdy HM, Abu Senna GM, Amin NE, El-Deshw OA. Radio-protective effect of silymarin against radiation induced hepatotoxicity. Pharmacol Res 2002; 45:447–454.
35. Boon H, Smith M. The Pharmacology of 47 Common Herbs. Kingston: Quarry Health, 1999.
36. Agency for Healthcare Research and Quality. Milk Thistle: Effects on Liver Disease and Cirrhosis and Clinical Adverse Effects. Rockville, MD: Summary, Evidence Report/Technology Assessment: Number 21, 2000. http://www.ahrq.gov/clinic/epcsums/milktsum.htm
37. Venkataramanan R, Ramachandran V, Komoroski BJ et al. Milk thistle, a herbal supplement, decreases the activity of CYP3A4 and uridine diphosphoglucuronosyl transferase in human hepatocyte cultures. Drug Metab Dispos 2000; 28:1270–1273.
38. Kim DH, Jin YH, Park JB, Kobashi K. Silymarin and its components are inhibitors of beta-glucuronidase. Biol Pharm Bull 1994; 17:443–445.
39. Budzinski JW, Foster BC, Vandenhoek S, Arnason JT. An in vitro evaluation of human cytochrome P450 3A4 inhibition by selected commercial herbal extracts and tinctures. Phytomedicine 2000; 7:273–282.
40. Beckmann-Knopp S, Rietbrock S, Weyhenmeyer R et al. Inhibitory effects of silibinin on cytochrome P-450 enzymes in human liver microsomes. Pharmacol Toxicol 2000; 86:250–256.

MONKSHOOD
Aconitum napellus

Synonyms and common names[1]

Wolfsbane, aconiti tuber, autumn monkshood, blue monkshood root, chuan-wu, monkshood tuber, friar's cap, mousebane, aconite

Indications

Analgesic:[2,3]	Evidence grade E
Neuralgia:[4]	Evidence grade E
Ovarian cysts (as part of the Turska formula (Aconite, Bryonia, Phytolacca and Gelsemium)):[5]	Evidence grade F

Pregnancy

Possible central nervous system effects:[6]	Evidence level 4

An animal study was conducted on the effects of an alkaloid similar to aconitine, i.e. methyllycaconitine (derived from *Delphinium brownii*).[6] The researchers reported that methyllycaconitine was a potent antagonist of *N*-acetylcholine receptors in the hippocampal neurons of rats.[6]

Anovulatory effects:[7]	Evidence level 4

A review article on the potential value of plants as sources of anti-fertility agents reported that aconite had anovulatory effects in vitro.[7]

Lactation

Possible central nervous system effects:[6]	Evidence level 4

An animal study was conducted on the effects of an alkaloid similar to aconitine, i.e. methyllycaconitine (derived from *D. brownii*).[6] The researchers reported that methyllycaconitine was a potent antagonist of *N*-acetylcholine receptors in the hippocampal neurons of rats.[6]

Unknown:	Evidence level 5

Despite the apparent toxicity of this herb, there were no reports in the scientific literature of monkshood being either safe or contraindicated during lactation.

Constituents

- Diterpene alkaloids:[8,9] aconitine (acetylbenzoylaconine), picraconitine (benzoylaconine), aconine, mesaconitine, napelline (isoaconitine, pseudoaconitine), hypaconitine, 3-acetylaconitine, lappaconitine, benzaconine
- Diterpenoid-ester alkaloids[8,9]

Toxicity

- Monkshood is one of the most poisonous plants known. There are a number of case reports of accidental poisonings.[10–16]
- Lethal dose:[8,9,17] 1 g (powdered herb), 5 mL (tincture), 3–6 mg of aconitine

Pharmacology

- Monkshood alkaloids have anti-nociceptive effects and can be useful analgesics.[2]
- Monkshood alkaloids have muscarinic effects where they stimulate the parasympathetic nervous system, causing bradycardia and hypotension.[8]
- The constituent lappaconitine is an antagonist of both sodium and calcium channels, thereby causing anti-arrhythmia and bradycardia-like effects.[2,8]

Part used[8]

Whole herb

References

1. Jellin JM, Batz F, Hitchens K. Natural Medicines Comprehensive Database, 3rd ed. Stockton, CA: Therapeutic Research Faculty, 2002:1530.
2. Gutser UT, Friese J, Heubach JF et al. Mode of antinociceptive and toxic action of alkaloids of Aconitum spec. Naunyn Schmiedebergs Arch Pharmacol 1998; 357:39–48.
3. Ameri A. The effects of Aconitum alkaloids on the central nervous system. Prog Neurobiol 1998; 56:211–235.
4. Blumenthal M, Goldberg A, Brinckmann J. Herbal Medicine Expanded Commission E Monographs. Newton, MA: Integrative Medicine Communications, 2000.
5. Hudson T. Women's Encyclopedia of Natural Medicine: Alternative Therapies and Integrative Medicine. Los Angeles, CA: Lowell House Contemporary Books, 1999:358.
6. Alkondon M, Pereira EF, Wonnacott S, Albuquerque EX. Blockade of nicotinic currents in hippocampal neurons defines methyllycaconitine as a potent and specific receptor antagonist. Mol Pharmacol 1992; 41:802–808.
7. Farnsworth NR, Bingel AS, Cordell GA, Crane FA, Fong HH. Potential value of plants as sources of new antifertility agents I. J Pharm Sci 1975; 64:535–598.
8. Brinker F. The Toxicology of Botanical Medicines. Sandy, OR: Eclectic Medical Publications, 2000:296.
9. Leung AY, Foster S. Encyclopedia of Common Natural Ingredients Used in Food, Drugs and Cosmetics. New York, NY: John Wiley & Sons, 1996:649.
10. Fatovich DM. Aconite: a lethal Chinese herb. Ann Emerg Med 1992; 21:309–311.
11. Tai YT, But PP, Young K, Lau CP. Cardiotoxicity after accidental herb-induced aconite poisoning. Lancet 1992; 340:1254–1256.

12. Chan TY, Tomlinson B, Critchley JA. Aconitine poisoning following the ingestion of Chinese herbal medicines: a report of eight cases. Aust N Z J Med 1993; 23:268–271.
13. Tomlinson B, Chan TY, Chan JC, Critchley JA. Herb-induced aconitine poisoning. Lancet 1993; 341:370–371.
14. Chan TY, Tomlinson B, Chan WW, Yeung VT, Tse LK. A case of acute aconitine poisoning caused by chuanwu and caowu. J Trop Med Hyg 1993; 96:62–63.
15. Chan TY, Tomlinson B, Critchley JA, Cockram CS. Herb-induced aconitine poisoning presenting as tetraplegia. Vet Hum Toxicol 1994; 36:133–134.
16. Elliott SP. A case of fatal poisoning with the aconite plant: quantitative analysis in biological fluid. Sci Justice 2002; 42:111–115.
17. But PP, Tai YT, Young K. Three fatal cases of herbal aconite poisoning. Vet Hum Toxicol 1994; 36:212–215.

OREGON GRAPE
Berberis aquifolium

Synonyms/common names/related substances[1]

Blue barberry, creeping barberry, holly barberry, holly-leaved berberis, holly mahonia, mountain-grape, Oregon barberry, Oregon grape-holly, scraperoot, trailing mahonia, water-holly

Indications

Chloroquine-resistant malaria (with pyrimethamine):[2]	Evidence grade B1
Infectious diarrhea:[3,4]	Evidence grade B1
Trachoma (*Chlamydia trachomatis* eye infection):[5,6]	Evidence grade B2
Psoriasis (topical):[7,8]	Evidence grade C
Congestive heart failure:[9]	Evidence grade C
Upper respiratory tract infections:[10,11]	Evidence grade E
Anti-*Helicobacter pylori*:[12]	Evidence grade E
Cancer prevention:[13–15]	Evidence grade E

Pregnancy

May cause newborn jaundice (kernicterus):[16]	Evidence level 3

In rats, berberine displaces bilirubin bound to albumin.[16] Berberine (10–20 μg/g) was administered intraperitoneally to adult rats on a daily basis for 1 week.[16] After 1 week, a significant decrease in mean bilirubin serum protein binding was observed, due to an in vivo displacement effect by berberine.[16] A persistent elevation in serum concentrations of unbound and total bilirubin was also observed.[16]

Uterine stimulant:[17,18]	Evidence level 4

A review article on the potential value of plants as sources of anti-fertility agents reported that Oregon grape contains the uterine stimulant berberine.[17,18]

Lactation

May cause or aggravate newborn jaundice (kernicterus):[16]	Evidence level 3

In rats, berberine displaces bilirubin bound to albumin.[16] Berberine (10–20 μg/g) was administered intraperitoneally to adult rats on a daily basis for 1 week.[16] After 1 week, a significant decrease in mean bilirubin serum protein binding was observed, due to an in vivo displacement effect by berberine.[16] A persistent elevation in serum concentrations of unbound and total bilirubin was also observed.[16]

Contraindication

Newborn jaundice (kernicterus)[16]

Toxic constituents

Isoquinoline alkaloids:[19,20] oxyacanthine, berbamine, berberine

Toxicity

LD_{50} of berberine in humans:[17] 27.5 mg/kg

Pharmacology

- Berberine was found to displace bilirubin bound to albumin in vitro.[16] Berberine was found to be about 10 times superior to phenylbutazone, a known potent displacer of bilirubin, and about 100 times superior to papaverine, a berberine-type alkaloid.[16]
- The constituents berberine and oxyacanthine have been shown to have antibacterial activity.[10,11,21,22]
- Berberine has been shown to have amebicidal, anti-parasitic (trypanocidal) and anti-fungal activity.[21,23–25]
- Berberine and β-hydrastine were shown to have anti-*Helicobacter pylori* activity in vitro.[12]
- In low doses, berberine may act as a cardiac and respiratory stimulant, whereas in high doses it may act as a cardiac and respiratory depressant.[17,19,21]
- Berberine was shown to have anti-platelet activity.[26]
- Berberine, oxyacanthine, and barbamine were shown to have anti-inflammatory effects.[27–30]
- Berberine was found to have antidiarrheal effects.[31]
- Berberine was found to inhibit parathyroid hormone-stimulated bone resorption, inhibit osteoclastic bone resorption and prevent a decrease in bone mineral density of the lumbar vertebrae.[32]

Drug interactions

Anticoagulant drugs[26]
Highly protein-bound drugs[16]

Parts used[1]

Root and rhizome

References

1. Jellin JM, Batz F, Hitchens K. Natural Medicines Comprehensive Database, 3rd ed. Stockton, CA: Therapeutic Research Faculty, 2002:1530.
2. Sheng WD, Jiddawi MS, Hong XQ, Abdulla SM. Treatment of chloroquine-resistant malaria using pyrimethamine in combination with berberine, tetracycline or cotrimoxazole. East Afr Med J 1997; 74:283–284.
3. Rabbani GH, Butler T, Knight J, Sanyal SC, Alam K. Randomized controlled trial of berberine sulfate therapy for diarrhea due to enterotoxigenic Escherichia coli and Vibrio cholerae. J Infect Dis 1987; 155:979–984.
4. Swabb EA, Tai YH, Jordan L. Reversal of cholera toxin-induced secretion in rat ileum by luminal berberine. Am J Physiol 1981; 241:G248–252.
5. Khosla PK, Neeraj VI, Gupta SK, Satpathy G. Berberine, a potential drug for trachoma. Rev Int Trach Pathol Ocul Trop Subtrop Sante Publique 1992; 69:147–165.
6. Mohan M, Pant CR, Angra SK, Mahajan VM. Berberine in trachoma. (A clinical trial). Indian J Ophthalmol 1982; 30:69–75.
7. Gieler U, von der Weth A, Heger M. Mahonia aquifolium – a new type of topical treatment for psoriasis. J Dermatol Treatment 1995; 6:31–34.
8. Wiesenauer M, Lydtke R. Mahonia aquifolium in patients with Psoriasis vulgaris; an intraindividual study. Phytomedicine 1996; 3:231–235.
9. Zeng X, Zeng X. Relationship between the clinical effects of berberine on severe congestive heart failure and its concentration in plasma studied by HPLC. Biomed Chromatogr 1999; 13:442–444.
10. Stermitz FR, Lorenz P, Tawara JN, Zenewicz LA, Lewis K. Synergy in a medicinal plant: antimicrobial action of berberine potentiated by 5′-methoxyhydnocarpin, a multidrug pump inhibitor. Proc Natl Acad Sci USA 2000; 97:1433–1437.
11. Stermitz FR, Tawara-Matsuda J, Lorenz P et al. 5′-Methoxyhydnocarpin-D and pheophorbide A: Berberis species components that potentiate berberine growth inhibition of resistant Staphylococcus aureus. J Nat Prod 2000; 63:1146–1149.
12. Mahady GB, Pendland SL, Stoia A, Chadwick LR. In vitro susceptibility of Helicobacter pylori to isoquinoline alkaloids from Sanguinaria canadensis and Hydrastis canadensis. Phytother Res 2003; 17:217–221.
13. Anis KV, Rajeshkumar NV, Kuttan R. Inhibition of chemical carcinogenesis by berberine in rats and mice. J Pharm Pharmacol 2001; 53:763–768.
14. Chung JG, Chen GW, Hung CF et al. Effects of berberine on arylamine N-acetyltransferase activity and 2-aminofluorene-DNA adduct formation in human leukemia cells. Am J Chin Med 2000; 28:227–238.
15. Fukuda K, Hibiya Y, Mutoh M et al. Inhibition by berberine of cyclooxygenase-2 transcriptional activity in human colon cancer cells. J Ethnopharmacol 1999; 66:227–233.
16. Chan E. Displacement of bilirubin from albumin by berberine. Biol Neonate 1993; 63:201–208.
17. McGuffin M, Hobbs C, Upton R, Goldberg A. American Herbal Products Association's Botanical Safety Handbook. Boca Raton, FL: CRC Press, 1997:231.
18. Farnsworth NR, Bingel AS, Cordell G, Crane FA, Fong HH. Potential value of plants as sources of new antifertility agents I. J Pharm Sci 1975; 64:535–598.
19. Foster S, Tyler VE. Tyler's Honest Herbal. Binghamton, NY: Haworth Herbal Press, 1999.
20. Gruenwald J, Brendler T, Jaenicke C. PDR for Herbal Medicines. Montvale, NJ: Medical Economics Company, 1998.

21. Leung AY, Foster S. Encyclopedia of Common Natural Ingredients Used in Food, Drugs and Cosmetics, 2nd ed. New York, NY: John Wiley & Sons, 1996:649.
22. Abel G. [Chromosome-damaging effect of beta-asaron on human lymphocytes]. Planta Med 1987; 53:251–253.
23. Ghosh AK, Bhattacharyya FK, Ghosh DK. Leishmania donovani: amastigote inhibition and mode of action of berberine. Exp Parasitol 1985; 60:404–413.
24. Ghosh AK, Rakshit MM, Ghosh DK. Effect of berberine chloride on Leishmania donovani. Indian J Med Res 1983; 78:407–416.
25. Mahajan VM, Sharma A, Rattan A. Antimycotic activity of berberine sulphate: an alkaloid from an Indian medicinal herb. Sabouraudia 1982; 20:79–81.
26. Huang CG, Chu ZL, Wei SJ, Jiang H, Jiao BH. Effect of berberine on arachidonic acid metabolism in rabbit platelets and endothelial cells. Thromb Res 2002; 106:223–227.
27. Ivanovska N, Philipov S. Study on the anti-inflammatory action of Berberis vulgaris root extract, alkaloid fractions and pure alkaloids. Int J Immunopharmacol 1996; 18:553–561.
28. Ivanovska N, Philipov S, Hristova M. Influence of berberine on T-cell mediated immunity. Immunopharmacol Immunotoxicol 1999; 21:771–786.
29. Kupeli E, Kosar M, Yesilada E, Husnu K, Baser C. A comparative study on the anti-inflammatory, antinociceptive and antipyretic effects of isoquinoline alkaloids from the roots of Turkish Berberis species. Life Sci 2002; 72:645–657.
30. Yesilada E, Kupeli E. Berberis crataegina DC. root exhibits potent anti-inflammatory, analgesic and febrifuge effects in mice and rats. J Ethnopharmacol 2002; 79:237–248.
31. Zhang MF, Shen YQ. [Antidiarrheal and anti-inflammatory effects of berberine]. Zhongguo Yao Li Xue Bao 1989; 10:174–176.
32. Li H, Miyahara T, Tezuka Y et al. The effect of kampo formulae on bone resorption in vitro and in vivo. II. Detailed study of berberine. Biol Pharm Bull 1999; 22:391–396.

PARSLEY

Petroselinum crispum, P. sativum

Synonyms/common names/related compounds[1]

Common parsley, garden parsley, hamburg parsley, persely, persil, petersylinge, *Petroselini herba*, *Petrosilini radix*, rock parsley

Indications

Antioxidant activity:[2]	Evidence grade B2
Abortifacient:[3]	Evidence grade C

Pregnancy

Whole plant

Abortifacient:[3–5]	Evidence level 1b

A descriptive retrospective survey was conducted on the calls received by the Montevideo Poison Center between 1986 and 1999 concerning the ingestion of herbal infusions with abortive intent. Parsley was reported as one of the most frequently used herbs for self-induced abortions. The authors also reported that abortion occurred in a number of cases after the ingestion of parsley. Also, there is a 1973 case report of abortion following the ingestion of parsley and naphthalene.[4] A review article on the potential value of plants as sources of anti-fertility agents reported that parsley was a potential abortifacient.[5]

Emmenagogue:[5]	Evidence level 4
Uterine stimulant constituent:[5]	Evidence level 4
Estrogenic:[6]	Evidence level 4

A review article on the potential value of plants as sources of anti-fertility agents reported that parsley was an emmenagogue, uterine stimulant and that its constituent, apiol, was a uterine stimulant.[5] This review article also reported that parsley has estrogenic activity.[6]

Aerial parts

Estrogenic activity:[6,7]	Evidence level 3

Extracts from the aerial parts of parsley showed potent estrogenic activity, which was equal to that of isoflavone glycosides from soybean.[7] The methanolic extract of parsley, apiin, and apigenin restored the uterus weight in ovariectomized mice when orally administered for consecutive 7 days.[7] A review article on the potential value of plants as sources of anti-fertility agents reported that parsley has estrogenic activity.[6]

Myristicin

Potentially mutagenic:[8]	Evidence level 3

Liver DNA adducts were detected in fetal liver when pregnant mice were intubated with myristicin.[8]

Lactation

Whole plant

Unknown:	Evidence level 5

There are no reports in the scientific literature of parsley being either safe or contraindicated during lactation.

Aerial parts

Estrogenic activity:[7]	Evidence level 3

Extracts from the aerial parts of parsley showed potent estrogenic activity.[7]

Contraindications

Kidney inflammation[9]

Constituents

- Leaf and root:[1,7] volatile oils (apiole, myristicin, furanocoumarins (psoralens)), flavone glycosides (apiin, apigenin), carotene, vitamin B_1, vitamin B_2, vitamin C, and vitamin K
- Seed:[1] volatile oils (apiole, myristicin, furanocoumarins (psoralens))

Toxicity

LD_{50} (oral) of volatile oil:[9] 1.52–3.96 g/kg

Pharmacology

Leaf and root

- Parsley has been reported as having anti-flatulent, antispasmodic, anti-rheumatic, expectorant, antimicrobial and aquaretic (increased urine volume without sodium loss) effects.[1,10–13]

- Parsley irritates the kidney epithelium, which increases renal blood flow and glomerular filtration rate and consequently increases urine output.[10]
- The constituent apiole may stimulate menstrual flow and smooth muscle contractibility in the bladder and intestines.[14]
- The constituents apiole and myristicin may have aquaretic and uterine stimulant effects.[10]

Seed

- Parsley seed may stimulate appetite and improve digestion due to its volatile oil content.[15]
- The volatile oil from the seed has mild aquaretic and laxative properties.[15,16]
- Parsley seed causes a laxative effect by inhibiting the Na–K pump and by stimulating the $NaKCl_2$ transporter.[16]
- Parsley seed oil may stimulate hepatic regeneration.[11]

Drug interactions[1]

Leaf and root

Anticoagulant/antiplatelet drugs[17]
Aspirin[18]
Diuretics[10]
Monoamine oxidase inhibitors[11]

Seed

Diuretics[10]
Monoamine oxidase inhibitors[11]

Parts used[1]

Leaf, root, and seed

References

1. Jellin JM, Batz F, Hitchens K. Natural Medicines Comprehensive Database, 3rd ed. Stockton, CA: Therapeutic Research Faculty, 2002:1530.
2. www.naturalstandard.com. Dandelion (Taraxacum officinale) Natural Standard Monograph, 2004.
3. Ciganda C, Laborde A. Herbal infusions used for induced abortion. J Toxicol Clin Toxicol 2003; 41:235–239.
4. Giusti GV, Moneta E. [A case of abortion using parsley extract and naphthalene]. Arch Kriminol 1973; 152:161–164.
5. Farnsworth NR, Bingel AS, Cordell G, Crane FA, Fong HH. Potential value of plants as sources of new antifertility agents I. J Pharm Sci 1975; 64:535–598.
6. Farnsworth NR, Bingel AS, Cordell GA, Crane FA, Fong HH. Potential value of plants as sources of new antifertility agents II. J Pharm Sci 1975; 64:717–753.
7. Yoshikawa M, Uemura T, Shimoda H et al. Medicinal foodstuffs. XVIII. Phytoestrogens from the aerial part of Petroselinum crispum MIll. (Parsley) and structures

of 6′-acetylapiin and a new monoterpene glycoside, petroside. Chem Pharm Bull (Tokyo) 2000; 48:1039–1044.

8. Randerath K, Putman KL, Randerath E. Flavor constituents in cola drinks induce hepatic DNA adducts in adult and fetal mice. Biochem Biophys Res Commun 1993; 192:61–68.
9. Brinker F. The Toxicology of Botanical Medicines. Sandy, OR: Eclectic Medical Publications, 2000:296.
10. Robbers JE, Tyler VE. Tyler's Herbs of Choice: The Therapeutic Use of Phytomedicinals. New York, NY: The Haworth Herbal Press, 1999.
11. Newall CA, Anderson LA, Phillipson JD. Herbal Medicines: A Guide for Health-care Professionals. London, UK: Pharmaceutical Press, 1996:296.
12. The Review of Natural Products by Facts and Comparisons. St. Louis, MO: Wolters Kluwer Co., 1999.
13. Gruenwald J et al. PDR for Herbal Medicines. Montvale, NJ: Medical Economics Company, 1998.
14. Leung AY, Foster S. Encyclopedia of Common Natural Ingredients Used in Food, Drugs and Cosmetics, 2nd ed. New York, NY: John Wiley & Sons, 1996:649.
15. Foster S, Tyler VE. Tyler's Honest Herbal: A Sensible Guide to the Use of Herbs and Related Remedies, 3rd ed. Binghamton, NY: Haworth Herbal Press, 1993.
16. Kreydiyyeh SI, Usta J, Kaouk I et al. The mechanism underlying the laxative properties of parsley extract. Phytomedicine 2001; 8:382–388.
17. Brinker F. Herb Contraindications and Drug Interactions, 2nd ed. Sandy, OR: Eclectic Medical Publications, 1998.
18. Eberhard P, Gall HM, Muller I, Moller R. Dramatic augmentation of a food allergy by acetylsalicylic acid. J Allergy Clin Immunol 2000; 105:844.

PASSION FLOWER

Passiflora incarnata

Synonyms/common names/related compounds[1]

Apricot vine, corona de cristo, fleischfarbige, fleur de la passion, flor de passion, madre selva, maracuja, maypop, maypop passion flower, passiflora, *Passiflorae herba*, passiflore, passiflorina, passionflower, passion vine, passionaria, passionblume, passionflower herb, passionsblumenkraut, purple passion flower, water lemon, wild passion flower

Indications

Anxiety associated with adjustment disorders (with hawthorn, black horehound, valerian, cola nut and guarana):[2]	Evidence grade B1
Anxiety:[3–6]	Evidence grade B2
Opiate withdrawal (with clonidine):[7]	Evidence grade B2
Increases exercise capacity in congestive heart failure (with hawthorn):[8]	Evidence grade B2

Pregnancy

Genotoxic constituents:[9]	Evidence level 3
Mutagenic constituents:[9]	Evidence level 3

Both harman and harmine, constituents of passion flower, increased aberrant cell frequency and induced DNA damage in vitro using single-cell gel assay.[9] The authors reported that harman and harmine are genotoxic and mutagenic.[9] Harmine was found to be more cytotoxic than harman.[9]

Uterine stimulant:[10]	Evidence level 4

A review article on the potential value of plants as sources of anti-fertility agents reported that passion flower was a uterine stimulant.[10]

Lactation

Genotoxic constituents:[9]	Evidence level 3
Mutagenic constituents:[9]	Evidence level 3

Both harman and harmine, constituents of passion flower, increased aberrant cell frequency and induced DNA damage in vitro using single-cell gel assay.[9] The authors reported that harman and harmine are genotoxic and mutagenic.[9] Harmine was found to be more cytotoxic than harman.[9]

Unknown:	Evidence level 5

There are no reports in the scientific literature of passion flower being either safe or contraindicated during lactation.

Constituents

- Flavonoids[1]: apigenin, luteolin, quercetin, kaempferol, vitexin
- β-Carboline alkaloids:[5,6] harmine, harmaline, harmalol, harman, harmin
- Cyanogenic glycoside:[5,11,12] gynocardine

Toxicity

LD_{50} of the closely related species *P. alata* was 456 mg/kg.[13]

Pharmacology

- Passion flower has been shown to have sedative, hypnotic, anxiolytic, anodyne and anti-spasmodic effects.[1,5,6,14]
- The alkaloid constituents have central nervous system stimulant activity via a monoamine oxidase mechanism.[14,15]
- The constituent apigenin binds to central benzodiazepine receptors, thereby causing anxiolytic effects without impairing memory or motor skills.[16]
- Passion flower may reduce amphetamine-induced hypermotility, aggressiveness, and restlessness, and may raise the pain threshold.[11,14,17]
- Passion flower may have anti-bacterial and antifungal activity.[14]
- The constituents harman and harmine are genotoxic and mutagenic, where harmine was found to be more cytotoxic than harman.[9]

Drug interactions[1]

Barbiturates[17]
Central nervous system depressants[12]
Monoamine oxidase inhibitors[14]

Parts used

Above ground parts[1]

References

1. Jellin JM, Batz F, Hitchens K. Natural Medicines Comprehensive Database, 3rd ed. Stockton, CA: Therapeutic Research Faculty, 2002:1530.
2. Bourin M, Bougerol T, Guitton B, Broutin E. A combination of plant extracts in the treatment of outpatients with adjustment disorder with anxious mood: controlled study versus placebo. Fundam Clin Pharmacol 1997; 11:127–132.

3. Dhawan K, Kumar S, Sharma A. Comparative biological activity study on Passiflora incarnata and P. edulis. Fitoterapia 2001; 72:698–702.
4. Akhondzadeh S, Naghavi HR, Vazirian M et al. Passionflower in the treatment of generalized anxiety: a pilot double-blind randomized controlled trial with oxazepam. J Clin Pharm Ther 2001; 26:363–367.
5. Dhawan K, Kumar S, Sharma A. Anti-anxiety studies on extracts of Passiflora incarnata Linneaus. J Ethnopharmacol 2001; 78:165–170.
6. Dhawan K, Kumar S, Sharma A. Anxiolytic activity of aerial and underground parts of Passiflora incarnata. Fitoterapia 2001; 72:922–926.
7. Akhondzadeh S, Kashani L, Mobaseri M et al. Passionflower in the treatment of opiates withdrawal: a double-blind randomized controlled trial. J Clin Pharm Ther 2001; 26:369–373.
8. Von Eiff M, Brunner H, Haegeli A et al. Hawthorn/passion flower extract and improvement in physical exercise capacity of patients with dyspnoea Class II of the NYHA functional classifications. Acta Ther 1994; 20:47–66.
9. Boeira JM, da Silva J, EB, Henriques JA. Genotoxic effects of the alkaloids harman and harmine assessed by comet assay and chromosome aberration test in mammalian cells in vitro. Pharmacol Toxicol 2001; 89:287–294.
10. Farnsworth NR, Bingel AS, Cordell G, Crane FA, Fong HH. Potential value of plants as sources of new antifertility agents I. J Pharm Sci 1975; 64:535–598.
11. Leung AY, Foster S. Encyclopedia of Common Natural Ingredients Used in Food, Drugs and Cosmetics, 2nd ed. New York, NY: John Wiley & Sons, 1996:649.
12. Brinker F. Herb Contraindications and Drug Interactions, 2nd ed. Sandy, OR: Eclectic Medical Publications, 1998.
13. Oga S, de Freitas PC, Gomes da Silva AC, Hanada S. Pharmacological trials of crude extract of Passiflora alata. Planta Med 1984; 50:303–306.
14. Newall CA, Anderson LA, Phillipson JD. Herbal Medicines: A Guide for Health-care Professionals. London, UK: Pharmaceutical Press, 1996:296.
15. Rommelspacher H, May T, Salewski B. (1-methyl-beta-carboline) is a natural inhibitor of monoamine oxidase type A in rats. Eur J Pharmacol 1994; 252:51–59.
16. Salgueiro JB, Ardenghi P, Dias M et al. Anxiolytic natural and synthetic flavonoid ligands of the central benzodiazepine receptor have no effect on memory tasks in rats. Pharmacol Biochem Behav 1997; 58:887–891.
17. Monographs on the medicinal uses of plant drugs. Exeter, UK: European Scientific Co-op Phytother, 1997.

PENNYROYAL
Hedeoma pulegioides, Mentha pulegium

Synonyms/common names/related compounds[1]

American pennyroyal, European pennyroyal, lurk-in-the-ditch, mosquito plant, penny royal, piliolerial, pudding grass, pulegium, run-by-the-ground, squaw balm, squawmint, stinking balm, tickweed

Indications

Potential abortifacient:[2–4]	Evidence grade E
Emmenagogue:[5]	Evidence grade E

Pregnancy

Potential abortifacient:[2–4,6]	Evidence level 2

Pennyroyal has a long tradition of use as an abortifacient.[5–8] In a 1904 case report, a woman ingested one-half ounce of pennyroyal oil and expulsed a dead fetus 4 days later.[2] In a 1955 case report, a 3-month pregnant woman ingested two bottles of an unknown amount of pennyroyal with the intention of inducing an abortion; several hours later, the fetus was aborted. A review article on the potential value of plants as sources of anti-fertility agents also reported that pennyroyal was an abortifacient.[6]

In two case reports from 1961 and 1985, however, two pregnant women consumed pennyroyal in combination with other herbs and this did not lead to an abortion.[5,9] One women experienced a severe psychotic episode and seizures, while the newborn of the other women was born with mild hyperbilirubinemia.[5,9]

Emmenagogue:[5,6,10]	Evidence level 2

In a 1996 case report, a 24-year-old woman drank glasses of pennyroyal tea with the intention of inducing menstruation.[5] After repeated intake of pennyroyal tea, the women experienced nausea, severe abdominal cramping for 4 days and eventually menses began.[5] In a 1983 case report, a 20-year-old woman took pennyroyal leaves and oil to induce menstruation.[10] The woman experienced some menstrual spotting from taking pennyroyal leaves and within hours of taking the oil, she was euphoric, vomited, and lost consciousness.[10] The woman was admitted to the hospital, received supportive treatment and recovered fully.[10] A review article on the potential value of plants as sources of anti-fertility agents also reported that pennyroyal was an emmenagogue.[6]

Hepatotoxicity:[5,11]	Evidence level 2
Neurotoxicity:[12]	Evidence level 2

Nephrotoxic:[5]	Evidence level 2
Pneumotoxic:[5]	Evidence level 2

Human and animal case reports found that pennyroyal use reduced liver glutathione levels and is hepatotoxic.[5,11–13] Neurologic injury developed in two infants after ingestion of pennyroyal tea.[12] A human case report also found that pennyroyal use may injure the kidneys and the lungs.[5]

Carachipita

Abortifacient:[4]	Evidence level 2
Multi-system organ failure:	Evidence level 2[4]
Death:[4]	Evidence level 2

The South American over-the-counter product called Carachipita, which contains pennyroyal, yerba de la perdiz (*Margiricarpus pinnatus*), oregano (*Origanum vulgare*), and guaycuri (*Statice brasiliensis*) was found to induce abortion, multi-system organ failure and, in one case, death of the mother.[4]

Lactation

Hepatotoxicity:[5,11]	Evidence level 2
Neurotoxicity:[12]	Evidence level 2
Nephrotoxic:[5]	Evidence level 2
Pneumotoxic:[5]	Evidence level 2

Human and animal case reports have documented liver, nerve, kidney and lung toxicity associated with the use of pennyroyal.[5,11,12] It is unclear if the toxic constituents of pennyroyal cross into breast milk.

Carachipita

Multi-system organ failure:[4]	Evidence level 2
Death:[4]	Evidence level 2

The South American over-the-counter product called Carachipita, which contains pennyroyal, yerba de la perdiz (*Margiricarpus pinnatus*), oregano (*Origanum vulgare*), and guaycuri (*Statice brasiliensis*) was found to induce multi-system organ failure and, in one case, death of the mother.[4]

Contraindications

Pregnancy[2,3]
Lactation[5,11,12]
Pre-existing kidney, liver, nerve or lung disease[5,15]
Children[12]

Caution

Alcoholism[16]
Acetominophen use[16]

Constituents

- Volatile oils:[14] hedeomal, pulegone, alpha-pinene, beta-pinene, limonene, 3-octanone, *p*-cymene, 3-octylacetate, 3-octanol, 1-octen-3-ol, 3-methylcyclohexanone, menthone, piperitenone
- Tannins[14]
- Paraffins[14]

Toxicity

Essential oil

- LD_{50} in rats (oral):[16,17] 0.4 g/kg
- LD_{50} in rabbits (dermal):[17] 4.2 g/kg

Pulegone

- LD_{50} in rats (oral):[18] 0.47 g/kg
- LD_{50} in rabbits (dermal):[18] 3.09 g/kg

Pharmacology

- The volatile oil pulegone and its metabolites, menthofuran and methofuran's metabolites, may cause hepatotoxicity, neurotoxicity, and bronchiolar epithelial cell destruction.[5,13,19]
- Metabolites of pulegone deplete hepatic glutathione levels.[5,12,13] This leads to metabolite accumulation and direct cellular damage similar to acetaminophen (paracetamol) toxicity.[12]
- Pulegone is isomerized to isopulegone, which can be toxic to the lungs and liver.[20]
- Excretion of the essential oil irritates the kidneys and the bladder, and reflexively excites uterine contractions.[16]

Drug interactions[14]

Acetominophen[21,22]
Antihistamines[23]
Drugs metabolized by cytochrome P450 enzymes[13,24–27]

Oral hypoglycemic drugs[12]
Hepatotoxic drugs[12,15,28]

Parts used[16]

Aerial parts, oil

References

1. Jellin JM, Batz F, Hitchens K. Natural Medicines Comprehensive Database, 3rd ed. Stockton, CA: Therapeutic Research Faculty, 2002:1530.
2. Runnalls HB. Report of a case of acute poisoning by oil of pennyroyal. Med Sentinel 1904; 12:325.
3. Vallance M. Pennyroyal poisoning. A fatal case. Lancet 1955; 269:850–853.
4. Ciganda C, Laborde A. Herbal infusions used for induced abortion. J Toxicol Clin Toxicol 2003; 41:235–239.
5. Anderson IB, Mullen WH, Meeker JE et al. Pennyroyal toxicity: measurement of toxic metabolite levels in two cases and review of the literature. Ann Intern Med 1996; 124:726–734.
6. Farnsworth NR, Bingel AS, Cordell G, Crane FA, Fong HH. Potential value of plants as sources of new antifertility agents I. J Pharm Sci 1975; 64:535–598.
7. Gold J, Cates W Jr. Herbal abortifacients. JAMA 1980; 243:1365–1366.
8. Conway GA, Slocumb JC. Plants used as abortifacients and emmenagogues by Spanish New Mexicans. J Ethnopharmacol 1979; 1:241–261.
9. Early DF. Pennyroyal: a rare cause of epilepsy. Lancet 1961:580–581.
10. Buechel DW, Haverlah VC, Gardner M. Pennyroyal oil ingestion: report of a case. J Am Osteopath Assoc 1983; 82:793–794.
11. Sudekum M, Poppenga RH, Raju N, Braselton WE Jr. Pennyroyal oil toxicosis in a dog. J Am Vet Med Assoc 1992; 200:817–818.
12. Bakerink JA, Gospe SMJ, Dimand RJ, Eldridge MW. Multiple organ failure after ingestion of pennyroyal oil from herbal tea in two infants. Pediatrics 1996; 98:944–947.
13. Thomassen D, Slattery JT, Nelson SD. Menthofuran-dependent and independent aspects of pulegone hepatotoxicity: roles of glutathione. J Pharmacol Exp Ther 1990; 253:567–572.
14. www.naturalstandard.com. American Pennyroyal (Hedeoma pulegioides L.), European Pennyroyal (Mentha pulegium L.) Natural Standard Monograph, 2003.
15. Sullivan JBJ, Rumack BH, Thomas HJ et al. Pennyroyal oil poisoning and hepatotoxicity. JAMA 1979; 242:2873–2874.
16. Brinker F. The Toxicology of Botanical Medicines. Sandy, OR: Eclectic Medical Publications, 2000:296.
17. Opdyke DLJ. Pennyroyal oil european. Food Cosmet Toxicol 1974; 12:949–950.
18. Opdyke DLJ. Fragrance raw materials monographs: d-pulegone. 1978:867–868.
19. The Review of Natural Products by Facts and Comparisons. St. Louis, MO: Wolters Kluwer Co., 1999.
20. MICROMEDEX. Micromedex Healthcare Series. Englewood, CO: MICROMEDEX.
21. Rumack BH. Acetaminophen overdose in young children. Treatment and effects of alcohol and other additional ingestants in 417 cases. Am J Dis Child 1984; 138:428–433.

22. Lieh-Lai MW, Sarnaik AP, Newton JF et al. Metabolism and pharmacokinetics of acetaminophen in a severely poisoned young child. J Pediatr 1984; 105:125–128.
23. Ortiz de Urbina AV, Martin ML, Montero MJ et al. Antihistaminic activity of pulegone on the guinea-pig ileum. J Pharm Pharmacol 1990; 42:295–296.
24. Madyastha P, Moorthy B, Vaidyanathan CS et al. In vivo and in vitro destruction of rat liver cytochrome P-450 by a monoterpene ketone, pulegone. Biochem Biophys Res Comm 1985; 128:921–927.
25. Khojasteh-Bakht SC, Koenigs LL, Peter RM et al. (R)-(+)-Menthofuran is a potent, mechanism-based inactivator of human liver cytochrome P450 2A6. Drug Metab Dispos 1998; 26:701–704.
26. Gordon WP, Huitric AC, Seth CL et al. The metabolism of the abortifacient terpene, (R)-(+)-pulegone, to a proximate toxin, menthofuran. Drug Metab Dispos 1987; 15:589–594.
27. Thomassen D, Pearson PG, Slattery JT et al. Partial characterization of biliary metabolites of pulegone by tandem mass spectrometry. Detection of glucuronide, glutathione, and glutathionyl glucuronide conjugates. Drug Metab Dispos 1991; 19:997–1003.
28. Molck AM, Poulsen M, Tindgard LS et al. Lack of histological cerebellar changes in Wistar rats given pulegone for 28 days. Comparison of immersion and perfusion tissue fixation. Toxicol Lett 1998; 95:117–122.

PEPPERMINT
Mentha piperita

Synonyms/common names/related compounds[1]
Brandy mint, lamb mint, *Menthae piperitae folium*, *Menthae piperitae Aetheroleum*, menthe poivree

Indications

Oral

Dyspepsia (with caraway oil):[2–4]	Evidence grade B1
Tension headaches:[5,6]	Evidence grade B1
Irritable bowel syndrome:[7–10]	Evidence grade B2
Post-operative nausea:[11]	Evidence grade B2
Dyspepsia (with bitter candy tuft, chamomile flower, lemon balm, caraway fruit, licorice root, angelica root, celandine herbs and milk thistle fruit):[8]	Evidence grade B2
Common cold (with juniper oil, cajeput oil, eucalyptus oil and methylquinolinium oil):[2]	Evidence grade C
Barium enema-related colonic spasm:[12–14]	Evidence grade C

Pregnancy

Used to treat pregnancy-induced nausea:[15]	Evidence level 1c
Safety unkown:[15]	Evidence level 1c

A qualitative study of self-care in pregnancy, birth and lactation was conducted on 27 women in British Columbia (Canada) where 20 women (74%) experienced pregnancy-induced nausea.[15] The authors reported that peppermint was one of the remedies used to treat nausea, but that there was no information on safety during pregnancy.[15]

Possibly unsafe:[16]	Evidence level 4

A literature review reported that seven of the 300 nonmedical sources reviewed cited peppermint as unsafe during pregnancy.[16] There are no reports in the scientific literature of peppermint being either safe or contraindicated during pregnancy.

Emmenagogue:[17]	Evidence level 4

A review article on the potential value of plants as sources of anti-fertility agents also reported that peppermint was an emmenagogue.[17]

Antigonadotrophic activity:[17]	Evidence level 4

A review article on the potential value of plants as sources of anti-fertility agents reported that peppermint had antigonadotrophic activity in rat.[17]

Food

Safe:[1]	Evidence level 4

Peppermint leaves and oil are believed to be safe during pregnancy if consumed in food amounts.[1]

Lactation

Unknown:	Evidence level 5

There are no reports in the scientific literature of peppermint being either safe or contraindicated during lactation.

Food

Safe:[1]	Evidence level 4

Peppermint leaves and oil are believed to be safe during lactation if consumed in food amounts.[1]

Caution

Large amounts of peppermint oil may cause interstitial nephritis and acute renal failure.[18]

Constituents[19]

- Essential oil:[18–22] cineol, isomenthone, liminene, menthofuran, menthol, menthone, menthyl acetate, terpenoids
- Leaf:[19–21] caffeic acid, chlorogenic acid, luteolin, hesperidin, rutin, volatile oil, flavonoids, azulene

Toxicity

- Acute oral LD_{50} of menthol:[23] 3.3 g/kg.
- Oral administration of a spray-dried infusion of peppermint (4 g/kg) did not result in any macroscopic signs of toxicity or death in mice over a 7-day period.[24]

Pharmacology

Leaf

Peppermint leaf has antispasmodic, antiflatulent, and bile stimulation activity.[20,25]

Oil

- The constituent menthol has direct antispasmodic activity on the smooth muscle of the digestive tract through calcium antagonist activity.[18,26,27]
- Peppermint oil increases salivation, which increases the swallowing reflex and suppresses the cough reflex.[18,28]
- Peppermint oil reduces bronchial secretions and has nasal decongestant activity.[26]
- Peppermint oil decreases gas and flatulence by relaxing the lower esophageal sphincter, thereby equalizing the intraluminal pressures between the stomach and esophagus.[22,29]
- Peppermint oil has antimicrobial and antiviral activity in vitro.[21]
- Peppermint oil may inhibit cytochrome P4503A.[4,30]
- The volatile oil azulene has anti-inflammatory and anti-ulcer activity.[21]
- Topically, peppermint oil is a counterirritant.[22]

Drug interactions

Leaf

Felodipine[19]
Simvastatin[19]
Cyclosporine[19]
5-Fluorouracil[19]
Drugs metabolized by cytochrome P4503A4[30]

Oil

Antacids[31]
Cyclosporine[32]
Drugs metabolized by cytochrome P4503A4[30]
H2-blockers[31]
Proton pump inhibitors[31]

Parts used1

Leaf, oil

References

1. Jellin JM, Batz F, Hitchens K. Natural Medicines Comprehensive Database, 3rd ed. Stockton, CA: Therapeutic Research Faculty, 2002:1530.
2. Madisch A, Heydenreich CJ, W V, Hufnagel R, Hotz J. Treatment of functional dyspepsia with a fixed peppermint oil and caraway oil combination preparation as

compared to cisapride. A multicenter, reference-controlled double-blind equivalence study. Arzneimittelforschung 1999; 49:925–932.
3. May B, Kuntz HD, Kieser M, Kohler S. Efficacy of a fixed peppermint oil/caraway oil combination in non-ulcer dyspepsia. Arzneimittelforschung 1996; 46:1149–1153.
4. May B, Kohler S, Schneider B. Efficacy and tolerability of a fixed combination of peppermint oil and caraway oil in patients suffering from functional dyspepsia. Aliment Pharmacol Ther 2000; 14:1671–1677.
5. Gobel H, Schmidt G, Soyka D. Effect of peppermint and eucalyptus oil preparations on neurophysiological and experimental algesimetric headache parameters. Cephalalgia 1994; 14:228–234; discussion 182.
6. Gobel H, Fresenius J, Heinze A, Dworschak M, Soyka D. [Effectiveness of Oleum menthae piperitae and paracetamol in therapy of headache of the tension type]. Nervenarzt 1996; 67:672–681.
7. Liu JH, Chen GH, Yeh H, Huang CK, Poon SK. Enteric-coated peppermint-oil capsules in the treatment of irritable bowel syndrome: a prospective, randomized trial. J Gastroenterol 1997; 32:765–768.
8. Kline RM, Kline JJ, Di Palma J, Barbero GJ. Enteric-coated, pH-dependent peppermint oil capsules for the treatment of irritable bowel syndrome in children. J Pediatr 2001; 138:125–128.
9. Dew MJ, Evans BK, Rhodes J. Peppermint oil for the irritable bowel syndrome: a multicentre trial. Br J Clin Pract 1984; 38:394–398.
10. Rees WD, Evans BK, Rhodes J. Treating irritable bowel syndrome with peppermint oil. Br Med J 1979; 2:835–836.
11. Tate S. Peppermint oil: a treatment for postoperative nausea. J Adv Nurs 1997; 26:543–549.
12. Leicester RJ, Hunt RH. Peppermint oil to reduce colonic spasm during endoscopy. Lancet 1982; ii:989.
13. Asao T, Kuwano H, Ide M et al. Spasmolytic effect of peppermint oil in barium during double-contrast barium enema compared with Buscopan. Clin Radiol 2003; 58:301–305.
14. Sparks MJ, O'Sullivan P, Herrington A, Morcos SK. Does peppermint oil relieve spasm during barium enema? Br J Radiol 1995; 68:841–843.
15. Westfall RE. Use of anti-emetic herbs in pregnancy: women's choices, and the question of safety and efficacy. Complement Ther Nurs Midwifery 2004; 10:30–36.
16. Wilkinson JM. What do we know about herbal morning sickness treatments? A literature survey. Midwifery 2000; 16:224–228.
17. Farnsworth NR, Bingel AS, Cordell G, Crane FA, Fong HH. Potential value of plants as sources of new antifertility agents I. J Pharm Sci 1975; 64:535–598.
18. Schulz V, Hansel R, Tyler VE, Terry C. Rational Phytotherapy: A Physician's Guide to Herbal Medicine, 3rd ed. Berlin: Springer, 1998.
19. www.naturalstandard.com. Peppermint (Mentha × piperita L.), 2003.
20. Gruenwald J, Brendler T, Jaenicke C. PDR for Herbal Medicines. Montvale, NJ: Medical Economics Company, 1998.
21. Leung AY, Foster S. Encyclopedia of Common Natural Ingredients Used in Food, Drugs and Cosmetics, 2nd ed. New York, NY: John Wiley & Sons, 1996:649.
22. Pizzorno JE, Murray MT. Textbook of Natural Medicine, 2nd ed. Edinburgh: Churchill Livingstone, 1999.
23. Opdyke DLJ. Monographs on fragrance raw materials. Food Cosmet Toxicol 1976; 14:471–472.

24. Della Loggia R, Tubaro A. Evaluation of some pharmacological activities of a peppermint extract. Fitoterapia 1990; 61:215–221.
25. Blumenthal M, Busse WR, Goldberg A et al. The Complete German Commission E Monographs: Therapeutic Guide to Herbal Medicines. Boston, MA: American Botanical Council, 1998.
26. Monographs on the medicinal uses of plant drugs. Exeter, UK: European Scientific Co-op Phytother, 1997.
27. Beesley A, Hardcastle J, Hardcastle PT, Taylor CJ. Influence of peppermint oil on absorptive and secretory processes in rat small intestine. Gut 1996; 39:214–219.
28. Tyler VE. Herbs of Choice. Binghamton, NY: Pharmaceutical Products Press, 1994.
29. Robbers JE, Tyler VE. Tyler's Herbs of Choice: The Therapeutic Use of Phytomedicinals. New York, NY: The Haworth Herbal Press, 1999.
30. Dresser GK, Wacher V, WS, Wong HT, Bailey DG. Evaluation of peppermint oil and ascorbyl palmitate as inhibitors of cytochrome P450 3A4 activity in vitro and in vivo. Clin Pharmacol Ther 2002; 72:247–255.
31. Foster S. Peppermint, Menta × piperita, botanical series #306. Austin, TX: American Botanical Council, 1990.
32. Wacher VJ, Wong S, Wong HT. Peppermint oil enhances cyclosporine oral bioavailability in rats: comparison with D-alpha-tocopheryl poly(ethylene glycol 1000) succinate (TPGS) and ketoconazole. J Pharm Sci 2002; 91:77–90.

RASPBERRY
Rubus idaeus

Synonyms/common names/related substances[1]

Red raspberry, *Rubi idaei folium*, rubus, framboise

Indications

Labor:[2,3]	Evidence grade B1

Pregnancy

Leaf

Minimal risk:[2,3]	Evidence level 1a
Shortens labor and reduces complications:[2,3]	Evidence level 1a
May decrease pre- and post-term births:[2]	Evidence level 1b
Less likely to receive an artificial rupture of the membranes or require a cesarean section, forceps, or vacuum birth:[2]	Evidence level 1b

A randomized controlled trial of 192 low-risk nulliparous women was conducted where one group consumed raspberry leaf tablets (2 × 1.2 g per day) from 32 weeks' gestation until labor and the other group received a placebo.[3] Raspberry leaf was found to cause no adverse effects for mother or baby.[3] The findings showed that raspberry leaf did not shorten the first stage of labor, but did shorten the second stage of labor and resulted in a lower rate of forceps deliveries.[3]

A retrospective cohort study of mothers who consumed raspberry leaf products during their pregnancy versus a control group found that raspberry leaf products shortened labor with no identified side effects for the women or their babies.[2] The findings suggested that ingestion of raspberry products might decrease the likelihood of pre- and post-term gestation.[2] The findings also suggested that women who ingested raspberry leaf might have been less likely to receive an artificial rupture of their membranes, or require a cesarean section, forceps, or vacuum birth than the women in the control group.[2]

Induces labor:[4]	Evidence level 4

A survey of midwives in the USA found that 63% use raspberry leaf to induce labor.[4] Raspberry leaf is part of a combination of herbal medicines that have been traditionally used in the third trimester to prepare a woman for delivery; this preparation is called 'mother's cordial' or 'partus preparatus'. In addition to raspberry leaf, mother's cordial may contain: squaw vine (*Mitchella ripens*), black cohosh (*Cimicifuga racemosa*), blue cohosh (*Caulophyllum thalictroides*) and false unicorn (*Chamaelirium luteum*).

Uterine stimulant:[5]	Evidence level 4

Estrogenic:[1]	Evidence level 4

A herb toxicology and drug interaction compendium reported that raspberry leaves have uterine stimulant properties.[5] A database of herbs and supplements reported that raspberry leaves may have estrogenic properties.[1] Raspberry was not reported in the scientific literature as having estrogenic properties.

Anti-gonadotrophic effects:[6]	Evidence level 4

A review article on the potential value of plants as sources of anti-fertility agents reported that raspberry had anti-gonadotrophic effects in vitro.[6]

Fruit

Minimal risk:[7]	Evidence level 4

Raspberry fruit is not believed to pose a risk to the mother or the baby during pregnancy.[7]

Lactation

Leaves

Unknown:	Evidence level 5

Raspberry leaves are not reported in the literature as being safe or contraindicated during lactation.

Fruit

Minimal risk:[7]	Evidence level 4

Raspberry fruit is not believed to pose a risk to the baby during lactation.[7]

Constituents

Leaf
Tannins[1]

Fruit
Anthocyanins[8]
Phenolic compounds:[9,10] ellagitannins, ellagic acid
Vitamin C[10]

Pharmacology

Leaf

- Raspberry leaf may decrease contraction of tonic tissues and increase contraction of relaxed tissues.[4,11]
- In animals, raspberry leaf extract was shown to relax smooth muscle.[12]

Fruit

- Raspberry fruit is an antioxidant.[9]
- Extracts of raspberry fruit were found to significantly inhibit mutagenesis on cervical and breast cancer cell lines by both direct-acting and metabolically activated carcinogens.[13]
- Raspberry cordial and juice were found to have anti-bacterial activity in vitro.[14]

Drug interactions

Metformin[1]

Part used[5]

Leaf

References

1. Jellin JM, Batz F, Hitchens K. Natural Medicines Comprehensive Database, 3rd ed. Stockton, CA: Therapeutic Research Faculty, 2002:1530.
2. Parsons M, Simpson M, Ponton T. Raspberry leaf and its effect on labour: safety and efficacy. Aust Coll Midwives Inc J 1999; 12:20–25.
3. Simpson M, Parsons M, Greenwood J, Wade K. Raspberry leaf in pregnancy: its safety and efficacy in labor. J Midwifery Womens Health 2001; 46:51–59.
4. McFarlin BL, Gibson MH, O'Rear J, Harman P. A national survey of herbal preparation use by nurse-midwives for labor stimulation. Review of the literature and recommendations for practice. J Nurse Midwifery 1999; 44:205–216.
5. Brinker F. The Toxicology of Botanical Medicines. Sandy, OR: Eclectic Medical Publications, 2000:296.
6. Farnsworth NR, Bingel AS, Cordell G, Crane FA, Fong HH. Potential value of plants as sources of new antifertility agents I. J Pharm Sci 1975; 64:535–598.
7. Newall CA, Anderson LA, Phillipson JD. Herbal Medicines: A Guide for Health-care Professionals. London, UK: Pharmaceutical Press, 1996:296.
8. Mullen W, Lean ME, Crozier A. Rapid characterization of anthocyanins in red raspberry fruit by high-performance liquid chromatography coupled to single quadrupole mass spectrometry. J Chromatogr A 2002; 966:63–70.

9. Kahkonen MP, Hopia AI, Heinonen M. Berry phenolics and their antioxidant activity. J Agric Food Chem 2001; 49:4076–4082.
10. de Ancos B, Gonzalez EM, Cano M. Ellagic acid, vitamin C, and total phenolic contents and radical scavenging capacity affected by freezing and frozen storage in raspberry fruit. J Agric Food Chem 2000; 48:4565–4570.
11. Bamford DS, Percival RC, Tothill AU. Raspberry leaf tea: a new aspect to an old problem. Br J Pharmacol 1970; 40:161P+.
12. Rojas-Vera J, Patel AV, Dacke C. Relaxant activity of raspberry (Rubus idaeus) leaf extract in guinea-pig ileum in vitro. Phytother Res 2002; 16:665–668.
13. Wedge DE, Meepagala KM, Magee JB et al. Anticarcinogenic activity of strawberry, blueberry, and raspberry extracts to breast and cervical cancer cells. J Med Food 2001; 4:49–51.
14. Ryan T, Wilkinson JM, Cavanagh H. Antibacterial activity of raspberry cordial in vitro. Res Vet Sci 2001; 71:155–159.

RED CLOVER
Trifolium pratense

Synonyms/common names/related compounds[1]

Beebread, clovone, cow clover, daidzein, genistein, isoflavone, isoflavones, meadow clover, phytoestrogen, phytoestrogens, purple clover, trefoil, trifolium, wild clover

Indications

Cyclic mastalgia:[2]	Evidence grade B2
Arterial compliance in menopause:[3]	Evidence grade B2
Prostate cancer:[4,5]	Evidence grade C
Menopausal symptoms:[6–8]	Evidence grade D
Osteoporosis:[9]	Evidence grade D
Hypercholesterolemia:[9,10]	Evidence grade D
Benign prostatic hyperplasia:[11]	Evidence grade D

Pregnancy

May cause infertility:[12]	Evidence level 3

During 1982–1983, serious fertility disturbances were observed in a herd of cattle.[13] The researchers determined that the cause was estrogenic stimulation from eating silage prepared almost entirely from pure red clover aftergrowth.[13] When feeding with the red clover silage was subsequently discontinued, the disturbances ceased to occur and the cows became pregnant more easily.[13]

Estrogenic activity:[14,15]	Evidence level 3
Anti-estrogenic activity:[16–23]	Evidence level 3

In human breast cancer cells, red clover was shown to bind to intracellular estrogen receptors and to enhance estrogenic effects.[14] A review article on the potential value of plants as sources of anti-fertility agents reported that red clover has estrogenic activity.[15]

In addition to having estrogenic activity, red clover was reported to have anti-estrogenic properties.[16–23]

Increases progesterone synthesis:[24]	Evidence level 3

The red clover constituent biochanin A was found to increase progesterone synthesis by 40–50% in bovine granulosa cells.[24]

Crosses the placenta:[25]	Evidence level 3

In a study of human amniotic fluid following phytoestrogen ingestion, dietary phytoestrogens were found in 96.2% of second trimester amniotic fluid samples tested.[25] The second trimester amniotic fluid contained quantifiable levels of formononetin, biochanin A and coumestrol, all constituents of red clover.[25]

Potential abortifacient:[12]	Evidence level 4

An evidence-based herbal monograph database reported that red clover has been implicated as a cause of abortion in grazing livestock.[12]

Food amounts

Minimal risk:[26]	Evidence level 4

Red clover was reported to be of minimal risk when consumed in food amounts.[26]

Lactation

Estrogenic activity:[14]	Evidence level 3
Increases progesterone synthesis:[24]	Evidence level 3

In human breast cancer cells, red clover was shown to bind to intracellular estrogen receptors and to enhance estrogenic effects.[14] The red clover constituent biochanin A was found to increase progesterone synthesis by 40–50% in bovine granulosa cells.[24]

Food amounts

Minimal risk:[26]	Evidence level 4

Red clover was reported to be of minimal risk when consumed in food amounts.[26]

Constituents

Isoflavones[1]: biochanin A, formononetin, coumestrol

Toxicity

- Insufficient human data available[12]
- In grazing animals, red clover ingestion has been associated with cachexia, bloating, infertility, growth disorders and abortion[12,27]

Pharmacology

- The phytoestrogens biochanin A and formononetin, and other isoflavones are metabolized to the isoflavones genistein and daidzein, respectively, when ingested.[16,28,29]
- Red clover has estrogenic and anti-estrogenic properties.[16–23]
- Isoflavones have a higher affinity for β-estrogen receptors (heart, vasculature, bone, and bladder) than α-estrogen receptors.[16,18,30–33]
- Red clover may prevent osteoporosis due to its weak estrogenic activity and to the osteoclast inhibitory activity of its metabolite genistein.[16,18,32,34]
- Red clovers improves systemic arterial compliance, thereby preventing cardiovascular disease.[3,28,32]
- Red clover increases bile acid excretion and up-regulates low-density lipoprotein receptors.[18,35,36]
- Red clover may have anti-carcinogenic activity, particularly in reducing the risk of endometrial cancer, due to estrogenic and anti-estrogenic activity.[37–40]
- Red clover may have anti-coagulant effects.[41]
- Red clover may interfere with the cytochrome P450 CYP3A4 enzyme.[42,43]

Drug interactions[1]

Anticoagulant/antiplatelet drugs[43]
Estrogen or oral contraceptives[43–45]
Tomoxifen[17]
Drugs metabolized by cytochrome P450 CYP3A4[42,43]

Part used[1]

Flower top

References

1. Jellin JM, Batz F, Hitchens K. Natural Medicines Comprehensive Database, 3rd ed. Stockton, CA: Therapeutic Research Faculty, 2002:1530.
2. Ingram DM, Hickling C, WL et al. A double-blind randomized controlled trial of isoflavones in the treatment of cyclical mastalgia. Breast 2002; 11:170–174.
3. Nestel PJ, Pomeroy S, Kay S et al. Isoflavones from red clover improve systemic arterial compliance but not plasma lipids in menopausal women. J Clin Endocrinol Metab 1999; 84:895–898.
4. Stephens FO. Phytoestrogens and prostate cancer: possible preventive role. Med J Aust 1997; 167:138–140.
5. Jarred RA, Keikha M, Dowling C et al. Induction of apoptosis in low to moderate-grade human prostate carcinoma by red clover-derived dietary isoflavones. Cancer Epidemiol Biomarkers Prev 2002; 11:1689–1696.
6. Nachtigall LB, La Grega L, Lee W et al. The effects of isoflavones derived from red clover on vasomotor symptoms and endometrial thickness. 9th International Menopause Society World Congress on the Menopause 1999:331–336.
7. Abernethy K, Brockie J, Suffling K et al. An open study of the effects of a 40mg isoflavone food supplement (derived from Red Clover), on menopausal symptoms. The British Menopause Society, 2001.

8. Jeri AR. The effect of isoflavone phytoestrogens in relieving hot flushes in Peruvian post menopausal women. 9th International Menopause Society World Congress on the Menopause, 1999.
9. Clifton-Bligh PB, Baber RJ, Fulcher G, Nery ML, Moreton T. The effect of isoflavones extracted from red clover (Rimostil) on lipid and bone metabolism. Menopause 2001; 8:259–265.
10. Baber R, Clifton Bligh P, Fulcher GR et al. The effect of an isoflavone extract (PO81) on serum lipids, forearm bone density and endometrial thickness in postmenopausal women. Proceedings of the North American Menopause Society, New York, 1999.
11. Gerber G, Lowe FC, Spigelman S. The use of a standardized extract of red clover isoflavones for the alleviation of BPH symptoms. The 82nd Annual Meeting of the Endocrine Society 2000; 82:2359.
12. www.naturalstandard.com. Red Clover (Trifolium pratense) Natural Standard Monograph.
13. Kallela K, Heinonen K, Saloniemi H. Plant oestrogens; the cause of decreased fertility in cows. A case report. Nord Vet Med 1984; 36(3–4):124–129.
14. Zava DT, Dollbaum CM, Blen M. Estrogen and progestin bioactivity of foods, herbs, and spices. Proc Soc Exp Biol Med 1998; 217:369–378.
15. Farnsworth NR, Bingel AS, Cordell GA, Crane FA, Fong HH. Potential value of plants as sources of new antifertility agents II. J Pharm Sci 1975; 64:717–753.
16. Umland EM, Cauffield JS, Kirk JK et al. Phytoestrogens as therapeutic alternatives to traditional hormone replacement in postmenopausal women. Pharmacotherapy 2000; 20:981–990.
17. This P, De La Rochefordiere A, Clough K et al. Phytoestrogens after breast cancer. Endocr Relat Cancer 2001; 8:129–134.
18. Setchell KD, Cassidy A. Dietary isoflavones: biological effects and relevance to human health. J Nutr 1999; 129:758S–767S.
19. Zand RS, Jenkins DJ, Diamandis EP. Steroid hormone activity of flavonoids and related compounds. Breast Cancer Res Treat 2000; 62:35–49.
20. Baird DD, Umbach DM, Lansdell L et al. Dietary intervention study to assess estrogenicity of dietary soy among postmenopausal women. J Clin Endocrinol Metab 1995; 80:1685–1690.
21. Duncan AM, Underhill KE, Xu X et al. Modest hormonal effects of soy isoflavones in postmenopausal women. J Clin Endocrinol Metab 1999; 84:3479–3484.
22. Ginsburg J, Prelevic GM. Lack of significant hormonal effects and controlled trials of phyto-oestrogens. Lancet 2000; 355:163–164.
23. Hargreaves DF, Potten CS, Harding C et al. Two-week dietary soy supplementation has an estrogenic effect on normal premenopausal breast. J Clin Endocrinol Metab 1999; 84:4017–4024.
24. Kaplanski O, Shemesh M, Berman A. Effects of phyto-oestrogens on progesterone synthesis by isolated bovine granulosa cells. J Endocrinol 1981; 89:343–348.
25. Foster WG, Chan S, Platt L, Hughes CL Jr. Detection of phytoestrogens in samples of second trimester human amniotic fluid. Toxicol Lett 2002; 129:199–205.
26. FDA. Center for Food Safety and Applied Nutrition, Office of Premarket Approval, EAFUS: A food additive database. vm.cfsan.fda.gov/~dms/eafus.html, 2004.
27. Frohne D, Pfander HJ. A colour atlas of poisonous plants. London: Wolfe, 1984.
28. Howes JB, Sullivan D, Lai N et al. The effects of dietary supplementation with isoflavones from red clover on the lipoprotein profiles of postmenopausal women with mild to moderate hypercholesterolemia. Atherosclerosis 2000; 152:143–147.

29. Setchell KD. Absorption and metabolism of soy isoflavones: from food to dietary supplements and adults to infants. J Nutr 2000; 130:654S–655S.
30. Barnes S, Kim H, Darley-Usmar V et al. Beyond ERalpha and ERbeta: estrogen receptor binding is only part of the isoflavone story. J Nutr 2000; 130:656S–657S.
31. Anthony MS. Soy and cardiovascular disease: Cholesterol lowering and beyond. J Nutr 2000; 130:662S–663S.
32. Anon. The role of isoflavones in menopausal health: consensus opinion of the North American Menopause Society. Menopause 2000; 7:215–229.
33. Vincent A, Fitzpatrick LA. Soy isoflavones: are they useful in menopause? Mayo Clin Proc 2000; 75:1174–1184.
34. Atkinson C, Compston JE, Robins SP, Bingham SA. The effects of isoflavone phytoestrogens on bone; preliminary results from a large randomized, controlled trial, 82nd Annual Meeting of the Endocrine Society, Toronto, 21–24 June 2000.
35. Lissin LW, Cooke JP. Phytoestrogens and cardiovascular health. J Am Coll Cardiol 2000; 35:1403–1410.
36. Hodgson JM, Puddey IB, Beilin LJ et al. Supplementation with isoflavonoid phytoestrogens does not alter serum lipid concentrations: a randomized controlled trial in humans. J Nutr 1998; 128:728–732.
37. Horn-Ross PL, John EM, Canchola AJ et al. Phytoestrogen intake and endometrial cancer risk. J Natl Cancer Inst 2003; 95:1158–1164.
38. Yanagihara K, Ito A, Toge T, Numoto M. Antiproliferative effects of isoflavones on human cancer cell lines established from the gastrointestinal tract. Cancer Res 1993; 53:5815–5821.
39. Cassady JM, Zennie TM, Chae YH et al. Use of a mammalian cell culture benzo(a)pyrene metabolism assay for the detection of potential anticarcinogens from natural products: inhibition of metabolism by biochanin A, an isoflavone from Trifolium pratense L. Cancer Res 1988; 48:6257–6261.
40. Le Bail JC, Champavier Y, Chulia AJ, Habrioux G. Effects of phytoestrogens on aromatase, 3beta and 17beta-hydroxysteroid dehydrogenase activities and human breast cancer cells. Life Sci 2000; 66:1281–1291.
41. Puschner B, Galey FD, Holstege DM et al. Sweet clover poisoning in dairy cattle in California. J Am Vet Med Assoc 1998; 212:857–859.
42. Budzinski JW, Foster BC, Vandenhoek S, Arnason JT. An in vitro evaluation of human cytochrome P450 3A4 inhibition by selected commercial herbal extracts and tinctures. Phytomedicine 2000; 7:273–282.
43. Nelsen J, Barrette E, Tsouronix C et al. Red clover (Trifolium pratense) monograph: a clinical decision support tool. J Herb Pharmacother 2002; 2:49–72.
44. Kurzer MS, Xu X. Dietary phytoestrogens. Annu Rev Nutr 1997; 17:353–381.
45. Anon. Phytoestrogens. Med Letter 2000; 42:17–18.

RYE ERGOT
Claviceps purpurea

Synonyms/common names/related substances[1]

Cockspur rye, hornseed, mother of rye, *Secale cornutum*, smut rye, spurred rye

Indications

Oxytoxin-ergot preparations

Prevention of post-partum hemorrhage:[2]	Evidence grade A

Ergot derivatives

Dementia and age-related cognitive impairment:[3,4]	Evidence grade A
Migraine headaches:[5,6]	Evidence grade B2

Pregnancy

Potentially teratogenic:[7]	Evidence level 4

A literature review on ergot and ergotamine reported that ergotamine is a suspected teratogen, where clinical reports in humans have been anecdotal, but in many the malformations are consistent with vascular injury.[7] The author reported that although epidemiologic studies have not shown any clear increase in malformations among exposed infants, this may reflect the limited exposure and toxicity when used episodically.[7] The author recommended that ergotamine be avoided in pregnancy.[7]

May cause convulsive ergotism:[8]	Evidence level 4

A historical review was conducted on the epidemics of 'convulsive ergotism' between 1085 and 1927 of the Rhine Valley in Europe.[8] The clinical features of convulsive ergotism are muscle twitching and spasms, changes in mental state, hallucinations, sweating, and fever lasting for several weeks.[8] The author suggested that these symptoms represented a serotonergic overstimulation of the central nervous system, i.e. the serotonin syndrome.[8]

Emmenagogue:[9]	Evidence level 4
Oxytoxic:[9]	Evidence level 4
Abortifacient:[9]	Evidence level 4

A herbal contraindication and drug interaction compendium reported that rye ergot is an emmenagogue, uterine stimulant, abortifacient and has oxytoxic properties.[9]

Cabergoline (ergot derivative)

No increased risk of malformations:[10]	Evidence level 1b

No increase in miscarriage weight:[10]	Evidence level 1b

A follow-up study on 204 live births to assess the reproductive safety of cabergoline, an ergot derivative, showed no increase in miscarriage rate, a distribution of birthweights and sex ratio within the expected range, and no increased rate of congenital malformations.[10] A further follow-up of babies, limited to 107 cases, indicated normal physical and mental development.[10]

Nonteratogenic:[11]	Evidence level 3

Does not impair fertility in males:[11]	Evidence level 3

Nontoxic to neonates:[11]	Evidence level 3

A study on the teratogenicity of cabergoline in animals concluded that cabergoline did not impair fertility in the male rat, was not teratogenic in mice and rabbits, did not affect the later phase of gestation or parturition in the rat, and was not toxic when administered directly to neonatal rats.[11]

C. purpurea *grown on wheat*

Reproductive problems:[12]	Evidence level 3

Ergot alkaloids from *C. purpurea* grown on wheat can cause reproductive problems in pigs.[12]

Lactation

Ergot derivatives

Inhibit lactation:[13,14]	Evidence level 1a

A number of randomized clinical trials reported that ergot derivatives inhibit post-partum lactation.[13,14]

C. purpurea *grown on wheat*

Lactational failure:[12]	Evidence level 3

Ergot alkaloids from *C. purpurea* grown on wheat are associated with lactational failure in pigs.[12]

Contraindications[9]

Peripheral blood flow disorders
Coronary insufficiency
Slow gastrointestinal absorption
Preexisting vascular pathology
Hypertonia
Liver disease
Infection
Fever

Constituents

Indole alkaloids:[9] ergonovine, ergocornine, ergotamine, ergocryptine, ergosine, ergocristine

Toxicity

- Toxic dose of rye ergot extract:[9] 1.0–3.9 g
- Lethal dose of rye ergot alkaloids:[9] 1 g (adults) and 12 mg (infants)
- Lethal dose of ergotamine tartrate:[9] 26 mg (oral) and 0.5–1.5 mg (intramuscular)
- LD_{50} of the rye ergot alkaloid elymoclavine:[15] 350 mg/kg (mice) and 145 mg/kg (rats)

Pharmacology

- Through α-adrenergic blocking and antagonism of 5-hydroxytryptamine, rye ergot stimulates smooth muscles and post-ganglionic synapses of the sympathetic nerves to the uterus, bladder, heart, blood vessels, and iris.[9]
- Ergot alkaloids produce vasoconstriction and myometrial stimulation.[16]
- The ergot alkaloids and derivatives have central, neurohumoral and peripheral effects.[1]
- The ergot alkaloids and derivatives bind to noradrenaline, serotonin, or dopamine receptor.[17]
- The ergot alkaloids are serotonin agonists.[8] Dihydroergotamine binds to serotonin receptors in the dorsal horn of the spinal cord, which is the site of neuropathological changes in convulsive ergotism.[8]

Drug interactions

Ergot alkaloids[1]
Sympathomimetics[16]

Parts used

Dried sclerotium grown on *Secale* (rye) kernels[9]

References

1. Jellin JM, Batz F, Hitchens K. Natural Medicines Comprehensive Database, 3rd ed. Stockton, CA: Therapeutic Research Faculty, 2002:1530.

2. Villar J, Gulmezoglu AM, Hofmeyr G, Forna F. Systematic review of randomized controlled trials of misoprostol to prevent postpartum hemorrhage. Obstet Gynecol 2002; 100:1301–1312.
3. Fioravanti M, Flicker L. Nicergoline for dementia and other age associated forms of cognitive impairment (Cochrane Review). Cochrane Library, Issue 1, 2004. Oxford: Update Software 2004.
4. Tsolaki M. Nimodipine vs dihydroergocristine in the treatment of old age dementias. Blind, randomized, cross-over, placebo-controlled study. Eur Neuropsychopharmacol 1995; 5:384.
5. Martucci N, Manna V, Mattesi P et al. Ergot derivatives in the prophylaxis of migraine: a multicentric study with a timed-release dihydroergotamine formulation. Cephalalgia 1983; 3:151–155.
6. Christie S, G'Bel H, Mateos V et al. Crossover comparison of efficacy and preference for rizatriptan 10 mg versus ergotamine/caffeine in migraine. Eur Neur 2003; 49:20–29.
7. Raymond GV. Teratogen update: ergot and ergotamine. Teratology 1995; 51:344–347.
8. Eadie MJ. Convulsive ergotism: epidemics of the serotonin syndrome? Lancet Neurol 2003; 2:429–434.
9. Brinker F. The Toxicology of Botanical Medicines. Sandy, OR: Eclectic Medical Publications, 2000:296.
10. Robert E, Musatti L, Piscitelli G, Ferrari CI. Pregnancy outcome after treatment with the ergot derivative, cabergoline. Reprod Toxicol 1996; 10:333–337.
11. Beltrame D, Longo M, Mazue G. Reproductive toxicity of cabergoline in mice, rats, and rabbits. Reprod Toxicol 1996; 10:471–483.
12. Diekman MA, Green ML. Mycotoxins and reproduction in domestic livestock. J Anim Sci 1992; 70:1615–1627.
13. Melis GB, Mais V, Paoletti A et al. Prevention of puerperal lactation by a single oral administration of the new prolactin-inhibiting drug, cabergoline. Obstet Gynecol 1988; 71(3 Pt 1):311–314.
14. Varga L, Lutterbeck PM, Pryor J, Wenner R, Erb H. Suppression of puerperal lactation with an ergot alkaloid: a double-blind study. Br Med J 1972; ii:743–744.
15. Petkov V, Georgiev V, Roussinov K et al. On the pharmacology of the ergot alkaloid elymoclavine. Biomed Biochim Acta 1984; 43:1305–1316.
16. Ellenhorn MJ, Schonwald S, Ordog G, Wasserberger J. Ellenhorn's Medical Toxicology: Diagnoses and Treatment of Human Poisoning, 2nd ed. Baltimore, MD: Williams & Wilkins, 1997.
17. Mantegani S, Brambilla E, Varasi M. Ergoline derivatives: receptor affinity and selectivity. Farmaco 1999; 54:288–296.

SENNA

Cassia acutifolia, C. angustifolia, C. senna, C. lanceolata

Synonyms/common names/related compounds[1]

Alexandrian senna, alexandrinische senna, casse, Indian senna, khartoum senna, sena alejandrina, séné d'Egypte, *Sennae folium, Sennae fructus, Sennae fructus acutifoliae, Sennae fructus angustifolia*, tinnevelly senna, true senna

Indications

Constipation:[2–4]	Evidence grade B1

Pregnancy

Minimal risk:[5]	Evidence level 3
Does not stimulate uterine motility:[5]	Evidence level 3

A study was conducted to evaluate the effects of sennosides on uterine motility in the pregnant ewe.[5] The experiments showed that sennosides did not stimulate uterine motility in the pregnant ewe, but slightly depressed it in some ewes.[5] Cervix motility was never influenced and pregnancy maintenance was normal in all ewes.[5]

Minimal risk:[6]	Evidence level 4

A review article reported that senna would appear to be the stimulant laxative of choice during pregnancy.[6]

Potential abortifacient:[7]	Evidence level 4
Emmenagogue:[7]	Evidence level 4

A toxicology and drug interaction compendium reported that senna is an emmenagogue and potential abortifacient.[7] There are no reports in the scientific literature of senna being an emmenagogue or potential abortifacient.

Conflicting evidence

Nongenotoxic:[8,9]	Evidence level 4
Genotoxic:[7]	Evidence level 3

A toxicology and drug interaction compendium reported that senna is genotoxic due to its aloe-emodin content.[7] A review study on the potential genotoxic and mutagenic properties of senna reported that human clinical trials and animal data do not support concerns that senna laxatives pose a genotoxic risk to humans when consumed under prescribed use conditions.[8,9]

Avoid during pregnancy:[10]	Evidence level 4

A compendium on herbal safety reported that senna should be avoided during pregnancy.[10] There are no reports in the literature of senna being contraindicated during pregnancy.

Lactation

Minimal risk:[4,11]	Evidence level 1a

Safe according to the American Association of Pediatrics (AAP):[11]	Evidence level 4

A clinical trial was conducted on the effectiveness of senna in the immediate postpartum period in white and black patients with matching placebo.[4] The author reported that it was well tolerated with minor abdominal cramps occurring in 13% of the patients treated with standardized senna.[4] The author reported that there was no evidence to suggest that standardized senna had any effect whatsoever on a breast-fed baby if taken by the mother.[4]

Senna is considered compatible by the American Association of Pediatrics (AAP) for breast-feeding.[11]

Low levels excreted in breast milk:[12,13]	Evidence level 1

A study was conducted on the excretion of rhein, a cathartic metabolite from sennosides, in breast milk samples of 15 post-partum women for at least 24 hours after the intake of a therapeutic dose (15 mg sennosides/day) of senna.[12] The authors observed that the amount of rhein transmitted to the infant was 0.3% of the rhein intake of the mother, which is far below the oral rhein dose necessary for inducing a laxative effect.[12] The authors also reported that none of the breast-fed infants showed any difference in stool consistency in comparison with the nonbreast-fed infants.[12] Another study in 100 breast milk samples found similar results.[13]

Contraindications[7]

Intestinal obstruction
Abdominal pain of unknown origin
Intestinal inflammation
Prolapsed rectum or anus
Kidney dysfunction
Children under 12 years

Caution

Avoid use for longer than 1–2 weeks as frequent use causes the colon to function poorly, creating laxative dependence.[10]

Constituents

Anthraquinones:[14,15] sennosides A and B (mostly), sennosides C and D (minor amounts)

Toxicity

LD_{50} (intraperitoneal):[16] 500–750 mg/kg

Pharmacology

- Senna leaf and fruit are stimulant laxatives, where the leaf is a stronger cathartic than the fruit.[17,18]
- The cathartic action is limited primarily to the colon.[17]
- Sennosides irritate the lining of the large intestine, causing contraction.[1]
- Sennosides A and B appear to induce fluid secretion in the colon.[1]
- Prostaglandins may be involved in the laxative effect.[14]
- Anthroquinones produce a laxative effect 8–12 hours after administration, though sometimes up to 24 hours can be required.[17]
- Anthroquinone laxative use is not associated with an increased risk of developing colorectal ademoma or carcinoma.[19]

Drug interactions

Cardiac glycoside drugs[1]

Parts used[7]

Leaf, fruit

References

1. Jellin JM, Batz F, Hitchens K. Natural Medicines Comprehensive Database, 3rd ed. Stockton, CA: Therapeutic Research Faculty, 2002:1530.
2. Ramesh PR, Kumar KS, Rajagopal MR, Balachandran P, Warrier PK. Managing morphine-induced constipation – a controlled comparison of an ayurvedic formulation and senna. J Pain Symptom Manage 1994; 9:240–244.
3. Passmore AP, Davies K, Flanagan PG, Stoker C, Scott MG. A comparison of Agiolax and lactulose in elderly patients with chronic constipation. Pharmacology 1993; 47:249–252.
4. Shelton MG. Standardized senna in the management of constipation in the puerperium: a clinical trial. S Afr Med J 1980; 57:78–80.
5. Garcia-Villar R. Evaluation of the effects of sennosides on uterine motility in the pregnant ewe. Pharmacology 1988; 36(Suppl 1):203–211.
6. Gattuso JM, Kamm MA. Adverse effects of drugs used in the management of constipation and diarrhoea. Drug Saf 1994; 10:47–65.
7. Brinker F. The Toxicology of Botanical Medicines. Sandy, OR: Eclectic Medical Publications, 2000:296.

8. Brusick D, Mengs U. Assessment of the genotoxic risk from laxative senna products. Environ Mol Mutagen 1997; 29:1–9.
9. Heidemann A, Miltenburger HG, Mengs U. The genotoxicity status of senna. Pharmacology 1993; 47(Suppl 1):178–186.
10. McGuffin M, Hobbs C, Upton R, Goldberg A. American Herbal Products Association's Botanical Safety Handbook. Boca Raton, FL: CRC Press, 1997:231.
11. Hagemann TM. Gastrointestinal medications and breastfeeding. J Hum Lact 1998; 14:259–262.
12. Faber P, Strenge-Hesse A. [Senna-containing laxatives: excretion in the breast milk?]. Geburtshilfe Frauenheilkd 1989; 49:958–962.
13. Faber P, Strenge-Hesse A. Relevance of rhein excretion into breast milk. Pharmacology 1988; 36(Suppl 1):212–220.
14. The Review of Natural Products by Facts and Comparisons. St. Louis, MO: Wolters Kluwer Co., 1999.
15. Leung AY, Foster S. Encyclopedia of Common Natural Ingredients Used in Food, Drugs and Cosmetics, 2nd ed. New York, NY: John Wiley & Sons, 1996:649.
16. Parry O, Matambo C. Some pharmacological actions of aloe extracts and Cassia abbreviata on rats and mice. Cent Afr J Med 1992; 38:409–414.
17. Covington TR, ed. Handbook of Nonprescription Drugs. Washington, DC: Amercian Pharmaceutical Association, 1996.
18. Newall CA, Anderson LA, Phillipson JD. Herbal Medicines: A Guide for Health-care Professionals. London, UK: Pharmaceutical Press, 1996:296.
19. Nusko G, Schneider B, Schneider I et al. Anthranoid laxative use is not a risk factor for colorectal neoplasia: results of a prospective case control study. Gut 2000; 46:651–655.

SIBERIAN GINSENG
Eleutherococcus senticosus

Synonyms/common names/related substances[1]

Ci wu jia, ciwujia, devil's bush, devil's shrub, eleuthera, eleuthero, eleuthero ginseng, eleutherococ, eleutherococc, *Eleutherococci radix*, eleutherococcus, ginseng, phytoestrogen, prickly eleutherococc, Russian root, shigoka, thorny bearer of free berries, touch-me-not, untouchable, ussuri, ussurian thorny pepperbrush, wild pepper, wu jia pi, wu-jia

Indications

Ventricular late potential (coronary artery disease and myocarditis):[2]	Evidence grade B1
Acute cerebral infarction:[3]	Evidence grade B2
Hyperlipidemia (with *Elscholtzia splendens*):[4]	Evidence grade C
Cognitive performance:[5]	Evidence grade C
Herpes simplex type II:[6]	Evidence grade C
Adaptogen:[7]	Evidence grade F

Pregnancy

No evidence to support androgenization:[8,9]	Evidence level 2

A case was reported of a 30-year-old woman who gave birth to a full-term baby boy with signs of androgenization following ingestion of 'ginseng' during the woman's pregnancy.[9] After further investigation, the herbal preparation used by the mother appeared to be adultered by the herb silk vine (*Periploca sepium*) and not Siberian ginseng (*E. senticosus*).[8]

Minimal risk:[10]	Evidence level 3
Prevents embryotoxic effects:[10]	Evidence level 3

Administration of Siberian ginseng extract during pre-natal and pre-embryonic periods of development prevented embryotoxic effects in pregnant rats treated with ethanol and sodium salicylate.[10]

Minimal risk:[11]	Evidence level 3
Anti-carcinogenic effects:[11]	Evidence level 3

Administration of Siberian ginseng inhibited the carcinogenesis induced by transplacental administration of *N*-nitrosoethylurea in rats.[11] This led to longer survival of the rats and lower occurrence and/or multiplicity of tumors (mainly those of the central nervous system).[11]

Unknown:	Evidence level 5

There are no reports in the literature of Siberian ginseng being either safe or contraindicated during pregnancy.

Lactation

Unknown:	Evidence level 5

There are no reports in the literature of Siberian ginseng being either safe or contraindicated during lactation.

Constituents

- Eleutherosides A through M[12]
- Saponins:[1] daucosterol, beta-sitosterol, hederasaponin B
- Coumarins:[1] isofraxidin
- Lignans:[1] sesamin, syringaresinol
- Phenylpropanoids:[1] syringin, caffeic acid, sinapyl alcohol, coniferyl aldehyde, protocatechuic acid
- Betulinic acid[1]
- Vitamin E[1]

Toxicity

- LD_{50} of root: 31 g/kg[13]
- LD_{50} of liquid extract: 10 mL/kg[14]

Pharmacology

- Siberian ginseng inhibits the alarm reaction to stress and decreases the activation of the adrenal cortex.[15]
- Siberian ginseng has anti-viral activity, where it inhibits human rhinovirus, respiratory syncytial virus, and influenza A virus.[16]
- Siberian ginseng increases lymphocyte count, particularly T lymphocytes, and increases phagocyte activity.[12,17,18]
- Several constituents of Siberian ginseng have antioxidant and possible anticancer effects, particularly on leukemia cells.[12,19]
- The constituent coniferyl aldehyde protects DNA against breakage caused by ultraviolet light.[12]
- The constituent protocatechuic acid may inhibit platelet aggregation.[20]
- Siberian ginseng eleutheroside G and saponins may have hypoglycemic activity.[20–22]
- Siberian ginseng may have anti-tubercular activity.[23]

- Intravenous Siberian ginseng may reduce myocardial infarct size.[24]
- Siberian ginseng may inhibit cytochrome P450 CYP1A2 and CYP2C9 enzymes.[25,26] It does not appear to inhibit drug metabolism by CYP2D6 and CYP3A4 enzymes in humans.[25,27]

Drug interactions[1]

Alcohol (ethanol)[26]
Anti-coagulant/anti-platelet drugs[20]
Anti-diabetic drugs[21]
Central nervous system depressants[26]
Drugs metabolized by cytochrome P450 1A2 (CYP1A2) and P450 2C9 (CYP2C9) enzymes[25,26]
Digoxin (Lanoxin)[9,28]

Parts used[1]

Root, rhizome

References

1. Jellin JM, Batz F, Hitchens K. Natural Medicines Comprehensive Database, 3rd ed. Stockton, CA: Therapeutic Research Faculty, 2002:1530.
2. Shang SY, Ma YS, Wang S. [Effect of eleutherosides on ventricular late potential with coronary heart disease and myocarditis]. Zhong Xi Yi Jie He Za Zhi 1991; 11:280–281, 261.
3. Han L, Cai D. [Clinical and experimental study on treatment of acute cerebral infarction with Acanthopanax Injection]. Zhongguo Zhong Xi Yi Jie He Za Zhi 1998; 18:472–474.
4. Shi Z, Liu C, Li R. [Effect of a mixture of Acanthopanax senticosus and Elsholtzia splendens on serum-lipids in patients with hyperlipemia]. Zhong Xi Yi Jie He Za Zhi 1990; 10:155–6, 132.
5. Winther K, Ranlov C, Rein E, Mehlsen J. Russian root (Siberian ginseng) improves cognitive functions in middle-aged people, whereas Ginkgo biloba seems effective only in the elderly. J Neurological Sci 1997; 150:S90.
6. Williams M. Immuno-protection against herpes simplex type II infection by eleutherococcus root extract. Int J Altern Complem Med 1995; 13:9–12.
7. Fulder S. The drug the builds Russians. New Science 1980; 21:576–579.
8. Awang DV. Maternal use of ginseng and neonatal androgenization. JAMA 1991; 266:363.
9. Koren G, Randor S, Martin S, Danneman D. Maternal ginseng use associated with neonatal androgenization. JAMA 1990; 264:2866.
10. Gordeichuk TN, Chebotar' NA, Konopistseva LA, Puchkov VF. [The prevention of congenital developmental anomalies in rats]. Ontogenez 1993; 24:48–55.
11. Bespalov VG, Aleksandrov VA, Iaremenko K et al. [The inhibiting effect of phytoadaptogenic preparations from bioginseng, Eleutherococcus senticosus and Rhaponticum carthamoides on the development of nervous system tumors in rats induced by N-nitrosoethylurea]. Vopr Onkol 1992; 38:1073–1080.
12. Davydov M, Krikorian AD. Eleutherococcus senticosus (Rupr. & Maxim.) Maxim. (Araliaceae) as an adaptogen: a closer look. J Ethnopharmacol 2000; 72:345–393.

13. Farnsworth NR, Kinghorn AD, Soefarto DD et al. Siberian Ginseng; current status as an adaptogen. In: Wagner H, Farnsworth NR, eds. Economic and medicinal plant research, vol 1. London: Academic Press, 1985:164–166.
14. Kaemmerer K, Fink J. Prakt Tierarzt 1980; 61:748, 750–752, 754, 759–760.
15. Brekhman II, Kirillox OI. Effect of eleutherococcus on alarm-phase of stress. Life Sci 1969; 8:113–121.
16. Glatthaar-Saalmuller B, Sacher F, Esperester A. Antiviral activity of an extract derived from roots of Eleutherococcus senticosus. Antiviral Res 2001; 50:223–228.
17. Bohn B, Nebe CT, Birr C. Low-cytometric studies with Eleuthrococcus senticosus extract as an immunomodulatory agent. Arzneimittelforschung 1987; 37:1193–1196.
18. Szolomicki S, Samochowiec L, Wojcicki J, Drozdzik M. The influence of active components of Eleutherococcus senticosus on cellular defense and physical fitness in man. Phytother Res 2000; 14:30–35.
19. Hacker B, Medon PJ. Cytotoxic effects of Eleutherococcus senticosus aqueous extracts in combination with N6-(delta 2-isopentenyl)-adenosine and 1-beta-D-arabinofuranosylcytosine against L1210 leukemia cells. J Pharm Sci 1984; 73:270–272.
20. Yun-Choi HS, Kim JH, Lee JR. Potential inhibitors of platelet aggregation from plant sources, III. J Nat Prod 1987; 50:1059–1064.
21. Hikino H, Takahashi M, Otake K, Konno C. Isolation and hypoglycemic activity of eleutherans A, B, C, D, E, F, and G: glycans of Eleutherococcus senticosus roots. J Nat Prod 1986; 49:293–297.
22. Sui DY, Lu ZZ, Li SH, Cai Y. [Hypoglycemic effect of saponin isolated from leaves of Acanthopanax senticosus (Rupr. et Maxin.) Harms]. Zhongguo Zhong Yao Za Zhi 1994; 19:683–685, 703.
23. Shen ML, Zhai SK, Chen HL. Immunomopharmacological effects of polysaccharides from Acanthopanax senticosus on experimental animals. Int J Immunopharmacol 1991; 13:549–554.
24. Sui DY, Lu ZZ, Ma LN, Fan ZG. [Effects of the leaves of Acanthopanax senticosus (Rupr. et Maxim.) Harms. On myocardial infarct size in acute ischemic dogs]. Zhongguo Zhong Yao Za Zhi 1994; 19:746–747, 764.
25. Harkey MR, Henderson GL, Zhou L et al. Effects of Siberian ginseng (Eleutherococcus senticosus) on c-DNA-expressed P450 drug metabolizing enzymes. Alt Ther 2001; 7:S14.
26. Medon PJ, Ferguson PW, Watson CF. Effects of Eleutherococcus senticosus extracts on hexobarbital metabolism in vivo and in vitro. J Ethnopharmacol 1984; 10:235–241.
27. Donovan JL, DeVane CL, Chavin KD et al. Siberian Ginseng (Eleutheroccus senticosus) effects on CYP2D6 and CYP3A4 activity in normal volunteers. Drug Metab Dispos 2003; 31:519–522.
28. Awang DVC. Siberian ginseng toxicity may be case of mistaken identity. CMAJ 1996; 155:1237.

SQUAW VINE
Mitchella repens

Synonyms/common names/related compounds[1]
Checkerberry, deerberry, hive vine, noon kie oo nah yeah, one-berry, partridge-berry, running box, squaw berry, squawvine, twinberry, two-eyed berry, winter clover

Indications

Induces labor	Evidence grade F

Pregnancy

Induces labor	Evidence level 4

Squaw vine is part of a combination of herbal medicines that have been traditionally used in the third trimester to prepare a woman for delivery; this preparation is called 'mother's cordial' or 'partus preparatus'. In addition to squaw vine, mother's cordial typically contains: black cohosh *(Cimicifuga racemosa)*, raspberry (*Rubus idaeus*), blue cohosh *(Caulophyllum thalictroides)* and false unicorn (*Chamaelirium luteum*).

Abortifacient:[2]	Evidence level 4

A botanical safety compendium reported that squaw vine is a potential abortificaint.[2] There are no reports in the scientific literature of squaw vine being either safe or contraindicated during pregnancy.

Lactation

Unknown:	Evidence level 5

There are no reports in the scientific literature of squaw vine being either safe or contraindicated during lactation.

Constituents[1,3]
Resin, wax, mucilages, dextrin, saponins, alkaloids, glycosides, tannins

Pharmacology
No available information

Drug interactions
None documented

Part used

Above ground parts[1]

References

1. Jellin JM, Batz F, Hitchens K. Natural Medicines Comprehensive Database 3rd ed. Stockton, CA: Therapeutic Research Faculty, 2002:1530.
2. McGuffin M, Hobbs C, Upton R, Goldberg A. American Herbal Products Association's Botanical Safety Handbook. Boca Raton, FL: CRC Press, 1997:231.
3. Grieve M. Squawvine Monograph. Vol. 1999: A Modern Herbal website, 1999.

ST JOHN'S WORT
Hypericum perforatum

Synonyms/common names/related substances[1]
Amber, amber touch-and-heal, demon chaser, *fuga daemonum*, goatweed, hardhay, hypereikon, hyperici herba, hypericum, Johns wort, klamath weed, millepertuis, Rosin rose, Saint Johns wort, Saint John's wort, Saynt Johannes wort, SJW, St Johns wort, St John's wort, tipton weed

Indications

Mild to moderate depression:[2–6]	Evidence grade A
Anxiety (with valerian):[7]	Evidence grade B2
Acute otitis media (with *Verbascum thapsus, Calendula flores* and *Allium sativum*):[30]	Evidence grade B2
Obsessive compulsive disorder :[8]	Evidence grade C
Psychological menopause symptoms:[9]	Evidence grade C
Premenstrual syndrome:[10]	Evidence grade C
Chronic colitis (with *Taraxacum officinale, Melissa officinalis, C. officinalis* and *Foeniculum vulgare*):[9]	Evidence grade C
Seasonal affective disorder:[11–13]	Evidence grade C

Pregnancy

Minimal risk:[14]	Evidence level 2

A case of a 38-year-old women who started taking St John's wort at 24 weeks gestation was reported in a letter to the editor.[14] The woman's pregnancy was unremarkable, with the exception of late onset of thrombocytopenia (the author did not attribute this to St John's wort).[14] The offspring was born healthy, had a normal birthweight and APGAR scores, and physical examination and laboratory results were normal.[14] Behavioral assessment at 4 and 23 days was within normal.[15]

Minimal risk:[16]	Evidence level 3
Does not affect cognitive development:[16]	Evidence level 3

A study on the cognitive impact of prenatal exposure to St John's wort in mice for 2 weeks before mating and throughout gestation found that prenatal exposure to a therapeutic dose of St John's wort did not have a major impact on certain cognitive tasks in mice offspring.[16]

Minimal risk:[17]	Evidence level 3

Lower offspring weight:[17]	Evidence level 3

A study was conducted where Sprague-Dawley rats were exposed to dietary doses of St John's wort 1–25 times the recommended human dose.[17] St John's wort had no effect on maternal weight gain or duration of gestation.[17] Offspring body weights were similar to controls, but for some treated groups, offspring weighed significantly less than the control.[17] There were no St John's wort-related behavioral alterations on any measure.[17] Whole and regional brain weights of offspring at adulthood indicated no significant effects of St John's wort.[17]

Minimal risk:[18]	Evidence level 3

Lower birthweights:[18]	Evidence level 3

No long-term behavioral deficits:[18]	Evidence level 3

A behavioural study on mice offspring exposed antenatally to St John's wort found that birthweights of male offspring were less in the St John's wort group than in the placebo group.[18] Offspring in both treatment groups showed no long-term statistical differences in early developmental tasks, locomotor activity, and exploratory behavior throughout development.[18] Performances on a depression task and on anxiety tasks revealed no differences between treatment groups.[18]

Minimal risk:[19]	Evidence level 3

Does not affect long-term growth and physical maturation:[19]	Evidence level 3

St John's wort was administered to mice to determine whether pre-natal exposure to the herb affects long-term growth and physical maturation of mouse offspring.[19] Maternal administration of St John's wort before and throughout gestation did not affect long-term growth and physical maturation of exposed mouse offspring.[19]

Conflicting evidence

Nonmutagenic:[20]	Evidence level 3

Teratogenic:[21]	Evidence level 3

A study on organogenesis found that hypericin induced teratogenic effects in whole rat embryo cultures.[21] A study on mammalian cells, however, showed that a standardized aqueous ethanolic of St John's wort did not induce any mutagenic effects.[20]

Increases uterine tone:[22]	Evidence level 3

St John's wort was shown to increase uterine tone in animals.[22]

Emmenagogue:[23]	Evidence level 4
Uterine stimulant:[23]	Evidence level 4
Abortifacient:[23]	Evidence level 4

A review article on the potential value of plants as sources of anti-fertility agents reported that St John's wort is an abortifacient, emmenagogue and uterine stimulant.[23]

Homeopathic H. perforatum *(Hypericum)*

Minimal risk:[24]	Evidence level 1

A homeopathic preparation of *H. perforatum*, called Hypericum, beyond the potency (dilution) of 12C, does not contain any molecules of the original substance. Although the principles of homeopathy are difficult to apply to evidence-based medicine research, a systematic review determined that homeopathic preparations do not significantly differ from placebo.[24]

Lactation

May cause colic, drowsiness or lethargy:[25]	Evidence level 1
Minimal risk:[25]	Evidence level 1

A prospective observational cohort study was conducted on 33 breast-feeding women receiving St John's wort (group 1) and for comparison, 101 disease-matched (group 2) and 33 age- and parity-matched controls with no disease (group 3).[25] In the group receiving St John's wort, there were two cases of colic, two cases of drowsiness and one case of lethargy.[25] Specific medical treatment was not required for the infants.[25] No significant difference was observed in the frequency of maternal report of decreased milk production among the groups, nor was a difference found in infant weight over the first year of life.[25]

Crosses into breast milk:[26]	Evidence level 2
Minimal risk:[26]	Evidence level 2

An analysis was performed on four breast-milk samples (fore and hind milk) during an 18-hour period from a mother with post-natal depression who had taken St John's wort during pregnancy in order to measure concentration of hypericin and hyperforin.[26] Only hyperforin was excreted into breast milk at a low level.[26] No side effects were seen in the mother or infant.[26]

Homeopathic H. perforatum *(Hypericum)*

Minimal risk:[24]	Evidence level 1

A homeopathic preparation of *H. perforatum*, called Hypericum, beyond the potency (dilution) of 12C, does not contain any molecules of the original substance. Although the principles of homeopathy are difficult to apply to evidence-based medicine research, a systematic review determined that homeopathic preparations do not significantly differ from placebo.[24]

Constituents

- Naphthodianthrones:[27] hypericin, pseudohypericin
- Flavonoids:[27] quercetin, quercetrin, amentoflavone, hyperin
- Phloroglucinols:[27] hyperforin, adhyperforin
- Essential oil[27]

Toxicity

- Delayed hypersensitivity photodermatitis.[28–30]
- Hypericin is believed to be the photosensitizing agent present in St John's wort.[31,32]

Pharmacology

- St John's wort effects on serotonin may be primarily responsible for its anti-depressant activity.[33]
- Extracts of St John's wort inhibit the reuptake of serotonin, norepinephrine, and dopamine in vitro.[33–35]
- Hyperforin and adhyperforin were shown to modulate the effects of serotonin, dopamine, and norepinephrine, and to act as serotonergic 5-hydroxytryptamine (5-HT)3 and 5-HT4 receptor antagonists.[35–38]
- Hypericin inhibits in vitro almost irreversibly both type A and B monoamine oxidase in rat brain mitochondria.[39]
- St John's wort induces some of the cytochrome P450 (CYP) enzymes and may interfere with drug metabolism.[40]
- Topical application of St John's wort inhibits the proliferation of T lymphocytes in inflammatory skin disorders.[41]
- St John's wort has anti-bacterial activity.[42]
- In human and animal cancer cells, hyperforin inhibited tumor cell growth by induction of apoptosis.[43]

Drug interactions

5-HT1 agonists[44,45]
Alprozolam[46]
Aminolaevulinic acid[47]
Amitriptyline[48–50]
Analagesics with serotonergic activity[33–35,45]
Antidepressants[45,51–53]
Barbituates[54]
Carbamazepine[55]
Cyclosporine[44,49,50,56–66]
Digoxin[44,50,67–69]
Dextromethorphan[33–35,45]
Fenfluramine[53]
Fexofenadine[70]
Irinotecan[71,72]
Monoamine oxidase inhibitors[35,37]
Mycophenolate mofetil[73]
Narcotics[54,74]
Nelazodone[75]
Nonnucleoside reverse transcriptase inhibitors[49,76,77]
Nortriptyline[48,50]
Oral contraceptives[44,78–80]
Paroxetine[45,52,53]
Phenobarbital[44]
Phenprocoumon[44]
Phenytoin[44]
Photosensitizing drugs[51]
Protease inhibitors[44,50,76]
Reserpine[54]
Sertraline[75]
Simvastatin[81]
Tacrolimus[73,82]
Theophylline[44,50,83]
Warfarin[44,78,84]
Drugs metabolized by cytochrome P450 enzymes[40,44,46,50,59,68,69,76,78,85]

Parts used

Whole plant[86]

References

1. Jellin JM, Batz F, Hitchens K. Natural Medicines Comprehensive Database, 3rd ed. Stockton, CA: Therapeutic Research Faculty, 2002:1530.
2. Linde K, Ramirez G, Mulrow C et al. St John's wort for depression – an overview and meta-analysis of randomised clinical trials. BMJ 1996; 313:253–258.

3. Linde K, Mulrow CD. St John's wort for depression. Cochrane Database Syst Rev 2000; CD000448.
4. Kim HL, Streltzer J, Goebert D. St. John's wort for depression: a meta-analysis of well-defined clinical trials. J Nerv Ment Dis 1999; 187:532–538.
5. Whiskey E, Werneke U, Taylor D. A systematic review and meta-analysis of Hypericum perforatum in depression: a comprehensive clinical review. Int Clin Psychopharmacol 2001; 16:239–252.
6. Gaster B, Holroyd J. St John's wort for depression: a systematic review. Arch Intern Med 2000; 160:152–156.
7. Panijel M. [Treatment of moderately severe anxiety states]. Therapiewoche 1985; 35:4659–4668.
8. Taylor LH, Kobak A. An open-label trial of St. John's Wort (Hypericum perforatum) in obsessive-compulsive disorder. J Clin Psychiatry 2000; 61:575–578.
9. Grube B, Walper A, Wheatley D. St. John's Wort extract: efficacy for menopausal symptoms of psychological origin. Adv Ther 1999; 16:177–186.
10. Stevinson C, Ernst E. A pilot study of Hypericum perforatum for the treatment of premenstrual syndrome. BJOG 2000; 107:870–876.
11. Martinez B, Kasper S, Rurhmann S, Moller HJ. Hypericum in the treatment of seasonal affective disorders. J Geriatr Psychiatry Neurol 1994; 7(Suppl 1):S29–33.
12. Kasper S. Treatment of seasonal affective disorder (SAD) with hypericum extract. Pharmacopsychiatry 1997; 30(Suppl 2):89–93.
13. Wheatley D. Hypericum in seasonal affective disorder (SAD). Curr Med Res Opin 1999; 15:33–37.
14. Grush LR, Nierenberg A, Keefe B, Cohen LS. St John's wort during pregnancy. JAMA 1998; 280:1566.
15. Farnsworth NR, Bingel AS, Cordell GA, Crane FA, Fong HH. Potential value of plants as sources of new antifertility agents II. J Pharm Sci 1975; 64:717–753.
16. Rayburn WF, Gonzalez CL, Christensen H, Harkins TL, Kupiec TC. Impact of hypericum (St.-John's-wort) given prenatally on cognition of mice offspring. Neurotoxicol Teratol 2001; 23:629–637.
17. Cada AM, Hansen DK, LaBorde J, Ferguson SA. Minimal effects from developmental exposure to St. John's wort (Hypericum perforatum) in Sprague-Dawley rats. Nutr Neurosci 2001; 4:135–141.
18. Rayburn WF, Christensen HD, Gonzalez C. Effect of antenatal exposure to Saint John's wort (Hypericum) on neurobehavior of developing mice. Am J Obstet Gynecol 2000; 183:1225–1231.
19. Rayburn WF, Gonzalez CL, Christensen H, Stewart JD. Effect of prenatally administered hypericum (St John's wort) on growth and physical maturation of mouse offspring. Am J Obstet Gynecol 2001; 184:191–195.
20. Okpanyi SN, Lidzba H, Scholl BC, Miltenburger HG. [Genotoxicity of a standardized Hypericum extract]. Arzneimittelforschung 1990; 40:851–855.
21. Chan LY, Chiu PY, Lau T. A study of hypericin-induced teratogenicity during organogenesis using a whole rat embryo culture model. Fertil Steril 2001; 76:1073–1074.
22. Shipochliev T. [Uterotonic action of extracts from a group of medicinal plants]. Vet Med Nauki 1981; 18:94–98.
23. Farnsworth NR, Bingel AS, Cordell G, Crane FA, Fong HH. Potential value of plants as sources of new antifertility agents I. J Pharm Sci 1975; 64:535–598.

24. Ernst E. A systematic review of systematic reviews of homeopathy. Br J Clin Pharmacol 2002; 54:577–582.
25. Lee A, Minhas R, Matsuda N, Lam M, Ito S. The safety of St. John's wort (Hypericum perforatum) during breastfeeding. J Clin Psychiatry 2003; 64:966–968.
26. Klier CM, Schafer MR, Schmid-Siegel B, Lenz G, Mannel M. St. John's wort (Hypericum perforatum) – is it safe during breastfeeding? Pharmacopsychiatry 2002; 35:29–30.
27. Upton R. St Johns wort – Hypericum perforatum. American Herbal Pharmacopoeia–American Botanical Council, 1996.
28. Duke JA. Handbook of Medicinal Herbs. Boca Raton: CRC, 1985.
29. Benner MH, Lee HJ. Toxic reactions to plant products sold in health food stores. Med Lett 1979; 21:29–32.
30. Mitchell J, Rook A. Botanical dermatology – plants and plant products injurious to the skin. Vancouver: Greengrass, 1979.
31. Frohne D, Pfander HJ. A Colour Atlas of Poisonous Plants. London: Wolfe, 1984.
32. Newall CA, Anderson LA, Phillipson JD. Herbal Medicines: A Guide for Health-care Professionals. London, UK: Pharmaceutical Press, 1996:296.
33. Calapai G, Crupi A, Firenzuoli F et al. Serotonin, norepinephrine and dopamine involvement in the antidepressant action of hypericum perforatum. Pharmacopsychiatry 2001; 34:45–49.
34. Kleber E, Obry T, Hippeli S et al. Biochemical activities of extracts from Hypericum perforatum. Arzneimittelforschung 1999; 49:106–109.
35. Muller WE, Singer A, Wonnemann M, Hafner U et al. Hyperforin represents the neurotransmitter reuptake inhibiting constituent of hypericum extract. Pharmacopsychiatry 1998; 31:16–21.
36. Chatterjee SS, Noldner M, Koch E, Erdelmeier C. Antidepressant activity of hypericum perforatum and hyperforin: the neglected possibility. Pharmacopsychiatry 1998; 31(Suppl 1):7–15.
37 Singer A, Wonnemann M, Muller WE. Hyperforin, a major antidepressant constituent of St. John's wort, inhibits serotonin uptake by elevating free intracellular Na+11. J Pharmacol Exp Ther 1999; 290:1363–1368.
38. Jensen AG, Hansen SH, Nielsen E. Adhyperforin as a contributor to the effect of Hypericum perforatum L. in biochemical models of antidepressant activity. Life Sci 2001; 68:1593–1605.
39. Suzuki O, Katsumata Y, Oya M, Bladt S, Wagner H. Inhibition of monoamine oxidase by hypericin. Planta Med 1984; 50:272–274.
40. Wang Z, Gorski JC, Hamman MA et al. The effects of St. John's wort (Hyericum perforatum) on human cytochrome P450 activity. Clin Pharmacol Ther 2001; 70:317–326.
41. Schempp CM, Winghofer B, Ludtke R et al. Topical application of St John's wort (Hypericum perforatum L.) and of its metabolite hyperforin inhibits the allostimulatory capacity of epidermal cells. Br J Dermatol 2000; 142:979–984.
42. Schempp CM, Pelz K, Wittmer A, Schopf E, Simon JC. Antibacterial activity of hyperforin from St John's wort, against multiresistant Staphylococcus aureus and gram-positive bacteria. Lancet 1999; 353(9170):2129.
43. Schempp CM, Kirkin V, Simon-Haarhaus B et al. Inhibition of tumour cell growth by hyperforin, a novel anticancer drug from St. John's wort that acts by induction of apoptosis. Oncogene 2002; 21:1242–1250.

44. Henderson L, Yue QY, Bergquist C et al. St John's wort (Hypericum perforatum): drug interactions and clinical outcomes. Br J Clin Pharmacol 2002; 54:349–356.
45. Singhal AB, Caviness VS, Begleiter AF et al. Cerebral vasoconstriction and stroke after use of serotonergic drugs. Neurology 2002; 58:130–133.
46. Markowitz JS, Donovan JL, DeVane CL et al. Effect of St. John's wort on drug metabolism by induction of cytochrome P450 3A4 enzyme. JAMA 2003; 290:1500–1504.
47. Ladner DP, Klein SD, Steiner RA, Walt H. Synergistic toxicity of delta-aminolaevulinic acid-induced protoporphyrin IX used for photodiagnosis and hypericum extract, a herbal antidepressant. Br J Dermatol 2001; 144:916–918.
48. Roots I, Johne A, Schmider J, Brockmoller J et al. Interaction of a herbal extract from St. John's wort with amitriptyline and its metabolites. Clin Pharmacol Ther 2000; 67:159.
49. Durr D, Stieger B, Kullak-Ublick GA et al. St. John's Wort induces intestinal P-glycoprotein/MDR1 and intestinal and hepatic CYP3A4. Clin Pharmacol Ther 2000; 68:598–604.
50. Schulz V. Incidence and clinical relevance of the interactions and side effects of Hypericum preparations. Phytomedicine 2001; 8:152–160.
51. Miller LG. Herbal medicinals: selected clinical considerations focusing on known or potential drug-herb interactions. Arch Intern Med 1998; 158:2200–2211.
52. Gordon JB. SSRIs and St. John's Wort: possible toxicity? Am Fam Physician 1998; 57:950–953.
53. Beckman SE, Sommi RW, Switzer J. Consumer use of St. John's wort: a survey of effectiveness, safety, and tolerability. Pharmacotherapy 2000; 20:568–574.
54. Upton R. St. John's wort, Hypericum perforatum: quality control, analytical and therapeutic monograph. American Herbal Pharmacopoeia. Santa Cruz, CA, 1997:1–32.
55. Burstein AH, Horton RL, Dunn T et al. Lack of effect of St John's Wort on carbamazepine pharmacokinetics in healthy volunteers. Clin Pharmacol Ther 2000; 68:605–612.
56. Abul-Ezz SR, Barone GW, Gurley BJ et al. Effect of herbal supplements on cyclosporine blood levels and associated acute rejection. American Society of Nephrology Annual Meeting, Toronto, 13–16 October 2000.
57. Mai I, Kruger H, Budde K et al. Hazardous pharmacokinetic interaction of Saint John's wort (Hypericum perforatum) with the immunosuppressant cyclosporin. Int J Clin Pharmacol Ther 2000; 38:500–502.
58. Gurley BJ, Barone GW. Herb-drug interaction involving St. John's wort and cyclosporine. AAPS Annual Meeting and Expo, Indianapolis, IN, 29 Oct–2 Nov 2000. Vol. presentation #3443.
59. Ruschitzka F, Meier PJ, Turina M et al. Acute heart transplant rejection due to Saint John's wort. Lancet 2000; 355:548–549.
60. Barone GW, Gurley BJ, Ketel BL et al. Drug interaction between St. John's wort and cyclosporin. Ann Pharmacother 2000; 34:1013–1016.
61. Breidenbach T, Hoffmann MW, Becker T et al. Drug interaction of St John's wort with ciclosporin. Lancet 2000; 355:1912.
62. Moschella C, Jaber BL. Interaction between cyclosporine and Hypericum perforatum (St. John's wort) after organ transplantation. Am J Kidney Dis 2001; 38:1105–1107.

63. Karliova M, Treichel U, Malago M et al. Interaction of Hypericum perforatum (SJW) with cyclosporin A metabolism in a patient after liver transplantation. J Hepatol 2000; 33:853–855.
64. Mandelbaum A, Pertzborn F, Martin-Facklam M, Wiesel M. Unexplained decrease of cyclosporin trough levels in a compliant renal transplant patient. Nephrol Dial Transplant 2000; 15:1473–1474.
65. Ernst E. St. John's Wort supplements endanger the success of organ transplantation. Arch Surg 2002; 137:316–319.
66. Bauer S, Stormer E, Johne A et al. Alterations in cyclosporin A pharmacokinetics and metabolism during treatment with St John's wort in renal transplant patients. Br J Clin Pharmacol 2003; 55:203–211.
67. Johne A, Brockmoller J, Bauer S et al. Pharmacokinetic interaction of digoxin with an herbal extract from St John's wort (Hypericum perforatum). Clin Pharmacol Ther 1999; 66:338–345.
68. Cheng TO. St. John's wort interaction with digoxin [letter]. Arch Intern Med 2000; 160:2548.
69. Hennessy M, Kelleher D, Spiers JP et al. St Johns wort increases expression of P-glycoprotein: implications for drug interactions. Br J Clin Pharmacol 2002; 53:75–82.
70 Wang Z, Hamman MA, Huang SM et al. Effect of St. John's wort on the pharmacokinetics of fexofenadine. Clin Pharmacol Ther 2002; 71:414–420.
71. Mathijssen RH, Verweij J, de Bruijn P et al. Effects of St. John's wort on irinotecan metabolism. J Natl Cancer Inst 2002; 94:1247–1249.
72. Mathijssen RHJ, Verweij J, De Bruijn P et al. Modulation of irinotecan (CPT-11) metabolism by St. John's wort in cancer patients. American Association for Cancer Research Annual Meeting, San Francisco, April 2002. Vol. Abstract 2443.
73. Mai I, Stormer E, Bauer S et al. Impact of St John's wort treatment on the pharmacokinetics of tacrolimus and mycophenolic acid in renal transplant patients. Nephrol Dial Transplant 2003; 18:819–822.
74. Hussain MD, Teixeira MG. Saint John's wort and analgesia: effect of Saint John's wort on morphine induced analgesia. AAPS Annual Meeting and Expo, Indianapolis, IN, 29 Oct–2 Nov 2000. Vol. presentation #3453.
75. Lantz MS, Buchalter E, Giambanco V. St. John's wort and antidepressant drug interactions in the elderly. J Geriatr Psychiatry Neurol 1999; 12:7–10.
76. Piscitelli SC, Burstein AH, Chaitt D et al. Indinavir concentrations and St. John's wort. Lancet 2000; 355:547–548.
77. de Maat M, Hoetelmans R, Mathot R et al. Drug interaction between St. John's wort and nevirapine. AIDS 2001; 15:420–421.
78. Yue QY, Bergquist C, Gerden B. Safety of St John's wort (Hypericum perforatum). Lancet 2000; 355:576–577.
79. Schwarz UI, Buschel B, Kirch W. Unwanted pregnancy on self-medication with St John's wort despite hormonal contraception. Br J Clin Pharmacol 2003; 55:112–113.
80. Gorski JC, Hamman MA, Wang Z et al. The effect of St. John's wort on the efficacy of oral contraceptives. Clin Pharmacol Ther 2001; 71:P.25.
81. Sugimoto K, Ohmori M, Tsuruoka S. Different effects of St John's wort on the pharmacokinetics of simvastatin and pravastatin. Clin Pharmacol Ther 2001; 70:518–524.
82. Mai I, Bauer S, Krueger H et al. Wechselwirkungen von Johaniskraut mit tacrolismus bei nierentransplantierten patienten. Symposium Phytopharmaka VII, Berlin, October 2001. Forschung und Klinische Anwendung.

83. Nebel A, Schneider BJ, Baker RA et al. Potential metabolic interaction between St. John's wort and theophylline. Ann Pharmacother 1999; 33:502.
84. Groning R, Breitkreutz J, Muller RS. Physico-chemical interactions between extracts of Hypericum perforatum L. and drugs. Eur J Pharm Biopharm 2003; 56:231–236.
85. Roby CA, Anderson GD, Kantor E et al. St. John's wort: effect on CYP3A4 activity. Clin Pharmacol Ther 2000; 67:451–457.
86. Brinker F. The Toxicology of Botanical Medicines. Sandy, OR: Eclectic Medical Publications, 2000:296.

STINGING NETTLE
Urtica dioica, U. urens

Synonyms/common names/related compounds[1,2]

Common nettle, dwarf nettle, great stinging nettle, nettle, nettles, ortie, small nettle, urtica, *Urticae herba et folium*

Indications

Above ground parts

Allergic rhinitis:[3]	Evidence grade B2
Osteoarthritis:[4,5]	Evidence grade B2

Root

Benign prostatic hyperplasia (with saw palmetto):[6,7]	Evidence grade B1
Benign prostatic hyperplasia:[8]	Evidence grade B2

Pregnancy

Above ground parts

Potential abortifacient:[9]	Evidence level 4
Emmenagogue:[9]	Evidence level 4
Uterine stimulant constituent:[9]	Evidence level 4
Estrogenic:[10]	Evidence level 4

A review article on the potential value of plants as sources of anti-fertility agents reported that stinging nettle was a potential abortifacient, emmenagogue and that its constituent, 5-hydroxytryptamine, was a uterine stimulant.[9] This review article also reported that singing nettle has estrogenic activity.[10]

Root

Interferes with human sex hormone-binding globulin:[11]	Evidence level 3

Stinging nettle root has been shown to interfere with human sex hormone-binding globulin.[11] The root is principally used in the treatment of prostate disorders and as such, would not likely be used during pregnancy. There are no reports in the scientific literature of stinging nettle root being either safe or contraindicated during pregnancy.

Lactation

Above ground parts

Unknown:	Evidence level 5

There are no reports in the scientific literature of stinging nettle leaf being either safe or contraindicated during lactation.

Root

Interferes with human sex hormone-binding globulin:[11]	Evidence level 3

Stinging nettle root has been shown to interfere with human sex hormone-binding globulin.[11] The root is principally used in the treatment of prostate disorders and as such, would not likely be used during lactation. There are no reports in the scientific literature of stinging nettle root being either safe or contraindicated during lactation.

Constituents

- Leaf:[1,2,12–16] β-sitosterol, flavonoids (quercetin, rutin, kaempferol), carotene, vitamin C, vitamin K, potassium, calcium, chlorophyll, 5-hydroxytryptamine
- Root:[1] polysaccharides

Toxicity

- LD_{50} (leaf infusion): 1.92 g/kg[4]
- LD_{50} (leaf decoction): 1.72 g/kg[4]

The stinging nettle hairs on the leaf contain histamine, acetylcholine and serotonin; these hairs cause skin irritation when touched.[13–15,17–19]

Pharmacology

Above ground parts

- Stinging nettle leaf has analgesic, anti-inflammatory, local anesthetic, hemostatic, antibacterial, antiviral, and hyperglycemic effects.[1,13,16,18–20]
- Stinging nettle contains the uterotropic constituent 5-hydroxytryptamine.[2]
- The constituent quercetin decreases histamine release from basophils and mast cells.[21]
- The leaf has been shown to have diuretic properties where it increases urine output and to slightly decrease systolic blood pressure and body weight in people with venous insufficiency.[13,18]

- Stinging nettle may inhibit adrenergic stimulation, tumor necrosis factor, and platelet activation factor.[18]
- Stinging nettle lowers body temperature and may act as a central nervous system depressant.[13,19,20]
- Stinging nettle may have anti-seizure activity.[19]
- Stinging nettle may decrease blood pressure and heart rate.[18,19]
- Stinging nettle contains a large amount of vitamin C and carotene.[17]

Root

- Stinging nettle root has immunomodulating and weak anti-inflammatory properties.[15,18,22]
- Root extracts have been shown to decrease binding capacity of sex hormone-binding globulin and to suppress prostatic cell metabolism.[14,18,22]
- Root extracts have been shown to increase urine output, decreased nocturia, and decreased urinary frequency.[12,13,18,20,22]

Drug interactions[1]

Anti-coagulants[16]
Anti-diabetic drugs[19]
Anti-hypertensive agents[19]
Central nervous system depressants[19]

Parts used[1]

Above ground parts, leaf

References

1. Jellin JM, Batz F, Hitchens K. Natural Medicines Comprehensive Database, 3rd ed. Stockton, CA: Therapeutic Research Faculty, 2002:1530.
2. Brinker F. The Toxicology of Botanical Medicines. Sandy, OR: Eclectic Medical Publications, 2000:296.
3. Mittman P. Randomized, double-blind study of freeze-dried Urtica dioica in the treatment of allergic rhinitis. Planta Med 1990; 56:44–47.
4. Mills S, Bone K. Principles and Practice of Phytotherapy: Modern Herbal Medicine. London: Churchill Livingstone, 2000.
5. Randall C, Randall H, Dobbs F, Hutton C, Sanders H. Randomized controlled trial of nettle sting for treatment of base-of-thumb pain. J R Soc Med 2000; 93:305–309.
6. Sokel J. Combined sabal and urtica extract compared with finasteride in men with benign prostatic hyperplasia: analysis of prostate volume and therapeutic outcome. BJU Int 2000; 86:439–442.
7. Sokel J, Albrecht J. [Combination of Sabal and Urtica extract vs. finasteride in benign prostatic hyperplasia (Aiken stages I to II). Comparison of therapeutic effectiveness in a one year double-blind study]. Urologe A 1997; 36:327–333.
8. Marks LS, Partin AW, Epstein J et al. Effects of a saw palmetto herbal blend in men with symptomatic benign prostatic hyperplasia. J Urol 2000; 163:1451–1456.
9. Farnsworth NR, Bingel AS, Cordell G, Crane FA, Fong HH. Potential value of plants as sources of new antifertility agents I. J Pharm Sci 1975; 64:535–598.

10. Farnsworth NR, Bingel AS, Cordell GA, Crane FA, Fong HH. Potential value of plants as sources of new antifertility agents II. J Pharm Sci 1975; 64:717–753.
11. Gansser D, Spiteller G. Plant constituents interfering with human sex hormone-binding globulin. Evaluation of a test method and its application to Urtica dioica root extracts. Z Naturforsch [C] 1995; 50:98–104.
12. Blumenthal M, Busse WR, Goldberg A et al. The Complete German Commission E Monographs: Therapeutic Guide to Herbal Medicines. Boston, MA: American Botanical Council, 1998.
13. Leung AY, Foster S. Encyclopedia of Common Natural Ingredients Used in Food, Drugs and Cosmetics, 2nd ed. New York, NY: John Wiley & Sons, 1996:649.
14. Wichtl M, Czygan FC, Frohne D et al. Herbal drugs and phytopharmaceuticals. Stuttgart, DE: Medpharm-CRC Press, 1994:566.
15. Gruenwald J, Brendler T, Jaenicke C. PDR for Herbal Medicines. Montvale, NJ: Medical Economics Company, 1998.
16. Brinker F. Herb Contraindications and Drug Interactions, 2nd ed. Sandy, OR: Eclectic Medical Publications, 1998.
17. Foster S, Tyler VE. Tyler's Honest Herbal: A Sensible Guide to the Use of Herbs and Related Remedies, 3rd ed. Binghamton, NY: Haworth Herbal Press, 1993.
18. Monographs on the medicinal uses of plant drugs. Exeter, UK: European Scientific Co-op Phytother, 1997.
19. Newall CA, Anderson LA, Phillipson JD. Herbal Medicines: A Guide for Health-care Professionals. London, UK: Pharmaceutical Press, 1996:296.
20. The Review of Natural Products by Facts and Comparisons. St. Louis, MO: Wolters Kluwer Co., 1999.
21. Anon. Quercetin. Alt Med Rev 1998; 3:140–143.
22. Schulz V, Hansel R, Tyler VE, Terry C. Rational Phytotherapy: A Physician's Guide to Herbal Medicine, 3rd ed. Berlin: Springer, 1998.

TURMERIC

Curcuma longa, C. aromatica

Synonyms/common names/related substances[1]

Curcuma, *Curcumae longae rhizoma*, curcumin, Indian saffron, tumeric, turmeric root

Indications

Oral

Anti-inflammatory:[2]	Evidence grade B1
Dyspepsia:[3]	Evidence grade B1
Biliary dyskinesia (with celandine):[4]	Evidence grade B2
Gallstone prevention (cholagogue):[5,6]	Evidence grade B2
Osteoarthritis (with *Withania somnifera*, *Boswellia serrata*, and a zinc complex):[7]	Evidence grade B2
Human immunodeficiency virus:[8]	Evidence grade B2
Peptic ulcers:[9]	Evidence grade C
Rheumatoid arthritis:[10]	Evidence grade C
Uveitis:[11]	Evidence grade C
Cancer prevention:[12–17]	Evidence grade D
Hyperlipidemia:[18]	Evidence grade D

Topical

Cancer prevention:[19]	Evidence grade D
Scabies:[20]	Evidence grade D

Pregnancy

Therapeutic doses

Nonteratogenic:[21–23]	Evidence level 3

Nonmutagenic in high doses:[24,25] Evidence level 3

Nontoxic in high doses:[24,25] Evidence level 3

Animal experiments reported that oral turmeric was not teratogenic in mice or rats.[21–23] Turmeric was reported as nonmutagenic and nontoxic at high doses in rats and monkeys.[24,25]

Inhibits uterine stretching:[26] Evidence level 3

An animal experiment of the stretch of the uterus imposed by the growing fetus, which contributes to the onset of labor, showed that curcumin inhibited one of the signalling pathways (c-Jun NH2-terminal kinase (JNK)) necessary for optimal stretching of the uterus.[26]

Minimal risk:[27] Evidence level 4

A retrospective explorative study was conducted to ascertain the knowledge, attitudes, and practices regarding diet patterns during pregnancy and lactation among non-Bengali Muslim mothers.[27] Turmeric was believed to improve the baby's complexion and to protect the baby and mother from cough and cold.[27] No adverse effects associated with the ingestion of turmeric during pregnancy were reported.[27]

Potential abortifacient:[28] Evidence level 4

Emmenagogue:[28] Evidence level 4

Uterine stimulant:[28] Evidence level 4

A review article on the potential value of plants as sources of anti-fertility agents reported that turmeric was a potential abortifacient, emmenagogue, and uterine stimulant.[28]

Spice

Minimal risk:[1] Evidence level 4

A natural medicine compendium reported that turmeric is of minimal risk during pregnancy if used as a spice.[1]

Lactation

Therapeutic doses

Crosses into breast milk:[29,30] Evidence level 3

Animal experiments reported the passage of active constituents and/or metabolites of turmeric and curcumin via the translactational route into breast milk.[29,30] There is no report in the literature of turmeric being either safe or contraindicated during lactation.

Minimal risk:[27]	Evidence level 4

A retrospective explorative study was conducted to ascertain the knowledge, attitudes and practices regarding diet patterns during pregnancy and lactation among non-Bengali Muslim mothers.[27] Turmeric was believed to improve the baby's complexion and to protect the baby and mother from cough and cold.[27] No adverse effects associated with the ingestion of turmeric during lactation were reported.[27]

Spice

Minimal risk:[1]	Evidence level 4

A natural medicine compendium reported that turmeric is of minimal risk during lactation if used as a spice.[1]

Constituents[1,31]

- Diarylheptanoids: curcumin
- Volatile oils: turmerone, zingiberene, bisabalona, guaiane, curlone
- Sugars: glucose, fructose, arabinose
- Vitamin C

Toxicity

- LD_{50} of curcumin in mice (oral):[32] >2 g/kg
- Turmeric was reported as nonmutagenic and nontoxic at high doses:[24,25] 300 mg/kg in rats and 2.5 g/kg in monkeys

Pharmacology

- In clinical trials, curcumin is a potent anti-inflammatory agent where its action is reported to be comparable to phenylbutazone.[2]
- In vitro, curcumin was shown to inhibit interleukin (IL)-8, MIP-1α, MCP-1, IL-1β, tumor necrosis factor (TNF) α, 5-lipoxygenase activity, cyclooxygenase activity and 5-hydroxy-eicosatetraenoic acid (5-HETE) formation, leukotriene formation and platelet aggregation, and to increase the breakdown of fibrin.[32–38]
- Curcumin was shown to significantly decrease the level of serum lipid peroxides (33%), increase high-density lipoprotein cholesterol (29%) and decrease total serum cholesterol, thereby having a preventive effect on arterial disease.[18]

- Turmeric increases bile secretion and bile flow, and induces contraction of the human gallbladder (cholagogue).[6,39,40]
- Turmeric has significant anti-oxidant activity and may protect DNA against free radical damage.[17,41,42]
- Turmeric may significantly increase gastric wall mucus and restore the non-protein sulfhydryl (NP-SH) content in the stomach.[43]
- Curcumin and turmeric were shown to inhibit human immunodeficiency virus (HIV)-1, HIV-2, and HIV-integrase.[44–46]
- Curcumin was shown to have anti-mutagen activity, anti-carcinogen activity, chemopreventive activity in colon carcinogenesis, reduce urinary excretion of mutagens in smokers, and inhibit and/or induce apoptosis in prostate cancer cells, skin and gastric tumors, colonic epithelial cell dysplasia, and others.[12–16]
- Curcumin is a potent inhibitor of cytochrome P450 (CYP) 1A1/1A2, a less potent inhibitor of CYP 2B1/2B2, and a weak inhibitor of CYP 2E1.[47]
- Turmeric may decrease hepatocyte glutathione levels and curcumin appears to induce glutathione-*S*-transferase activity in mice.[48,49]

Drug interactions

Anti-platelet drugs[50]
Reserpine and indometacin[50]
Drugs metabolized by cytochrome P450 (CYP) 1A1/1A2, CYP 2B1/2B2, and CYP 2E1 enzymes.[47]

Part used[51]

Rhizome

References

1. Jellin JM, Batz F, Hitchens K. Natural Medicines Comprehensive Database, 3rd ed. Stockton, CA: Therapeutic Research Faculty, 2002:1530.
2. Satoskar RR, Shah SJ, Shenoy S. Evaluation of anti-inflammatory property of curcumin (diferuloyl methane) in patients with postoperative inflammation. Int J Clin Pharmacol Ther Toxicol 1986; 24:651–654.
3. Thamlikitkul V, Bunyapraphatsara N, Dechatiwongse T et al. Randomized double blind study of Curcuma domestica Val. for dyspepsia. J Med Assoc Thai 1989; 72:613–620.
4. Niederau C, Gopfert E. [The effect of chelidonium- and turmeric root extract on upper abdominal pain due to functional disorders of the biliary system. Results from a placebo-controlled double-blind study]. Med Klin (Munich) 1999; 94:425–430.
5. Hussain MS, Chandrasekhara N. Effect on curcumin on cholesterol gall-stone induction in mice. Indian J Med Res 1992; 96:288–291.
6. Rasyid A, Lelo A. The effect of curcumin and placebo on human gall-bladder function: an ultrasound study. Aliment Pharmacol Ther 1999; 13:245–249.
7. Kulkarni RR, Patki PS, Jog V, Gandage SG, Patwardhan B. Treatment of osteoarthritis with a herbomineral formulation: a double-blind, placebo-controlled, cross-over study. J Ethnopharmacol 1991; 33(1–2):91–95.

8. Copeland R. Curcumin therapy in HIV-infected patients initially increased CD-4 and CD-8 cell counts. 10th International AIDS Conference, Yokohama, Japan, 7–10 August 1994, Vol. 10.
9. Kositchaiwat C, Kositchaiwat S, Havanondha J. Curcuma longa Linn. in the treatment of gastric ulcer comparison to liquid antacid: a controlled clinical trial. J Med Assoc Thai 1993; 76:601–605.
10. Deodhar SD, Sethi R, Srimal R. Preliminary study on antirheumatic activity of curcumin (diferuloyl methane). Indian J Med Res 1980; 71:632–634.
11. Lal B, Kapoor AK, Asthana O et al. Efficacy of curcumin in the management of chronic anterior uveitis. Phytother Res 1999; 13:318–322.
12. Polasa K, Raghuram TC, Krishna T, Krishnaswamy K. Effect of turmeric on urinary mutagens in smokers. Mutagenesis 1992; 7:107–109.
13. Azuine MA, Bhide SV. Chemopreventive effect of turmeric against stomach and skin tumors induced by chemical carcinogens in Swiss mice. Nutr Cancer 1992; 17:77–83.
14. Kawamori T, Lubet R, Steele V et al. Chemopreventive effect of curcumin, a naturally occurring anti-inflammatory agent, during the promotion/progression stages of colon cancer. Cancer Res 1999; 59:597–601.
15. Dorai T, Cao YC, Dorai B, Buttyan R, Katz AE. Therapeutic potential of curcumin in human prostate cancer. III. Curcumin inhibits proliferation, induces apoptosis, and inhibits angiogenesis of LNCaP prostate cancer cells in vivo. Prostate 2001; 47:293–303.
16. Huang MT, Deschner EE, Newmark H et al. Effect of dietary curcumin and ascorbyl palmitate on azoxymethanol-induced colonic epithelial cell proliferation and focal areas of dysplasia. Cancer Lett 1992; 64:117–121.
17. Subramanian M, Sreejayan RM, Devasagayam TP, Singh BB. Diminution of singlet oxygen-induced DNA damage by curcumin and related antioxidants. Mutat Res 1994; 311:249–255.
18. Soni KB, Kuttan R. Effect of oral curcumin administration on serum peroxides and cholesterol levels in human volunteers. Indian J Physiol Pharmacol 1992; 36:273–275.
19. Kuttan R, Sudheeran PC, Josph C. Turmeric and curcumin as topical agents in cancer therapy. Tumori 1987; 73:29–31.
20. Charles V, Charles SX. The use and efficacy of Azadirachta indica ADR ('Neem') and Curcuma longa ('Turmeric') in scabies. A pilot study. Trop Geogr Med 1992; 44:178–181.
21. Chandra D, Gupta SS. Anti-inflammatory and anti-arthritic activity of volatile oil of Curcuma longa (Haldi). Indian J Med Res 1972; 60:138–142.
22. Garg SK. Effect of Curcuma longa (rhizomes) on fertility in experimental animals. Planta Med 1974; 26:225–227.
23. Vijayalaxmi. Genetic effects of turmeric and curcumin in mice and rats. Mutat Res 1980; 79:125–132.
24. Nagabhushan M, Amonkar AJ, Bhide SV. In vitro antimutagenicity of curcumin against environmental mutagens. Food Chem Toxicol 1987; 25:545–547.
25. Shankar TN, Murthy VS. Effect of turmeric (Curcuma longa) fractions on the growth of some intestinal and pathogenic bacteria in vitro. J Exper Biol 1979; 17:1363–1366.
26. Oldenhof AD, Shynlova OP, Liu M, Langille BL, Lye SJ. Mitogen-activated protein kinases mediate stretch-induced c-fos mRNA expression in myometrial smooth muscle cells. Am J Physiol Cell Physiol 2002; 283:C1530–1539.

27. Chaudhuri RN, Ghosh BN, Chatterjee B. Diet intake patterns of non-Bengali Muslim mothers during pregnancy and lactation. Indian J Public Health 1989; 33:82–83.
28. Farnsworth NR, Bingel AS, Cordell G, Crane FA, Fong HH. Potential value of plants as sources of new antifertility agents I. J Pharm Sci 1975; 64:535–598.
29. Singh A, Singh SP, Bamezai R. Postnatal modulation of hepatic biotransformation system enzymes via translactational exposure of F1 mouse pups to turmeric and curcumin. Cancer Lett 1995; 96:87–93.
30. Singh A, Singh SP, Bamezai R. Effect of arecoline on the curcumin-modulated hepatic biotransformation system enzymes in lactating mice and translactationally exposed F1 pups. Nutr Cancer 1996; 25:101–110.
31. Leung AY, Foster S. Encyclopedia of Common Natural Ingredients Used in Food, Drugs and Cosmetics, 2nd ed. New York, NY: John Wiley & Sons, 1996:649.
32. Srimal RC, Dhawan BN. Pharmacology of diferuloyl methane (curcumin), a non-steroidal anti-inflammatory agent. J Pharm Pharmacol 1973; 25:447–452.
33. Abe Y, Hashimoto S, Horie T. Curcumin inhibition of inflammatory cytokine production by human peripheral blood monocytes and alveolar macrophages. Pharmacol Res 1999; 39:41–47.
34. Chan MM. Inhibition of tumor necrosis factor by curcumin, a phytochemical. Biochem Pharmacol 1995; 49:1551–1556.
35. Ammon HP, Safayhi H, Mack T, Sabieraj J. Mechanism of antiinflammatory actions of curcumine and boswellic acids. J Ethnopharmacol 1993; 38:113–119.
36. Flynn DL, Rafferty MF, Boctor AM. Inhibition of 5-hydroxy-eicosatetraenoic acid (5-HETE) formation in intact human neutrophils by naturally-occurring diarylheptanoids: inhibitory activities of curcuminoids and yakuchinones. Prostaglandins Leukot Med 1986; 22:357–360.
37. Mukhopadhyay A, Basu N, Ghatak N, Gujral P. Anti-inflammatory and irritant activities of curcumin analogues in rats. Agents Actions 1982; 12:508–515.
38. Srivastava R, Srimal RC. Modification of certain inflammation-induced biochemical changes by curcumin. Indian J Med Res 1985; 81:215–223.
39. Murray MT. The Healing Power of Herbs. Rocklin, CA: Prima Publishing, 1992.
40. Ramprassad C, Sirsi RC. Curcuma longa and bile secretion: quantitative changes in the bile constituents induced by sodium curcuminate. J Sci Ind Res 1957; 16C:108–110.
41. Selvam R, Subramaniam L, Gayathri R, Angayarkanni N. The anti-oxidant activity of turmeric (Curcuma longa). J Ethnopharmacol 1995; 47:59–67.
42. Osawa T, Sugiyama Y, Inayoshi M, Kawakishi S. Antioxidative activity of tetrahydrocurcuminoids. Biosci Biotechnol Biochem 1995; 59:1609–1612.
43. Rafatullah S, Tariq M Al-Yahya M, Mossa JS, Ageel AM. Evaluation of turmeric (Curcuma longa) for gastric and duodenal antiulcer activity in rats. J Ethnopharmacol 1990; 29:25–34.
44. Barthelemy S, Vergnes L, Moynier M et al. Curcumin and curcumin derivatives inhibit Tat-mediated transactivation of type 1 human immunodeficiency virus long terminal repeat. Res Virol 1998; 149:43–52.
45. Sui Z, Salto R, Li J, Craik C, Ortiz de Montellano PR. Inhibition of the HIV-1 and HIV-2 proteases by curcumin and curcumin boron complexes. Bioorg Med Chem 1993; 1:415–422.

46. Mazumder A, Raghavan K, Weinstein J, Kohn KW, Pommier Y. Inhibition of human immunodeficiency virus type-1 integrase by curcumin. Biochem Pharmacol 1995; 49:1165–1170.
47. Oetari S, Sudibyo M, Commandeur JN, Samhoedi R, Vermeulen NP. Effects of curcumin on cytochrome P450 and glutathione S-transferase activities in rat liver. Biochem Pharmacol 1996; 51:39–45.
48. Mathews S, Rao MNA. Interaction of curcumin with glutathione. Int J Pharmaceut 1991; 76:257–259.
49. Susan M, Rao MN. Induction of glutathione S-transferase activity by curcumin in mice. Arzneimittelforschung 1992; 42:962–964.
50. Brinker F. Herb Contraindications and Drug Interactions, 2nd ed. Sandy, OR: Eclectic Medical Publications, 1998.
51. Brinker F. The Toxicology of Botanical Medicines. Sandy, OR: Eclectic Medical Publications, 2000:296.

VALERIAN
Valeriana officinalis

Synonyms/common names/related compounds[1]

Amantilla, all-heal, baldrian, baldrianwurzel, Belgium valerian, common valerian, fragrant valerian, garden heliotrope, garden valerian, Indian valerian, Mexican valerian, Pacific valerian, valeriana, *Valeriana officinalis*, *Valeriana rhizome*, *Valerianae radix*, valeriane

Indications

Insomnia:[2–6]	Evidence grade B1
Anxiety:[7–9]	Evidence grade B2
Sedation:[7,10]	Evidence grade B2
Sleep quality and quantity (with lemon balm)[11]	Evidence grade B2
Mental stress (with kava):[11]	Evidence grade B2
Fibromyalgia (as a bath):[12]	Evidence grade B2
Anxiety (with passion flower):[14]	Evidence grade C
Anxiety (with St John's wort):[15]	Evidence grade C
Coronary heart disease:[16]	Evidence grade C

Pregnancy

Nonteratogenic:[17]	Evidence level 2

According to a study on adverse effects of intoxication during pregnancy, there are no reports of teratogenic activity from valerian intoxication during pregnancy.[17]

Minimal risk:[18]	Evidence level 3
May retard ossification:[18]	Evidence level 3

In rats, 30-day administration of the valepotriate constituents of valerian did not change the average length of estral cycle, nor the number of estrous phases during this period, nor the fertility index.[18] No changes were detected in the development of the offspring after treatment during pregnancy.[18] No signs of fetotoxicity or external malformations were observed, although internal examination revealed an increase in number of retarded ossification at higher doses.[18]

Cytotoxic and mutagenic:[19,20]	Evidence level 3

Valepotriates have been shown to be cytotoxic and mutagenic in vitro.[19,20]

Lactation

Unknown:	Evidence level 5

There are no reports in the scientific literature of valerian being either safe or contraindicated during lactation.

Contraindication

Surgery[21]

Caution

Driving or operating heavy machinery[22]
Liver disease[23]

Constituents

- Valepotriates:[23] valtrate, isovaltrate, didrovaltrate
- Volatile oils:[23] kessanes, valerenal, valeranone, valerenic acid
- Monoterpenes:[24,25] berneol
- Sesquiterpenes:[24,25] valerenic acid, valerenone, kessyl glycol
- Lignans[24]
- γ-Aminobutyric acid (GABA)[24]

Toxicity

- LD_{50} of essential oil (intraperitoneal):[26] 15 g/kg
- LD_{50} of valerenic acid (intraperitoneal):[26] 300 mg/kg
- LD_{50} of valepotriate constituents (intraperitoneal):[22] 64–150 mg/kg
- Valepotriates were not found to be toxic at 4.6 g/kg orally in mice[22]
- Valepotriates are poorly absorbed and subject to a significant first pass effect.[27] As such, they are quickly degraded to less toxic metabolites and are not likely to cause acute adverse reactions.[24]

Pharmacology

- Valerian has sedative, anxiolytic, antidepressant, anticonvulsant, hypotensive and antispasmodic effects.[12,25,28]
- The valepotriate constituents were shown to decrease benzodiazepine withdrawal and to bind dopamine receptors.[24,25]
- The constitiuents valerenic acid and kessyl glycol were shown to cause sedation in animals.[24]
- Valerenic acid may inhibit the enzyme system responsible for the catabolism of GABA, thereby increasing GABA concentrations and decreasing central nervous system activity.[24]

- The lignans and GABA constituents in valerian may contribute to its sedative effect.[24]
- Valerian does not appear to cause adverse effects with respect to reaction time, alertness, and concentration the morning after intake.[10]
- In healthy elderly people, valerian does not appear to affect psychomotor performance.[29]
- Valerian may affect the cytochrome P450 CYP3A4 enzyme.[30]

Drug interactions[1]

Alcohol[31]
Barbiturates[24]
Benzodiazepines[24]
Drugs metabolized by cytochrome CYP3A4[30]
Sedative drugs[24]

Part used[1]

Root

References

1. Jellin JM, Batz F, Hitchens K. Natural Medicines Comprehensive Database, 3rd ed. Stockton, CA: Therapeutic Research Faculty, 2002:1530.
2. Ziegler G, Ploch M, Miettinen-Baumann A, Collet W. Efficacy and tolerability of valerian extract LI 156 compared with oxazepam in the treatment of non-organic insomnia – a randomized, double-blind, comparative clinical study. Eur J Med Res 2002; 7:480–486.
3. Dorn M. [Efficacy and tolerability of Baldrian versus oxazepam in non-organic and non-psychiatric insomniacs: a randomised, double-blind, clinical, comparative study]. Forsch Komplementarmed Klass Naturheilkd 2000; 7:79–84.
4. Leathwood PD, Chauffard F, Heck E, Munoz-Box R. Aqueous extract of valerian root (Valeriana officinalis L.) improves sleep quality in man. Pharmacol Biochem Behav 1982; 17:65–71.
5. Schulz H, Stolz C, Muller J. The effect of valerian extract on sleep polygraphy in poor sleepers: a pilot study. Pharmacopsychiatry 1994; 27:147–151.
6. Vorbach EU, Gortelmeyer R, Brunin J. Therapie von Insomnien. Psychopharmakotherapie 1996; 3:109–115.
7. Kohnen R, Oswald WD. The effects of valerian, propranolol, and their combination on activation, performance, and mood of healthy volunteers under social stress conditions. Pharmacopsychiatry 1988; 21:447–448.
8. Sousa MP, Pacheco P, Roldao V. Double-blind comparative study of the efficacy and safety of Valdispert vs. clobazepam. KaliChemi Med Research Info (Report) 1992; 1992.
9. Delsignore R, Orlando S, Costi D et al. Placebo controlled clinical trial with valerian. Settimana Medica 1980; 68:437–447.
10. Kuhlmann J, Berger W, Podzuweit H, Schmidt U. The influence of valerian treatment on 'reaction time, alertness and concentration' in volunteers. Pharmacopsychiatry 1999; 32:235–241.

11. Cerny A, Shmid K. Tolerability and efficacy of valerian/lemon balm in healthy volunteers (a double blind, placebo-controlled, multicentre study). Fitoterapia 1999; 70:221–8.
12. Cropley M, Cave Z, Ellis J, Middleton RW. Effect of kava and valerian on human physiological and psychological responses to mental stress assessed under laboratory conditions. Phytother Res 2002; 16:23–27.
13. Ammer K, Melnizky P. [Medicinal baths for treatment of generalized fibromyalgia]. Forschende Komplementarmedizin 1999; 6:80–85.
14. Schellenberg R, Schwartz A, SV et al. Quantitative EEG-monitoring and psychometric evaluation of the therapeutic efficacy of Biral N in psychosomatic diseases. Naturamed 1994; 4:9.
15. Panijel M. [Treatment of moderately severe anxiety states]. Therapiewoche 1985; 35:4659–4668.
16. Yang GY, Wang W. Clinical studies on the treatment of coronary heart disease with Valeriana officinalis var latifolia. Zhongguo Zhong Xi Yi Jie He Za Zhi Zhongguo Zhongxiyi Jiehe Zazhi 1994; Sep 14:540–542.
17. Czeizel A, Szentesi I, Szekeres I et al. A study of adverse effects on the progeny after intoxication during pregnancy. Arch Toxicol 1988; 62:1–7.
18. Tufik S, Fujita K, Seabra Mde L, Lobo LL. Effects of a prolonged administration of valepotriates in rats on the mothers and their offspring. J Ethnopharmacol 1994; 41(1–2):39–44.
19. Bounthanh C, Bergmann C, Beck J, Haag-Berrurier M, Anton R. Valepotriates, a new class of cytotoxic and antitumor agents. Planta Med 1981; 41:21–28.
20. Bounthanh C, Richert L, Beck J, Haag-Berrurier M, Anton R. The action of valepotriates on the synthesis of DNA and proteins of cultured hepatoma cells. Planta Med 1983; 49:138–142.
21. Ang-Lee MK, Moss J, Yuan C. Herbal medicines and perioperative care. JAMA 2001; 286:208–216.
22. Brinker F. The Toxicology of Botanical Medicines. Sandy, OR: Eclectic Medical Publications, 2000:296.
23. www.naturalstandard.com. Valerian (Valeriana officinalis L.) Natural Standard Monograph.
24. Houghton PJ. The scientific basis for the reputed activity of Valerian. J Pharm Pharmacol 1999; 51:505–512.
25. Klepser TB, Klepser ME. Unsafe and potentially safe herbal therapies. Am J Health Syst Pharm 1999; 56:125–138.
26. Hendriks H, Bos R, Woerdenbag HJ et al. Central nervous depressant activity of valerenic acid in the mouse. Planta Med 1985; 1:28–31.
27. Braun R, Dittmar W, Hubner G, Maurer HR. [In vivo effect of valtrate/isovaltrate on bone marrow cells and the metabolic activity of the liver in mice]. Planta Med 1984; 1–4.
28. Plushner SL. Valerian: Valerian officinalis. Am J Health Syst Pharm 2000; 57:333–335.
29. Glass JR, Sproule BA, Herrmann N et al. Acute pharmacological effects of temazepam, diphenhydramine, and valerian in healthy elderly subjects. J Clin Psychopharmacol 2003; 23:260–268.
30. Budzinski JW, Foster BC, Vandenhoek S, Arnason JT. An in vitro evaluation of human cytochrome P450 3A4 inhibition by selected commercial herbal extracts and tinctures. Phytomedicine 2000; 7:273–282.
31. Hadley S, Petry JJ. Valerian. Am Fam Physician 2003; 67:1755–1758.

WILD YAM
Dioscorea villosa

Synonyms/common names/related compounds[1]

Atlantic yam, barbasco, China root, colic root, devil's bones, dioscorea, *Dioscoreae*, Mexican yam, natural DHEA, phytoestrogen, rheumatism root, wild Mexican yam, yam, yuma

Indications

Oral

Menopausal symptoms (with burdock root, licorice root, motherwort, and angelica root):[2]	Evidence grade B2
Hyperlipidemia:[3,4]	Evidence grade D
Unproven hormonal effects:[4]	Evidence grade D

Topical

No effect on menopausal symptoms:[5]	Evidence grade B1
Unproved hormonal effects:[5]	Evidence grade B1

Pregnancy

Uterine stimulant:[6]	Evidence level 4

Wild yam is believed to induce uterine contractions.[6] There are no reports in the literature of wild yam causing uterine contractions.

Cream

Wild yam products may contain synthetic progesterone:[7]	Evidence level 4

Commercial wild yam products may contain synthetic progesterone and therefore have hormonal effects.[7]

Diosgenin

Nonteratogenic:[8,9]	Evidence level 3

Animal studies have reported that diosgenin, a constituent of wild yam, is nonteratogenic.[8,9]

Lactation

Unknown:	Evidence level 5

There are no reports in the literature of wild yam being either safe or contraindicated during lactation.

Cream

Wild yam products may contain synthetic progesterone:[7]	Evidence level 4

Commercial wild yam products may contain synthetic progesterone and therefore have hormonal effects.[7]

Constituents

- Saponins:[4,10] diosgenin, dioscin
- Alkaloid:[4,10] dioscorin

Toxicity

- LD_{50} of aqueous fraction: 1.4 g/kg (mice)[11]
- LD_{50} of dioscoretine: 0.58 g/kg (mice)[11]

Pharmacology

- Diosgenin is a steroid precursor that was used in the first pharmaceutical manufacture of oral contraceptives, topical hormones, systemic corticosteroids, androgens, estrogens, progesterone, and other sex hormones.[12–14]
- The chemical conversion of diosgenin into estrogen, progesterone, or any other steroidal compound has not been demonstrated in the human body.[12]
- Topical application of wild yam has not been shown to affect serum levels of follicule-stimulating hormone, estradiol, or progesterone.[5]
- Oral administration of wild yam did not increase serum dehydroepiandrosterone sulfate levels.[4,15]
- Wild yam has been shown to enhance estradiol binding to estrogen receptors and to induce transcription activity in estrogen-responsive cells.[16]
- Diosgenin may stimulate the growth of mammary tissue.[17]
- The saponins, namely dioscin, are gastrointestinal irritants.[18]

Drug interactions[7]

Nonsteroidal anti-inflammatory drugs[19]
Hormone replacement therapy/oral contraceptives[20]
insulin/oral hypoglycemic agents[11]
Fibric acid derivatives[21,22]
Cholesterol-lowering agents[4,10,21–29]

Parts used[1]

Root and rhizome

References

1. Jellin JM, Batz F, Hitchens K. Natural Medicines Comprehensive Database, 3rd ed. Stockton, CA: Therapeutic Research Faculty, 2002:1530.
2. Hudson T, Standish L, Breed C et al. Clinical and endocrinological effects of a menopausal botanical formula. J Naturopathic Med 1997; 7:73–77.
3. Malinow MR, Elliott WH, McLaughlin P, Upson B. Effects of synthetic glycosides on steroid balance in Macaca fascicularis. J Lipid Res 1987; 28:1–9.
4. Araghiniknam M, Chung S, Nelson-White T, Eskelson C, Watson RR. Antioxidant activity of dioscorea and dehydroepian drosterone (DHEA) in older humans. Life Sci 1996; 59:147–157.
5. Komesaroff PA, Black CV, Cable V et al. Effects of wild yam extract on menopausal symptoms, lipids and sex hormones in healthy menopausal women. Climacteric 2001; 4:144–150.
6. Boikova VV, Korkhov VV, Paseshnichenko VA. Contraceptive activity of deltonin isolated from Dioscorea-Deltoida wall. Rastitel'nye Resursy 1990; 26:85–88.
7. www.naturalstandard.com. Wild Yam (Dioscoreaceae) Natural Standard Monograph, 2003.
8. Keeler RF, Young S, Brown D. Spina bifida, exencephaly, and cranial bleb produced in hamsters by the solanum alkaloid solasodine. Res Commun Chem Pathol Pharmacol 1976; 13:723–730.
9. Keeler RF. Cyclopamine and related steroidal alkaloid teratogens: their occurrence, structural relationship, and biologic effects. Lipids 1978; 13:708–715.
10. Zakharov VN. [Hypolipemic effect of diosponine in ischemic heart disease depending on the type of hyperlipoproteinemia]. Kardiologiia 1977; 17:136–137.
11. Iwu MM, Okunji CO, Ohiaeri GO et al. Hypoglycaemic activity of dioscoretine from tubers of Dioscorea dumetorum in normal and alloxan diabetic rabbits. Planta Med 1990; 56:264–267.
12. Foster S, Tyler VE. Tyler's Honest Herbal. Binghamton, NY: Haworth Herbal Press, 1999.
13. Chevalier A. The Encyclopedia of Medicinal Plants. London: Reader's Digest, 1996.
14. Evans W. Trease and Evans' pharmacognosy, 13th ed. London: Bailliere Tindall, 1989.
15. Dollbaum C. Lab analyses of salivary DHEA and progesterone following ingestion of yam-containing products. Townsend Newsletter for Doctors 1996; 159:104.
16. Eagon PK, Elm MS, Hunter DS et al. Medicinal herbs: modulation of estrogen action. Breast Cancer Reseach Program, Era of Hope Meeting, Department of Defense, Atlanta, GA, 8–11 June 2000.
17. Aradhana, Rao AR, Kale RK. Diosgenin – a growth stimulator of mammary gland of ovariectomized mouse. Indian J Exp Biol 1992; 30:367–370.
18. Brinker F. The Toxicology of Botanical Medicines. Sandy, OR: Eclectic Medical Publications, 2000:296.
19. Yamada T, Hoshino M, Hayakawa T et al. Dietary diosgenin attenuates subacute intestinal inflammation associated with indomethacin in rats. Am J Physiol 1997; 273:G355–364.
20. Smolinske SC. Dietary supplement-drug interactions. J Am Med Womens Assoc 1999; 54:191–192, 195.
21. Cayen MN, Dvornik D. Effect of diosgenin on lipid metabolism in rats. J Lipid Res 1979; 20:162–174.

22. Cayen MN, Ferdinandi ES, Greselin E, Dvornik D. Studies on the disposition of diosgenin in rats, dogs, monkeys and man. Atherosclerosis 1979; 33:71–87.
23. Juarez-Oropeza MA, Diaz-Zagoya JC, Rabinowitz JL. In vivo and in vitro studies of hypocholesterolemic effects of diosgenin in rats. Int J Biochem 1987; 19:679–683.
24. Ulloa N, Nervi F. Mechanism and kinetic characteristics of the uncoupling by plant steroids of biliary cholesterol from bile salt output. Biochim Biophys Acta 1985; 837:181–189.
25. Nervi F, Bronfman M, Allalon W et al. Regulation of biliary cholesterol secretion in the rat. Role of hepatic cholesterol esterification. J Clin Invest 1984; 74:2226–2237.
26. Zagoya JCD, Laguna J, Guzman-Garcia J. Studies on the regulation of cholesterol metabolism by the use of structural analogue, diosgenin. Biochem Pharmacol 1971; 20:3471–3480.
27. Nervi F, Marinovic I, Rigotti A et al. Regulation of biliary cholesterol secretion. Functional relationship between the canalicular and sinusoidal cholesterol secretory pathways in the rat. J Clin Invest 1988; 82:1818–1825.
28. Uchida K, Takase H, Nomura Y et al. Changes in biliary and fecal bile acids in mice after treatments with diosgenin and beta-sitosterol. J Lipid Res 1984; 25:236–245.
29. Odumosu A. How vitamin C, clofibrate and diosgenin control cholesterol metabolism in male guinea-pigs. Int J Vitam Nutr Res Suppl 1982; 23:187–195.

YARROW
Achillea millefolium

Synonyms/common names/related substances[1]

Achilee, achillea, acuilee, band man's plaything, bauchweh, birangasifa, bloodwort, carpenter's weed, civan percemi, common yarrow, devil's nettle, devil's plaything, erba da cartentieri, erba da falegname, gemeine schafgarbe, green arrow, herbe aux charpentiers, katzenkrat, milefolio, milfoil, millefeuille, millefolii flos, millefolii herba, millefolium, millegoglie, noble yarrow, nosebleed, old man's pepper, roga mari, sanguinary, soldier's wound wort, staunchweed, tausendaugbram, thousand-leaf, wound wort

Indications

Rehabilitation following chronic hepatitis:[2]	Evidence grade E
Anti-inflammatory:[3]	Evidence grade E
Blood sugar regulation:[4]	Evidence grade E
Diuretic:[5]	Evidence grade E
Anti-bacterial:[6]	Evidence grade E
Anti-coagulant activity:[7]	Evidence grade E
Hypotensive:[8]	Evidence grade E

Pregnancy

Reduces fetal weight:[9]	Evidence level 3
Increases placental weight:[9]	Evidence level 3

When administered to pregnant rats at 56 times the human dose, yarrow was associated with reduced fetal weight and increased placental weight.[9]

Neurotoxic component (thujone):[10]	Evidence level 3

The yarrow constituent thujone is neurotoxic, where it was found to cause convulsions in the central nervous system of rats.[10]

Porphyrogenic component (thujone):[11]	Evidence level 3

The yarrow constituent thujone is porphyrogenic and may be hazardous to patients with underlying defects in hepatic heme synthesis.[11]

Weakly genotoxic:[12]	Evidence level 3

Yarrow tea was weakly genotoxic in a somatic mutation and recombination test using *Drosophila melanogaster.*[12]

May interfere with spermatogenesis:[13]	Evidence level 3

A study showed that when Swiss mice where exposed to ethanolic and hydro-alcoholic extracts of *Achillea* flowers, observations of spermatogenesis showed exfoliation of immature germ cells, germ cell necrosis and seminiferous tubule vacuolization.[13]

Potential abortifacient:[14,15]	Evidence level 4
Emmenagogue:[14]	Evidence level 4

A review article on the potential value of plants as sources of anti-fertility agents reported that yarrow was a potential abortifacient and an emmenagogue.[14]

Lactation

Neurotoxic component (thujone):[10]	Evidence level 3

The yarrow constituent thujone is neurotoxic, where it was found to cause convulsions in the central nervous system of rats.[10]

Porphyrogenic component (thujone):[11]	Evidence level 3

The yarrow constituent thujone is porphyrogenic and may be hazardous to patients with underlying defects in hepatic heme synthesis.[11]

Weakly genotoxic:[12]	Evidence level 3

Yarrow tea was weakly genotoxic in a somatic mutation and recombination test using *D. melanogaster.*[12]

Caution

Epilepsy[15]

Toxic constituents

- Volatile oils:[8,15] chamazulene, thujone (trace amounts) and other azulenes
- Polyunsaturated alkamides[16]
- Sesquiterpenoids:[17] achimillic acids (A, B C)
- Alkaloid:[7] achilleine

Toxicity

LD_{50} in mice (oral):[14] 3.65 g/kg

Pharmacology

- In diabetic mice and rats, yarrow was shown to have marked hypoglycemic and glycogen-sparing properties.[4]
- The polyunsaturated alkamides from *Achillea* species were shown to have anti-inflammatory activity where they inhibited cyclooxygenase and 5-lipoxygenase assays in vitro.[16]
- The sesquiterpenoids constituents achimillic acids A, B, and C from yarrow were shown to have anti-tumor activity against mouse P-388 leukemia cells in vivo.[17]
- The volatile oil of yarrow was reported to have a depressant activity on the central nervous system.[14]
- The alkaloid constituent achilleine was found to decrease blood clotting time in rabbits.[7]
- Yarrow showed some evidence of diuretic activity.[5]
- Yarrow has moderate anti-bacterial activity.[6]
- Persons allergic to the Asteraceae family may exhibit allergic reactions, such as contact dermatitis, when exposed to yarrow.[18–20] Alpha-peroxyachifolid was identified as the contact allergen in yarrow.[21]
- Yarrow alkaloids were reported to have hypotensive properties.[15]

Drug interactions

Antacids[22]
Anticoagulants and antiplatelets[7]
Barbiturates[14]
Hypertensive or hypotensive therapy[15]
Proton pump inhibitors[22]

Part containing toxins[14]

Flower head

References

1. Jellin JM, Batz F, Hitchens K. Natural Medicines Comprehensive Database, 3rd ed. Stockton, CA: Therapeutic Research Faculty, 2002:1530.
2. Harnyk TP. [The use of preparations of plant origin in treating and rehabilitating elderly patients with chronic hepatitis]. Lik Sprava 1999:168–170.
3. Koren G, Randor S, Martin S, Danneman D. Maternal ginseng use associated with neonatal androgenization. JAMA 1990; 264:2866.
4. Molokovskii DS, Davydov VV, Tiulenev VV. [The action of adaptogenic plant preparations in experimental alloxan diabetes]. Probl Endokrinol (Mosk) 1989; 35:82–87.
5. Goldberg AS, Mueller EC, Eigen E, Desalva SJ. Isolation of the anti-inflammatory principles from Achillea millefolium (Compositae). J Pharm Sci 1969; 58:938–941.
6. Moskalenko SA. Preliminary screening of far-Eastern ethno-medicinal plants for antibacterial activity. J Ethnopharmacol 1986; 15:231–259.
7. Miller FM, Chow LM. Alkaloids of Achillea millefolium L. Isolation and characterization of Achilleine. J Am Chem Soc 1954; 76:1353–1354.

8. Boswell-Ruys CL, Ritchie HE, Brown-Woodman PD. Preliminary screening study of reproductive outcomes after exposure to yarrow in the pregnant rat. Birth Defects Res B Dev Reprod Toxicol 2003; 68:416–420.
9. Millet Y, Jouglard J, Steinmetz MD et al. Toxicity of some essential plant oils – clinical and experimental study. Clin Toxicol 1981; 18:1485–1498.
10. Bonkovsky HL, Cable EE, Cable JW et al. Porphyrogenic properties of the terpenes camphor, pinene, and thujone (with a note on historic implications for absinthe and the illness of Vincent van Gogh). Biochem Pharmacol 1992; 43:2359–2368.
11. Graf U, Moraga AA, Castro R, Diaz Carrillo E. Genotoxicity testing of different types of beverages in the Drosophila wing Somatic Mutation And Recombination Test. Food Chem Toxicol 1994; 32:423–430.
12. Montanari T, de Carvalho JE, Dolder H. Antispermatogenic effect of Achillea millefolium L. in mice. Contraception 1998; 58:309–313.
13. Farnsworth NR, Bingel AS, Cordell G, Crane FA, Fong HH. Potential value of plants as sources of new antifertility agents I. J Pharm Sci 1975; 64:535–598.
14. Newall CA, Anderson LA, Phillipson JD. Herbal Medicines: A Guide for Health-care Professionals. London, UK: Pharmaceutical Press, 1996:296.
15. Leung AY, Foster S. Encyclopedia of Common Natural Ingredients Used in Food, Drugs and Cosmetics, 2nd ed. New York, NY: John Wiley & Sons, 1996:649.
16. Muller-Jakic B, Breu W, Probstle A et al. In vitro inhibition of cyclooxygenase and 5-lipoxygenase by alkamides from Echinacea and Achillea species. Planta Med 1994; 60:37–40.
17. Tozyo T, Yoshimura Y, Sakurai K et al. Novel antitumor sesquiterpenoids in Achillea millefolium. Chem Pharm Bull (Tokyo) 1994; 42:1096–1100.
18. Hausen BM. A 6-year experience with compositae mix. Am J Contact Dermat 1996; 7:94–99.
19. Hausen BM, Breuer J, Weglewski J, Rucker G. alpha-Peroxyachifolid and other new sensitizing sesquiterpene lactones from yarrow (Achillea millefolium L., Compositae). Contact Dermatitis 1991; 24:274–280.
20. Paulsen E, Andersen KE, Hausen BM. Compositae dermatitis in a Danish dermatology department in one year (I). Results of routine patch testing with the sesquiterpene lactone mix supplemented with aimed patch testing with extracts and sesquiterpene lactones of Compositae plants. Contact Dermatitis 1993; 29:6–10.
21. Rucker G, Neugebauer M, Kiefer A. [Quantitative determination of alpha-peroxyachifolide in yarrow by HPLC with amperometric detection]. Pharmazie 1994; 49:167–169.
22. Brinker F. Herb Contraindications and Drug Interactions, 3rd ed. Sandy, OR: Eclectic Medical Publications, 2001:432.

Chapter 5
VITAMINS

Vitamins are frequently taken by the general public to correct nutritional deficiencies and to prevent disease. In pregnancy, vitamins are often taken to help with the symptoms of pregnancy (vitamin B_6 for nausea), to help prevent anemia (vitamin B_{12}) and to support newborn blood clotting (vitamin K). In the case of some vitamins, such as vitamin A, too high a dose may be associated with teratogenic effects.

In selecting the six vitamins reviewed here, we focused on the vitamins that would support the common deficiencies of pregnancy and lactation and the vitamins that, in elevated doses, may have harmful effects on the mother or fetus. All eight reviews are presented as follows:

Vitamin name
Name of the vitamin.

Pregnancy
The safety of this herb during pregnancy. According to evidence-based medicine principles, the safety of this herb during pregnancy is evaluated based on levels of evidence (see Chapter 3).

Lactation
The safety of this herb during lactation. According to evidence-based medicine principles, the safety of this herb during lactation is evaluated based on levels of evidence (see Chapter 3).

VITAMIN A

Pregnancy

May reduce maternal mortality and morbidity:[1]	Evidence level 1a

A systematic review was conducted on the effect of vitamin A supplementation during pregnancy and how it improves maternal mortality and morbidity.[1] In five trials involving 23 426 women, weekly vitamin A supplementation resulted in a reduction in maternal mortality up to 12 weeks post-partum and a reduction in night blindness.[1]

Non-teratogenic at 6000 IU per day:[2]	Evidence level 1a

A clinical trial showed that daily intake of 6000 IU of vitamin A during pregnancy did not increase the incidence of fetal malformations.[2]

Conflicting evidence

Potentially teratogenic >10 000 IU per day:[3–5]	Evidence level 1b

Potentially non-teratogenic at doses >8000 IU or >10 000 IU per day:[5,6]	Evidence level 1c

There is conflicting evidence as to the teratogenicity of vitamin A during pregnancy.[5] A prospective cohort study of 22 748 pregnant women found that 339 had babies with birth defects; 121 of these babies had defects occurring in sites that originated in the cranial neural crest, which are associated with vitamin A teratogenicity.[4] A higher prevalence of cranial neural crest defects was found in women consuming >15 000 IU and >10 000 IU of vitamin A per day than in women consuming only 5000 IU.[4] The increased frequency of defects was concentrated among the babies born to women who had consumed high levels of vitamin A before the seventh week of gestation.[4] Among the babies born to women who took more than 10 000 IU of preformed vitamin A per day in the form of supplements, it was estimated that about 1 infant in 57 had a malformation attributable to the supplement.[4]

Another case–control study of 1000 live births reported that a teratogenic effect might exist for exposures to high doses of vitamin A (>40 000 IU), particularly during the first three months of pregnancy.[3]

On the other hand, a case–control study on 955 offspring with either major malformations or neural tube defects found no association between periconceptional vitamin A exposure at doses >8000 IU or >10 000 IU per day and malformations in general, cranial neural crest defects, or neural tube defects.[6]

Potential liver toxicity at 25 000 IU/day over long periods:[7]	Evidence level 1c

Vitamin A hepatoxicity was reported in 41 patients.[7] The smallest continuous daily consumption leading to cirrhosis was 25 000 IU during six years, whereas higher daily doses (greater than or equal to 100 000 IU) taken during 2.5 years resulted in liver damage.[7]

Retinoic acid

Teratogenic:[8]	Evidence level 1b
Retinoic acid syndrome:[8]	Evidence level 1b

Retinoic acid, an analogue of vitamin A, was shown to be teratogenic and led to a characteristic pattern of malformation involving craniofacial, cardiac, thymic, and central nervous system structures called 'retinoic acid syndrome'.[8] These malformations included microtia/anotia, micrognathia, cleft palate, conotruncal heart defects and aortic arch abnormalities, thymic defects, retinal or optic nerve abnormalities, and central nervous system malformations.[8] The malformations are believed to result from the action of retinoic acid on cranial neural crest cells.[9]

Mother-to-child human immunodeficiency virus (HIV) transmission

Vitamin A 5000 IU and 200 000 IU of β-carotene daily may reduce mother-to-child HIV transmission in preterm births:[10]	Evidence level 1a
Decreases incidence of preterm delivery:[10]	Evidence level 1a
Vitamin A 5000 IU daily No effect of preterm delivery:[11]	Evidence level 1a

A randomized controlled trial of 728 pregnant HIV-positive women found that a daily dose of 5000 IU of vitamin A and 200 000 IU of β-carotene reduced the incidence of preterm delivery.[10] Among the preterm deliveries, newborns born to mothers taking vitamin A were less likely to be infected with HIV.[10]

In a randomized controlled trial of 1075 HIV-positive pregnant women, vitamin A supplementation did not affect newborn death rate or preterm delivery.[11]

Conflicting evidence

May increase mother-to-child HIV transmission:[12]	Evidence level 1a
No effect on mother-to-child HIV transmission:[10,13,14]	Evidence level 1a
No effect of HIV immunologic markers (CD4, CD8, and CD3 counts):[11]	Evidence level 1a

A randomized controlled trial of 1078 HIV-infected pregnant African women found that vitamin A supplementation increased the risk of mother-to-child HIV transmission.[12]

Two randomized controlled trials, however, one involving 697 HIV-positive pregnant African women and another involving 728 HIV-positive African women, found that vitamin A supplementation (daily dose of 10 000 IU and 5000 IU, respectively) did not affect mother-to-child HIV transmission.[10,13] In a randomized controlled trial of 1075 HIV-positive pregnant African women, vitamin A supplementation did not affect immunologic markers (CD4, CD8, and CD3 counts) associated with HIV.[11]

A cohort study of 95 HIV-1-infected pregnant women living in the USA found that vitamin A deficiency was rare in the USA and that serum retinol levels were not associated with risk of vertical HIV-1 transmission.[14] The researchers recommended that pregnant HIV-1-infected women living in nations where vitamin A deficiency is not a public health problem should not be advised to take extra vitamin A supplements due to possible teratogenic effects.[14]

Deficiency

Low levels in habitual abortion:[15]	Evidence level 1a

A study of 40 women with habitual abortions showed that vitamin A levels were significantly lower in women with habitual abortions than in controls.[15]

Lactation

Minimal risk:[16,17]	Evidence level 1a

A randomized controlled trial of 100 mothers having uncomplicated deliveries showed that receiving 200 000 IU of vitamin A orally soon after delivery improved vitamin A intake of breast-fed infants during the first three months.[16] No adverse effects were reported.[16]

Another randomized controlled trial of 220 women showed that a single dose of 200 000 IU of vitamin A at 1–3 weeks post-partum did not result in any adverse effects.[17]

May increase HIV transmission via breastfeeding from HIV-positive mothers:[12]	Evidence level 1a

Did not affect infant mortality:[12]	Evidence level 1a

A randomized controlled trial of 1078 HIV-positive pregnant women found that vitamin A supplementation increased the risk of HIV breastfeeding transmission.[12] The study also found that vitamin A supplementation had no effect on infant mortality by 24 months.[12]

Potential liver toxicity at 25 000 IU/day over long periods:[7]	Evidence level 1c

Vitamin A hepatoxicity was reported in 41 patients.[7] The smallest continuous daily consumption leading to cirrhosis was 25 000 IU during six years, whereas higher daily doses (greater than or equal to 100 000 IU) taken during 2.5 years resulted in liver damage.[7]

VITAMIN D

Pregnancy

Not enough evidence to evaluate:[18]	Evidence level 1a

A systematic review was conducted to assess the effects of vitamin D supplementation on pregnancy outcome.[18] Two trials involving 232 women were included in this study where in one trial the mothers had higher mean daily weight gain and lower number of low-birthweight infants, and in the other trial the supplemented group had lower birthweights.[18] The researchers concluded that there is not enough evidence to evaluate the effects of vitamin D supplementation during pregnancy.[18]

Minimal risk:[19,20]	Evidence level 1a

A randomized controlled trial was conducted to evaluate the effects of single-dose (5 mg at the seventh month) and daily vitamin D supplementation (1000 IU/day) in pregnant women during the last trimester.[19] No adverse effects or significant modification of maternal calciuria or of the birthweight of term infants were observed.[19]

A randomized controlled trial of 30 low-birthweight infants, 35 infants with perinatal asphyxia, and 16 infants of diabetic mothers showed no adverse effects associated with vitamin D supplementation.[20]

Crosses the palcenta:[21]	Evidence level 4

According to one study, the fetus is entirely dependent on the mother for its supply of vitamin D (25 hydroxyvitamin D) which is believed to easily cross the placenta.[21]

Minimal risk when used below 2000 IU (50 μg) per day:[22]	Evidence level 4

According to the Institute of Medicine, vitamin D is safe during pregnancy when used in amounts below 2000 IU (50 μg) per day.[23]

Risk of hypercalcemia at >2000 IU (50 μg) per day:[23]	Evidence level 4

According to the Institute of Medicine, daily intake of vitamin D above 2000 IU (50 μg) may lead to hypercalcemia.[23] In pregnancy, hypercalcemia can lead to suppression of parathyroid hormone, hypocalcemia, tetany, seizures, aortic valve stenosis, retinopathy, and mental and/or physical retardation in the infant.[23]

Deficiency

May develop hypocalcemia:[24]	Evidence level 1b

In a study of 120 pregnant women, 75 women who did not take any vitamin D supplements during pregnancy showed statistically significant hypocalcemia, hypophosphatemia and elevation of heat-labile alkaline phosphatase (HLAP).[24]

Lactation

Minimum intake of 200 IU per day for infant:[25]	Evidence level 4

According to the National Academy of Sciences, it is recommended that all infants, including those who are exclusively breast-fed, have a minimum intake of 200 IU of vitamin D per day beginning during the first two months of life.[25] In addition, it is recommended that an intake of 200 IU of vitamin D per day be continued throughout childhood and adolescence, because adequate sunlight exposure is not easily determined for a given individual.[25]

Minimal risk when used below 2000 IU (50 μg) per day:[22]	Evidence level 4

According to the Institute of Medicine, vitamin D is safe during lactation when used in amounts below 2000 IU (50 μg) per day.[23]

Risk of hypercalcemia at >2000 IU (50 μg) per day:[23]	Evidence level 4

According to the Institute of Medicine, daily intake of vitamin D above 2000 IU (50 μg) may lead to hypercalcemia.[23]

VITAMIN E

Pregnancy

Minimal risk at 400 IU per day:[26]	Evidence level 1a

May prevent preeclampsia (with vitamin C):[26]	Evidence level 1a

A randomized controlled trial on the effect of supplementation with vitamin E and C in 283 pregnant women with preeclampsia showed no adverse effects with daily doses of 400 IU of vitamin E at weeks 16–22 of gestation.[26] The combination of vitamin E and C was also shown to be beneficial in the prevention of preeclampsia.[26]

Spontaneous abortion associated with blood levels above 0.50 mg/100 mL:[27]	Evidence level 1b

In a group of 50 spontaneously aborting women compared with the same number of pregnant women whose pregnancies terminated uneventfully, a significantly higher percentage of aborting women had individual values of serum α-tocopherol above the 0.50 mg/100 mL normal limit.[27]

Decreases malformations:[28–30]	Evidence level 3

Maternal dietary treatment with vitamin E markedly reduced the severity of malformations in diabetic rats.[28–30]

Non-teratogenic:[31,32]	Evidence level 3

Non-mutagenic:[31,32]	Evidence level 3

Non-carcinogenic:[31,32]	Evidence level 3

Few side effects at high doses in humans:[31,32]	Evidence level 4

Animal studies have shown that vitamin E does not have mutagenic, teratogenic nor carcinogenic properties.[31,32] In human studies, oral vitamin E supplementation resulted in few side effects even at doses as high as 3200 mg/day.[31,32]

Large doses may enlarge liver:[33]	Evidence level 3

Pregnant rats receiving large doses of vitamin E (22.5–2252 mg/kg per day) had larger livers, higher levels of lipids and vitamin E in plasma, and higher concentrations of vitamin E in the livers than did controls.[33] The researchers reported no obvious teratogenic effects in the newborn young of the vitamin E-supplemented rats, although some eye abnormalities were seen in the older pups of rats given extremely high amounts of the vitamin.[33] The survival rate, weight of the pups, and litter size were unaffected by vitamin E supplementation.[33]

Minimal risk at 600–900 IU per day:[34]	Evidence level 4

According to a compendium on the safety of drugs during pregnancy and lactation, no adverse effects were reported with oral intake of 600–900 IU of vitamin E daily during the last two months of pregnancy.[34]

Deficiency

Low levels in habitual abortion:[15]	Evidence level 1b

A study of 40 women with habitual abortion (HA) and controls showed that vitamin E levels were significantly lower in women with HA than in controls.[15]

Lactation

Crosses into breast milk:[33,35]	Evidence level 1c

Minimal risk:[36]	Evidence level 2

Orally administered α-tocopherol (1.1 g) reached a maximum value of 414 μg/100 g in human breast milk, which was 6.6-fold the pre-supplemental level, after three days and declined to the base line level after five days.[35] A case study of a pregnant women mega-dosing vitamin E showed breast milk vitamin E levels more than three times the upper range of normal.[36] No adverse effects were reported.[36] In a study of pregnant rats receiving large doses of vitamin E (22.5–2252 mg/kg per day), mammary transfer of vitamin E was found to be quite efficient.[33]

Does not interfere with milk production:[33,37–39]	Evidence level 3

Does not adversely affect milk composition:[33,37–39]	Evidence level 3

There are numerous animal studies on the transfer of vitamin E into breast milk and vitamin E supplementation in cattle. None of these studies reported that vitamin E supplementation interfered with milk production or negatively affected milk composition.[33,37–39]

VITAMIN K

Pregnancy

Hemolytic disease of the newborn:[40]	Evidence level 1a

Improves indices of coagulation:[40]	Evidence level 1a

A systematic review concluded that a single dose (1.0 mg) of intramuscular vitamin K after birth is effective in the prevention of classic hemolytic disease of the newborn.[40] Either intramuscular or oral (1.0 mg) vitamin K prophylaxis improves biochemical indices of coagulation status at 1–7 days.[40]

Does not prevent periventricular hemorrhage in preterm infants:[41]	Evidence level 1a

A systematic review found that vitamin K administered to women at risk of imminent preterm birth did not significantly prevent periventricular hemorrhage in preterm infants.[41]

In preterm pregnancies, slow and limited placental transport:[42]	Evidence level 1a

A randomized controlled trial of 78 women with preterm pregnancies showed that vitamin K_1 crosses the placenta slowly and to a limited degree.[42]

In low birthweight and <32 weeks' gestation infants, supplementation during pregnancy may not affect coagulation parameters:[43]	Evidence level 1b

A prospective cohort study of 33 women showed that maternal supplementation with vitamin K_1 had no significant effect on the level of vitamin K-dependent factors in low birthweight and <32 weeks' gestation infants.[43]

Conflicting evidence

No association with acute lymphoblastic leukemia or cancer:[44–46]	Evidence level 1b

Potential risk of acute lymphoblastic leukemia or cancer with *intramuscular* vitamin K:[47–49]	Evidence level 1b

Minimal risk of cancer with oral vitamin K:[48]	Evidence level 1b

A cohort study of 177 cases and 354 age- and sex-matched controls showed no relation between childhood acute lymphoblastic leukemia and neonatal administration of intramuscular vitamin K.[44] A case–control study found no significant association between parenteral vitamin K prophylaxis and leukemia or tumors.[45] Another case–control study of 54 795 children born from 1959 through 1966 found no association between exposure to vitamin K and an increased risk of any childhood cancer or of all childhood cancers combined.[46]

A retrospective case–control study on 16 193 infants delivered in Great Britain in one week of April 1970 showed an association between cancer incidence and the prophylactic administration of vitamin K.[49] A cohort study of 195 children diagnosed with cancer from 1971 to 1991, matched with 558 controls, found a significant association with intramuscular vitamin K and cancer when compared with oral vitamin K or no vitamin K therapy.[48] There was no significant increase in risk for children who had been given oral vitamin K when compared with no vitamin K.[48] The researchers concluded that the prophylactic benefits against hemorrhagic disease are unlikely to exceed the potential adverse effects from intramuscular vitamin K.[48] A review article reported that vitamin K administration to newborns may increase the risk of acute lymphoblastic leukemia in childhood.[47]

Poor transport to the fetus:[50,51]	Evidence level 2

Good transport to placenta:[50,51]	Evidence level 2

Intravenous injection of vitamin K_2 into mothers was shown to be actively incorporated into placental tissue, while transfer of vitamin K_2 to fetal blood (cord blood) was small.[51] An in vitro investigation of vitamin K_2 transport using human placental villous tissues found that the transport of vitamin K_1 into the fetus is not especially pronounced, but transport into the placental villous tissue is comparatively good.[50]

Non-mutagenic:[52]	Evidence level 3

High concentrations of vitamin K_1 did not induce primary DNA damage in cells from rat embryos grown in vitro.[52]

Minimal risk:[53]	Evidence level 4

According to the Food and Nutrition Board, Institute of Medicine, there is no evidence to suggest that vitamin K intake for pregnant women should be different to that for non-pregnant women.[53]

Deficiency

Vitamin K deficiency bleeding:[54]	Evidence level 1b

A stratified cluster sampling of 28 156 live newborns from five districts and six counties in China found that vitamin K deficiency bleeding (VKDB) was 3.27

per thousand.[54] VKDB was higher in the rural areas than in the urban areas, in breast-fed babies and in preterm babies.[54]

Anti-convulsant therapy may cause deficiency:[55]	Evidence level 1c

A multicenter observational case–control study of 25 pregnant women receiving anti-convulsant therapy and 25 pregnant controls found that the incidence of vitamin K deficiency was increased in neonates exposed to anti-convulsant drugs prenatally.[55]

May be secondary to hyperemesis gravidum:[56]	Evidence level 2

A case of a woman at 15 weeks gestation with hyperemesis gravidarum complicated by an episode of severe epistaxis was associated with a coagulopathy secondary to vitamin K deficiency.[56] The coagulopathy resolved after vitamin K replacement.[56]

Lactation

Breast-fed infants appear to be vitamin K deficient up to three months after birth:[57,58]	Evidence level 1b

In comparison with bottle-fed infants, breast-fed infants appear to be vitamin K deficient from 1 to 3 months after birth.[57,58] Breast-fed infants receiving no vitamin K at birth were more deficient in vitamin K at 3 months then breast-fed infants having received vitamin K prophylaxis.[58] Based on these results, routine vitamin K prophylaxis after birth for all breast-fed infants was recommended.[58]

Continuous menaquinone-4 (MK-4) administration increases vitamin K in breast milk:	Evidence level 1b

In an outcome study of 60 puerperal women, the continuous administration of MK-4 to mothers was shown to increase the concentration of vitamin K in milk, preventing idiopathic vitamin K deficient bleeding in infants.[59] MK-4 was shown to be accumulated and concentrated into breast milk.[59]

Phylloquinone administration may not affect breast milk concentration:[60]	Evidence level 1c

In a longitudinal study of 23 lactating mothers, there was no significant correlation between phylloquinone intake and breast milk concentration at 6, 12, and 26 weeks.[60]

Low levels in breast milk:[61–63]	Evidence level 1c

Vitamin K is present in very low concentrations in human milk.[62] A cross-sectional study of 15 mothers from day 1 to 6 months post-partum showed that vitamin K levels between colostrum and mature milk at 6 months were not statistically significant.[61] Because of significantly increased volumes of milk over the lactation period, however, approximately twice as much vitamin K was delivered in mature milk than in colostrum.[61] Based on these results, the researchers concluded that vitamin K in human milk is insufficient to meet recommended intakes for infants aged less than 6 months.[61]

Breast-fed infants may be at risk of late onset haemorrhagic disease of the newborn:[64,65]	Evidence level 2

Four cases of infants with acute bleedings due to vitamin K deficiency beyond the neonatal period were reported.[64] Two of these infants had intracranial hemorrhages and died.[64] All infants were breast-fed, born appropriate for date and did not receive vitamin K prophylaxis.[64] In a different study, another four cases of hemorrhage in breast-fed infants were reported.[65] In all cases, the infants were males, between 4 and 6 weeks old and in two of these cases, hemorrhage in the central nervous system was involved.[65] There was a prompt improvement after administration of vitamin K.[65]

Crosses into breast milk:[51]	Evidence level 2

Intravenous injection of vitamin K_2 into mothers was shown to increase the release of vitamin K_2 into milk with time even after the plasma vitamin K_2 concentration in maternal blood decreased.[51]

Non-mutagenic:[52]	Evidence level 3

High concentrations of vitamin K_1 did not induce primary DNA damage in cells from rat embryos grown in vitro.[52]

Minimal risk:[53]	Evidence level 4

According to the Food and Nutrition Board, Institute of Medicine, there is no evidence to suggest that vitamin K intake for breast-feeding women should be different from that of nonbreast-feeding women.[53]

Oral administration to infants

Prevents vitamin K deficiency bleeding in healthy breast-fed infants:[66,67]	Evidence level 1b

A prospective clinical trial found that 1 mg per week or 25 μg per day of vitamin K_1 proved to be effective in preventing vitamin K deficiency bleeding in healthy breast-fed infants.[66] The oral administration of vitamin K_1 1 mg, repeated weekly during the first three months of life, was shown to offer complete protection against vitamin K deficiency in 48 healthy breast-fed infants and did not result in an accumulation of vitamin K_1 in the blood.[67]

FOLIC ACID

Pregnancy

Improves hemoglobin levels and folate status:[68]	Evidence level 1a

A systematic review of 21 studies showed that folate supplementation during pregnancy appears to improve hemoglobin levels and folate status.[68]

Prevents neural tube defects:[69–71]	Evidence level 1a

Prevents recurrence of neural tube defects in woman with one child with neural tube defects:[69]	Evidence level 1a

The United States Food and Drug Administration (FDA) recommends folic acid supplementation at 800 μg daily in order to reduce the risk of neural tube defects.[71] A randomized controlled trial of 293 women found that a fortification program that delivered between 200 and 400 μg of folic acid daily to women would protect against neural tube defects.[70]

A randomized controlled trial of 111 women who had one child with a neural tube defect found that 4 mg of folic acid a day before and during early pregnancy prevented the recurrence of neural tube defects.[69]

Folic acid supplements may be more effective than increased dietary folic acid intake:[72]	Evidence level 1a

A randomized controlled trial of 62 women showed that compared with folic acid supplements and fortified foods, consumption of extra folic acid-containing natural food was relatively ineffective at increasing folic acid status.[72] The researchers concluded that the advice to women to consume folic acid-rich foods as a means of optimizing folic acid status is misleading.[72]

Deficiency

Low folic acid levels may be a risk factor for Down syndrome:[73]	Evidence level 1b

A cohort study of 31 women with pregnancies affected by Down syndrome and of 60 age-matched controls showed that plasma levels of homocysteine were significantly increased and serum levels of folic acid were significantly decreased in mothers with Down syndrome.[73]

Elevated homocysteine levels associated with recurrent spontaneous miscarrages:[74]	Evidence level 1b

Reduces plasma homocysteine levels:[75]	Evidence level 1a

A cohort study of 40 women with unexplained fetal loss showed an association with elevated serum homocysteine levels.[74] Homocysteine levels can be safely reduced with folic acid, vitamin B_6 and vitamin B_{12}.[74–76]

Elevated homocysteine levels associated with placental abruption or infarction:[77]	Evidence level 1b

A cohort study of 84 women with placental abruption or infarction and of 46 women with normal pregnancy outcome showed elevated homocysteine levels were associated with placental abruption or infarction.[77] Homocysteine levels can be safely reduced with folic acid, vitamin B_6 and vitamin B_{12}.[74–76]

Lactation

Folic acid levels can be depleted in the mother during lactation:[78]	Evidence level 1a

Breast milk folic acid levels may decline postpartum:[78]	Evidence level 1a

Plasma homocysteine levels may increase postpartum in women not taking folic acid supplements:[78]	Evidence level 1a

A double-blind, randomized, longitudinal study of 42 lactating women found that a dietary folate intake of approximately 380 µg daily may not be sufficient to prevent mobilization of maternal folate stores during lactation.[78] In women not taking folic acid supplements, breast milk folic acid decreased and plasma homocysteine increased.[78]

>300 µg daily of folic acid may prevent folic acid decline in adolescent pregnancies:[79]	Evidence level 1a

A randomized controlled trial of 71 breast-feeding adolescents (14–19 years) showed that 300 µg daily of folic acid was sufficient to prevent a postpartum decline in folic acid.[79]

VITAMIN B_6

Pregnancy

Reduces dental decay during pregnancy:[80]	Evidence level 1a

A systematic review on the effects of vitamin B_6 supplementation during pregnancy and labor found that vitamin B_6 supplementation was associated with decreased incidence of dental decay in pregnant women.[80]

Reduces nausea and vomiting of pregnancy:[81,82]	Evidence level 1a

Reduces nausea and vomiting of pregnancy (with ginger):[83]	Evidence level 1a

A randomized controlled trial of 59 pregnant women found that 25 mg of vitamin B_6 taken orally every 8 hours for 72 hours was effective in reducing the nausea and vomiting of pregnancy.[81] Another randomized controlled trial of 342 pregnant women receiving 30 mg per day of vitamin B_6 found that vitamin B_6 was effective in reducing the severity of nausea during pregnancy.[82]

A randomized controlled trial of 138 pregnant women found that vitamin B_6 given in combination with ginger was effective in reducing nausea and vomiting during pregnancy.[83]

Non-teratogenic:[84]	Evidence level 1b

Reduces congenital cardiovascular malformations:[84]	Evidence level 1b

A cohort study was conducted on 22 843 pregnant women with newborns or fetuses with congenital abnormalities and 38 151 matched controls of pregnant women who had newborn infants without any congenital abnormalities.[84] Treatment with vitamin B_6 during pregnancy was found to be of non-teratogenic risk to the fetus, but may provide some protective effect for cardiovascular malformations.[84]

Improves oxygenation of newborn at delivery:[85]	Evidence level 1b

A loading dose of vitamin B_6 (intramuscularly or per os) improved oxygen transport function of the newborn's blood when given to 24 non-supplemented pregnant women at term.[85]

High doses may cause neonatal seizures:[86–90]	Evidence level 2

There is some concern that high-dose maternal vitamin B_6 can cause neonatal seizures.[86–89] There have been anecdotal reports of neonatal seizures after use of vitamin B_6 by the mother for hyperemesis.[90] High-dose vitamin B_6 has also been shown to have a proconvulsant effect in mice and rats.[91,92]

Deficiency

Deficiency of vitamin B_6 may lead to slow growth in exclusively breast-fed infants:[93]	Evidence level 1b

An outcome study of 44 infants who were exclusively breast-fed for 6 months showed that low vitamin B_6 status was associated with reduced gain in length.[93]

Elevated homocysteine levels associated with recurrent spontaneous miscarrages:[74]	Evidence level 1b

A cohort study of 40 women with unexplained fetal loss showed an association with elevated serum homocysteine levels.[74] Homocysteine levels can be safely reduced with folic acid, vitamin B_6, and vitamin B_{12}.[74–76]

Elevated homocysteine levels associated with placental abruption or infarction:[77]	Evidence level 1b

A cohort study of 84 women with placental abruption or infarction and of 46 women with normal pregnancy outcome showed elevated homocysteine levels were associated with placental abruption or infarction.[77] Homocysteine levels can be safely reduced with folic acid, vitamin B_6 and vitamin B_{12}.[74–76]

Deficiency may be associated with oral lesions:[94]	Evidence level 1b

A comparative study of two groups of pregnant women of low socioeconomic status found an association between oral lesions and vitamin B_6 deficiency during pregnancy.[94]

Deficiency may be associated with lower APGAR scores:[95]	Evidence level 1b

A cohort study of 127 low-income pregnant adolescent and adult women found lower APGAR scores in infants whose mothers were vitamin B_6 deficient than those with adequate vitamin B_6 status.[95]

Lactation

Minimal risk:[96]	Evidence level 1b

A cohort study of 47 healthy full-term infants found that maternal supplementation of 2.5 mg/day of vitamin B_6 provided an adequate amount of vitamin B_6 in breast milk for the growth of breast-fed infants.[96]

Exclusive breast-feeding without vitamin B_6 supplementation may lead to deficiency after 6 months:[97]	Evidence level 1b

On cohort study of 118 nursing women found that by 6 months of exclusive breast-feeding, 30% of cases of low vitamin B_6 status in nursing mothers were reflected in their infants.[97] The study concluded that for some infants, human milk alone, without supplementary foods, may be insufficient to meet vitamin B_6 needs after 6 months of age.[97]

Does not interfere with breast milk production:[98,99]	Evidence level 1b

May suppress plasma prolactin:[98]	Evidence level 1b

An outcome study of 20 lactating women showed that although vitamin B_6 may suppress plasma prolactin, vitamin B_6 supplementation did not interfere with breast milk production.[98] An observational study of 11 full-term infants found that supplemental B_6 during pregnancy in ordinary doses does not have an antilactogenic effect.[99]

Vitamin B_6 crosses into breast milk:[99]	Evidence level 1b

An observational study of 11 full-term infants found that vitamin B_6 was transported into breast milk.[99]

References

1. van den Broek N, Kulier R, GA, Villar J. Vitamin A supplementation during pregnancy (Cochrane Review). Cochrane Library, Issue 3, 2004. Oxford: Update Software, 2004.
2. Dudas I, Czeizel AE. Use of 6000 IU vitamin A during early pregnancy without teratogenic effect. Teratology 1992; 45:335–336.
3. Martinez-Frias ML, Salvador J. Epidemiological aspects of prenatal exposure to high doses of vitamin A in Spain. Eur J Epidemiol 1990; 6:118–123.
4. Rothman KJ, Moore LL Singer MR et al. Teratogenicity of high vitamin A intake. N Engl J Med 1995; 333:1369–1373.
5. Azais-Braesco V, Pascal G. Vitamin A in pregnancy: requirements and safety limits. Am J Clin Nutr 2000; 71(5 Suppl):1325S–133S.
6. Mills JL, Simpson JL CG, Conley MR, Rhoads GG. Vitamin A and birth defects. Am J Obstet Gynecol 1997; 177:31–36.
7. Geubel AP, De Galocsy C, Alves N, Rahier J, Dive C. Liver damage caused by therapeutic vitamin A administration: estimate of dose-related toxicity in 41 cases. Gastroenterology 1991; 100:1701–1709.
8. Lammer EJ, Chen RH, Hoar RM et al. Retinoic acid embryopathy. N Engl J Med 1985; 313:837–841.
9. Werler MM, Lammer EJ, Rosenberg L, Mitchell AA. Maternal vitamin A supplementation in relation to selected birth defects. Teratology 1990; 42:497–503.
10. Coutsoudis A, Pillay K Spooner E, Kuhn L, Coovadia HM. Randomized trial testing the effect of vitamin A supplementation on pregnancy outcomes and early mother-to-child HIV-1 transmission in Durban, South Africa. South African Vitamin A Study Group. AIDS 1999; 13:1517–1524.

11. Fawzi WW, Msamanga GI, Spiegelman D et al. Randomised trial of effects of vitamin supplements on pregnancy outcomes and T cell counts in HIV-1-infected women in Tanzania. Lancet 1998; 351:1477–1482.
12. Fawzi WW, Msamanga GI, Hunter D et al. Randomized trial of vitamin supplements in relation to transmission of HIV-1 through breastfeeding and early child mortality. AIDS 2002; 16:1935–1944.
13. Kumwenda N, Miotti PG, Taha TE, et al. Antenatal vitamin A supplementation increases birth weight and decreases anemia among infants born to human immunodeficiency virus-infected women in Malawi. Clin Infect Dis 2002; 35:618–624. Epub 2002 Aug 02.
14. Burger H, Kovacs A, Weiser B et al. Maternal serum vitamin A levels are not associated with mother-to-child transmission of HIV-1 in the United States. J Acquir Immune Defic Syndr Hum Retrovirol 1997; 14:321–326.
15. Simsek M, Naziroglu MSH, Cay M, Aksakal M, Kumru S. Blood plasma levels of lipoperoxides, glutathione peroxidase, beta carotene, vitamin A and E in women with habitual abortion. Cell Biochem Funct 1998; 16:227–231.
16 Bhaskaram P, Balakrishnan N. Effect of administration of 200 000 IU of vitamin A to women within 24 hrs after delivery on response to PPV administered to the newborn. Indian Pediatr 1998; 217:217–222.
17. Rice AL, Stoltzfus RJ, de Francisco A et al. Maternal vitamin A or beta-carotene supplementation in lactating Bangladeshi women benefits mothers and infants but does not prevent subclinical deficiency. J Nutr 1999; 356:356–365.
18. Mahomed K, AM. G. Vitamin D supplementation in pregnancy. Cochrane Database Syst Rev, Issue 4 1999.
19. Mallet E, Gugi B, Brunell P et al. Vitamin D supplementation in pregnancy: a controlled trial of two methods. Obstet Gynecol 1986; 68:300–304.
20. Petersen S, Christensen NC, Fogh-Andersen N. Effect on serum calcium of a alpha-hydroxy-vitamin D3 supplementation in infants of low birth weight, infants with perinatal asphyxia, and infants of diabetic mothers. Acta Paediatr Scand 1981; 70:897–901.
21. Salle BL, Delvin E, Glorieux F. [Vitamin D and pregnancy]. Bull Acad Natl Med 2002; 186:369–376; discussion 376–377.
22. Medicine IoM. Dietary reference intakes for calcium, phosphorus, magnesium, vitamin D, and fluoride. Washington, DC: National Academy Press, 1997.
23. Medicine ASfR. Patient Fact Sheet: Prolactin Excess.
24. Marya RK, Rathee S, Lata V, Mudgil S. Effects of vitamin D supplementation in pregnancy. Gynecol Obstet Invest 1981; 12:155–161.
25. Gartner LM, Greer FR; Section on Breastfeeding and Committee on Nutrition. American Academy of Pediatrics. Prevention of rickets and vitamin D deficiency: new guidelines for vitamin D intake. Pediatrics 2003; 111(4 Pt 1):908–910.
26. Chappell LC, Seed PT, Briley AL et al. Effect of antioxidants on the occurrence of pre-eclampsia in women at increased risk: a randomised trial. Lancet 1999; 354:810–816.
27. Vobecky JS, Vobecky J, Shapcott D et al. Vitamins C and E in spontaneous abortion. Int J Vitam Nutr Res 1976; 46:291–296.
28. Siman CM, Gittenberger-De Groot AC, Wisse B, Eriksson UJ. Malformations in offspring of diabetic rats: morphometric analysis of neural crest-derived organs and effects of maternal vitamin E treatment. Teratology 2000; 61:355–367.

29. Siman M. Congenital malformations in experimental diabetic pregnancy: aetiology and antioxidative treatment. Minireview based on a doctoral thesis. Ups J Med Sci 1997; 102:61–98.
30. Viana M, Herrera E, Bonet B. Teratogenic effects of diabetes mellitus in the rat. Prevention by vitamin E. Diabetologia 1996; 39:1041–1046.
31. Kappus H, Diplock AT. Tolerance and safety of vitamin E: a toxicological position report. Free Radic Biol Med 1992; 13:55–74.
32. Bendich A, Machlin LJ. Safety of oral intake of vitamin E. Am J Clin Nutr 1988; 48:612–619.
33. Martin MM, Hurley LS. Effect of large amounts of vitamin E during pregnancy and lactation. Am J Clin Nutr 1977; 30:1629–1637.
34. Briggs GB, Freeman RK, Yaffe SJ. Drugs in Pregnancy and Lactation. 5th ed. Philadelphia: Lippincott Williams & Wilkins, 1998.
35. Kanno C, Kobayashi H, Yamauchi K. Transfer of orally administered alpha-tocopherol into human milk. J Nutr Sci Vitaminol (Tokyo) 1989; 35:649–653.
36. Anderson DM, Pittard WB 3rd. Vitamin E and C concentrations in human milk with maternal megadosing: a case report. J Am Diet Assoc 1985; 85:715–717.
37. Lundin PK, Palmquist DL. Vitamin E supplementation of high fat diets for dairy cows. J Dairy Sci 1983; 66:1909–1916.
38. Schingoethe DJ, Parsons JG, Ludens F, Schaffer LV, Shave HJ. Response of lactating cows to 300 mg of supplemental vitamin E daily. J Dairy Sci 1979; 62:333–338.
39. Al-Mabruk RM, Beck NF, Dewhurst R. Effects of silage species and supplemental vitamin E on the oxidative stability of milk. J Dairy Sci 2004; 87:406–412.
40. Puckett RM, Offringa M. Prophylactic vitamin K for vitamin K deficiency bleeding in neonates. Cochrane Database Syst Rev 2000, Issue 4. Art. No.: CD002776. DOI: 10.1002/14651858.CD002776 2004.
41. Crowther CA, Henderson-Smart DJ. Vitamin K prior to preterm birth for preventing neonatal periventricular haemorrhage. Cochrane Database Syst Rev 2000; CD000229.
42. Kazzi NJ, Ilagan NB, Liang K, et al. Placental transfer of vitamin K_1 in preterm pregnancy. Obstet Gynecol 1990; 75(3 Pt 1):334–337.
43. Dickson RC, Stubbs TM, Lazarchick J. Antenatal vitamin K therapy of the low-birth-weight infant. Am J Obstet Gynecol 1994; 170(1 Pt 1):85–89.
44. Roman E, Ansell P, Bull D. Leukaemia and non-Hodgkin's lymphoma in children and young adults: are prenatal and neonatal factors important determinants of disease? Br J Cancer 1997; 76:406–415.
45. Kaatsch P, Kaletsch U, Krummenauer F et al. Case–control study on childhood leukemia in Lower Saxony, Germany. Basic considerations, methodology, and summary of results. Klin Padiatr 1996; 208:179–185.
46. Klebanoff MA, Read JS, Mills J, Shiono PH. The risk of childhood cancer after neonatal exposure to vitamin K. N Engl J Med 1993; 329:905–908.
47. Autret-Leca E, Jonville-Bera AP. Vitamin K in neonates: how to administer, when and to whom. Paediatr Drugs 2001; 3:1–8.
48. Golding J, Greenwood R, Birmingham K, Mott M. Childhood cancer, intramuscular vitamin K, and pethidine given during labour. BMJ 1992; 305:341–346.
49. Golding J, Paterson M, Kinlen L. Factors associated with childhood cancer in a national cohort study. Br J Cancer 1990; 62:304–308.
50. Iioka H, Akada S, Hisanaga H et al. A study on the placental transport mechanism of vitamin K_2 (MK-4). Asia Oceania J Obstet Gynaecol 1992; 18:49–55.

51. Iioka H, Moriyama IS, Morimoto K et al. Pharmacokinetics of vitamin K in mothers and children in the perinatal period: transplacental transport of vitamin K_2 (MK-4). Asia Oceania J Obstet Gynaecol 1991; 17:97–100.
52. Webster WS, Vaghef H, Ryan B, Dencker L, Hellman B. Measurement of DNA damage by the comet assay in rat embryos grown in media containing high concentrations of vitamin K. Toxicol In Vitro 2000; 14:95–99.
53. Food and Nutrition Board IoM. Dietary reference intakes for vitamin A, vitamin K, arsenic, boron, chromium, copper, iodine, iron, manganese, molybdenum, nickel, silicon, vanadium, and zinc. Washington, DC: National Academy Press, 2002.
54. Zhou F, He S, Wang X. [An epidemiological study on vitamin K deficiency bleeding in infants under six months]. Zhonghua Yu Fang Yi Xue Za Zhi 2002; 36:305–307.
55. Cornelissen M, Steegers-Theunissen R, Kollee L, et al. Increased incidence of neonatal vitamin K deficiency resulting from maternal anticonvulsant therapy. Am J Obstet Gynecol 1993; 168(3 Pt 1):923–928.
56. Robinson JN, Banerjee R, Thiet M. Coagulopathy secondary to vitamin K deficiency in hyperemesis gravidarum. Obstet Gynecol 1998; 92(4 Pt 2):673–675.
57. Goldschmidt B, Benedek L, Golan Z, Bukovszky M, Marko I. [Latent vitamin K deficiency in breast-fed infants]. Orv Hetil 1990; 131:235–238.
58. Widdershoven J, Lambert W, Motohara K et al. Plasma concentrations of vitamin K_1 and PIVKA-II in bottle-fed and breast-fed infants with and without vitamin K prophylaxis at birth. Eur J Pediatr 1988; 148:139–142.
59. Saga K, Terao T. [Studies on transfer of vitamin K into human breast milk]. Nippon Sanka Fujinka Gakkai Zasshi 1989; 41:1713–1719.
60. Greer FR, Marshall S, Cherry J, Suttie JW. Vitamin K status of lactating mothers, human milk, and breast-feeding infants. Pediatrics 1991; 88:751–756.
61. Canfield LM, Hopkinson JM, Lima A, Silva B, Garza C. Vitamin K in colostrum and mature human milk over the lactation period – a cross-sectional study. Am J Clin Nutr 1991; 53:730–735.
62. Greer FR. Vitamin K status of lactating mothers and their infants. Acta Paediatr Suppl 1999; 88:95–103.
63. Greer FR. Vitamin K in human milk – still not enough. Acta Paediatr 2004; 93:449–450.
64. Dremsek PA, Sacher M. [Life-threatening hemorrhage caused by vitamin K deficiency in breast-fed infants]. Wien Klin Wochenschr 1987; 99:314–316.
65. Sutor AH, Pancochar H, Niederhoff H et al. [Vitamin K deficiency hemorrhages in 4 exclusively breast-fed infants 4 to 6 weeks of age]. Dtsch Med Wochenschr 1983; 108:1635–1639.
66. Cornelissen EA, Monnens LA. [Evaluation of various forms of vitamin-K prophylaxis in breast-fed infants]. Ned Tijdschr Geneeskd 1993; 137:2205–2208.
67. Cornelissen EA, Kollee LA, De Abreu RA, Motohara K, Monnens LA. Prevention of vitamin K deficiency in infancy by weekly administration of vitamin K. Acta Paediatr 1993; 82:656–659.
68. Mahomed K. Folate supplementation in pregnancy. Cochrane Database Syst Rev 1997, Issue 3.
69. Laurence KM, James N, Miller M, Tennant GB, Campbell H. Double-blind randomised controlled trial of folate treatment before conception to prevent recurrence of neural-tube defects. Br Med J (Clin Res Ed) 1981; 282:1509–1511.
70. Daly S, Mills JL, Molloy A et al. Minimum effective dose of folic acid for food fortification to prevent neural-tube defects. Lancet 1997; 350:1666–1669.

71. US Food and Drug Administration CfFS, and Applied Nutrition, Office of Nutritional Products, Labeling, and Dietary Supplements. Letter regarding dietary supplement health claim for folic acid with respect to neural tube defects. http://vm.cfsan.fda.gov/~dms/ds-ltr.7html.
72. Cuskelly GJ, McNulty H, Scott J. Effect of increasing dietary folate on red-cell folate: implications for prevention of neural tube defects. Lancet 1996; 347:657–659.
73. Takamura N, Kondoh T, Ohgi S et al. Abnormal folic acid-homocysteine metabolism as maternal risk factors for Down syndrome in Japan. Eur J Nutr 2004; 43:285–287.
74. Del Bianco A, Maruotti G, Fulgieri AM et al. [Recurrent spontaneous miscarriages and hyperhomocysteinemia]. Minerva Ginecol 2004; 56:379–383.
75. Venn BJ, Mann JI, Williams S et al. Assessment of three levels of folic acid on serum folate and plasma homocysteine: a randomised placebo-controlled double-blind dietary intervention trial. Eur J Clin Nutr 2002; 56:748–754.
76. Mayer EL, Jacobsen DW, Robinson K. Homocysteine and coronary atherosclerosis. J Am Coll Cardiol 1996; 27:517–527.
77. Goddijn-Wessel TA, Wouters MG, van de Molen EF et al. Hyperhomocysteinemia: a risk factor for placental abruption or infarction. Eur J Obstet Gynecol Reprod Biol 1996; 66:23–29.
78. Mackey AD, Picciano MF. Maternal folate status during extended lactation and the effect of supplemental folic acid. Am J Clin Nutr 1999; 69:285–292.
79. Keizer SE, Gibson RS, O'Connor D. Postpartum folic acid supplementation of adolescents: impact on maternal folate and zinc status and milk composition. Am J Clin Nutr 1995; 62:377–384.
80. Mahomed K, Gulmezoglu AM. Pyridoxine (vitamin B_6) supplementation in pregnancy. Cochrane Database Syst Rev 2000; 2.
81. Sahakian V, Rouse D, Sipes S, Rose N, Niebyl J. Vitamin B_6 is effective therapy for nausea and vomiting of pregnancy: a randomized, double-blind placebo-controlled study. Obstet Gynecol 1991; 78:33–36.
82. Vutyavanich T, Wongtra-ngan S, Ruangsri R. Pyridoxine for nausea and vomiting of pregnancy: a randomized, double-blind, placebo-controlled trial. Am J Obstet Gynecol 1995; 173(3 Pt 1):881–884.
83. Sripramote M, Lekhyananda N. A randomized comparison of ginger and vitamin B_6 in the treatment of nausea and vomiting of pregnancy. J Med Assoc Thai 2003; 86:846–853.
84. Czeizel AE, Puho E, Banhidy F, Acs N. Oral pyridoxine during pregnancy: potential protective effect for cardiovascular malformations. Drugs R D 2004; 5:259–269.
85. Temesvari P, Szilagyi I, Eck E, Boda D. Effects of an antenatal load of pyridoxine (vitamin B_6) on the blood oxygen affinity and prolactin levels in newborn infants and their mothers. Acta Paediatr Scand 1983; 72:525–529.
86. Gordon N. Pyridoxine dependency: an update. Dev Med Child Neurol 2000; 42:174–181.
87. Baxter P, Aicardi J. Neonatal seizures after pyridoxine use. Lancet 1999; 354:2082–2083.
88. South M. Neonatal seizures after pyridoxine use – reply. Lancet 1999; 354:2083.
89. Bernstein AL. Vitamin B_6 in clinical neurology. Ann N Y Acad Sci 1990; 585:250–260.
90. Barness L. Nutrition and nutritional disorders. In: Behrman RE, Kliegman RM, Arvin AM, eds. Philadelphia: WB Saunders, 1992.
91. Dolina S, Peeling J, Sutherland G, Pillay N, Greenberg A. Effect of sustained pyri-

doxine treatment on seizure susceptibility and regional brain amino acid levels in genetically epilepsy-prone BALB/c mice. Epilepsia 1993; 34:33–42.

92. Veresova S, Kabova R, Vellsek L. Proconvulsant effects induced by pyridoxine in young rats. Epilepsy Res 1998; 29:259–264.
93. Heiskanen K, Siimes MA, Salmenpera L, Perheentupa J. Low vitamin B_6 status associated with slow growth in healthy breast-fed infants. Pediatr Res 1995; 38:740–746.
94. Bapurao S, Raman L, Tulpule PG. Biochemical assessment of vitamin B_6 nutritional status in pregnant women with orolingual manifestations. Am J Clin Nutr 1982; 36:581–586.
95. Schuster K, Bailey LB, Mahan CS. Vitamin B_6 status of low-income adolescent and adult pregnant women and the condition of their infants at birth. Am J Clin Nutr 1981; 34:1731–1735.
96. Chang SJ, Kirksey A. Vitamin B_6 status of breast-fed infants in relation to pyridoxine HCl supplementation of mothers. J Nutr Sci Vitaminol (Tokyo) 2002; 48:10–17.
97. Heiskanen K, Siimes MA, Perheentupa J, Salmenpera L. Risk of low vitamin B_6 status in infants breast-fed exclusively beyond six months. J Pediatr Gastroenterol Nutr 1996; 23:38–44.
98. Andon MB, Howard MP, Moser PB, Reynolds RD. Nutritionally relevant supplementation of vitamin B_6 in lactating women: effect on plasma prolactin. Pediatrics 1985; 76:769–773.
99. Ejderhamn J, Hamfelt A. Pyridoxal phosphate concentration in blood in newborn infants and their mothers compared with the amount of extra pyridoxol taken during pregnancy and breast feeding. Acta Paediatr Scand 1980; 69:327–330.

Chapter 6
SUPPLEMENTS

The use of supplements is fairly widespread among the general public. Over-the-counter use of supplements is most common for joint support (arthritis and arthralgia), depression, insomnia, seasonal allergies, and so on.

For this chapter, we selected 10 supplements that are more commonly used by the general public. Our assumption is that given their frequency of use, pregnant and lactating mothers would likely continue administrating these supplements throughout gestation and lactation.

Each of the nine supplement monographs are outlined as follows.

Supplement name

The name of the supplement, e.g. glucosamine sulfate.

Description

A brief description of the supplement, where it is derived from and what type of constituent it is (oil, amino acid, flavonoid).

Main indications

The main therapeutic indications for this herb. According to evidence-based medicine principles, the indications for this herb have been evaluated based on grades/levels of evidence (see Chapter 3).

Pregnancy

The safety of this herb during pregnancy. According to evidence-based medicine principles, the safety of this herb during pregnancy has been evaluated based on grades/levels of evidence (see Chapter 3).

Lactation

The safety of this herb during lactation. According to evidence-based medicine principles, the safety of this herb during lactation has been evaluated based on grades/levels of evidence (see Chapter 3).

METHYL-SULFONYL-METHANE

Methyl-sulfonyl-methane (MSM) is a naturally occurring compound found in plants, algae and human milk.[1] MSM is an odorless metabolite of dimethyl sulfoxide (DMSO) and a source of sulfur for cysteine and methionine.[2]

Main indications

Hayfever:[1]	Evidence grade C
Joint disorders:*	Evidence grade E

*MSM is frequently used in the treatment of joint disorders and is often used in combination with glucosamine sulfate. Preliminary research shows that MSM inhibits degenerative changes in arthritic joints.[3]

Pregnancy

Unknown:	Evidence level 5

Although the safety of MSM during pregnancy is unknown, it should be noted that there were no reports in the evidence-based medical literature of MSM supplementation associated with abortion, teratogenicity, mutagenicity, uterine stimulation, menstrual stimulation (emmenagogue) or hormonal (estrogen, progesterone) activity.

Lactation

Unknown:	Evidence level 5

Although the safety of MSM is unknown during lactation, it should be noted that there are no reports in the evidence-based medical literature of MSM supplementation associated with decreased lactation, hormonal activity, or mutagenicity.

GLUCOSAMINE SULFATE

Glucosamine sulfate is an amino sugar with a sulfate group attached. Glucosamine sulfate is a constituent of cartilage proteoglycans and can be synthetically derived or derived from marine exoskeletons.[4]

Main indications

Knee osteoarthritis:[5]	Evidence grade A
Osteoarthritis:[6]	Evidence grade A

Pregnancy

Avoid:[7]	Evidence level 4
Unknown:	Evidence level 5

A natural products evidence-based database reported that glucosamine sulfate should be avoided in pregnancy and in women wishing to become pregnant.[7] The database does not provide an explanation for this caution.[7]

Although the safety of glucosamine during pregnancy is unknown, it should be noted that there were no reports in the evidence-based medical literature of glucosamine supplementation associated with abortion, teratogenicity, mutagenicity, uterine stimulation, menstrual stimulation (emmenagogue), or hormonal (estrogen, progesterone) activity.

Use with caution in gestational diabetes:	Evidence level 4
Does not affect type 2 diabetes mellitus:[8]	Evidence level 1a
Does not affect insulin sensitivity:[9]	Evidence level 1a

Although the research indicates that glucosamine does not affect blood sugar metabolism in people with type 2 diabetes and does not affect insulin sensitivity, it should be used with caution until more is known of its effects during gestational diabetes.

A randomized controlled trial of people with type 2 diabetes demonstrated that oral glucosamine sulfate supplementation does not result in clinically significant alterations in glucose metabolism.[8] A randomized controlled trial on 18 healthy subjects showed that glucosamine supplementation did not affect the regulation of insulin sensitivity in humans.[9]

Lactation

Uptake by mammary glands:[10]	Evidence level 3

Unknown:	Evidence level 5

Intravenous infusion of glucosamine through the jugular vein of a lactating cow lead to the isolation of lactosamine.[10] The researchers concluded that these results showed the uptake of glucosamine in bovine mammary gland, and also indicated that a part of glucosamine was metabolized to the product lactosamine.[10] No adverse effects were reported with respect to glucosamine adminstration.[10]

Despite this study, there are no reports in the evidence-based medical literature of glucosamine supplementation being either safe or contraindicated during lactation. As such, the safety of glucosamine sulfate during lactation is unknown.

QUERCETIN

Quercetin is a dietary bioflavonoid found in many plants.[11]

Main indications

Prostatitis:[11]	Evidence grade B2
Hayfever*:	Evidence grade E

* Quercetin is frequently used in the treatment of seasonal allergies. In vitro studies have shown that quercetin reduces histamine release from nasal scrapings by 46% to 96%.[12]

Pregnancy

Uterine relaxant:[13]	Evidence level 3

In the rat uterus, quercetin was shown to relax the tonic contractions induced by potassium chloride.[13]

Anti-estrogenic activity:[14–16]	Evidence level 3

Quercetin was shown have anti-estrogenic activity where it inhibited growth in cultures of breast cancer cells.[14] Quercetin was also shown to act as a potent inhibitor of estrone sulfatase in vitro and thus has the potential to express anti-estrogenic activity in vivo by decreasing estrogenic production in human liver cells.[15]

Non-teratogenic:[17]	Evidence level 3
May lower fetus body weight:[17]	Evidence level 3

Doses of up to 2000 mg/kg of quercetin were administered to pregnant rats on the morning of day 9 of gestation.[17] On day 20 of gestation, some quercetin-treated groups showed a significant decrease in the average weight of the fetuses compared with the corresponding control weight.[17] The fetuses recovered on day 30 of gestation and failed to reveal any reproducible dose-related syndrome of teratogenic effects attributable to quercetin treatment.[17]

Non-embryotoxic:[18]	Evidence level 3

Quercetin was shown to enhance the survival of purified rat spinal embryonic motor neurons after they have been sampled.[18]

May interfere with transplacental calcium transport:[19]	Evidence level 3

Quercetin was shown to inhibit the enzyme Ca^{2+}-activated ATPase in the mouse chorioallantoic placenta, thereby affecting transplacental calcium transport during mouse embryonic development.[19]

Non-mutagenic:[20]	Evidence level 3

May cause infertility in males (inconclusive):[20]	Evidence level 3

At doses of up to 400 mg/kg, quercetin did not induce any postimplantation losses in mice and rats, thereby a reliable measure of non-lethal mutagenic activity.[20] In male mice, however, there was a profound reduction in fertility at 300 mg/kg and 400 mg/kg of quercetin; this relation was not observed in male rats.[20] The researchers hypothesized that the loss of fertility could be due to germinal cytotoxicity, oligospermia, or impairment of fertilizing ability by quercetin.[20]

May interfere with tissue proliferation in the uterus:[21]	Evidence level 3

In rats, quercetin was shown to interfere with a protein kinase enzyme responsible for tissue proliferation in the uterus.[21]

Lactation

Blocks binding of prolactin:[22]	Evidence level 3

Quercetin was shown to block prolactin action on milk protein genes in the mammary gland.[22]

May interfere with growth of mammary gland cells:[21,23]	Evidence level 3

Quercetin was shown to inhibit the activity of a protein kinase enzyme responsible for the growth of mammary gland cells in lactating mice.[21,23]

5-HYDROXYTRYPTOPHAN

5-Hydroxytryptophan (5-HTP) is an amino acid that readily crosses the blood–brain barrier and increases central nervous system (CNS) synthesis of serotonin.[24]

Main indications

Depression:[24]	Evidence grade A
Fibromyalgia:[25]	Evidence grade B2

Pregnancy

Increases serum levels of prolactin:[26]	Evidence level 1b

Oral administration of 5-HTP in 10 obese but otherwise healthy women was shown to increase serum levels of prolactin.[26] During pregnancy and lactation, prolactin levels normally increase.[27] High levels of prolactin, as in the case of hyperprolactinemia, may be associated with reproductive dysfunctions due to menstrual irregularities and amenorrhea.[28]

May contain impurities associated with eosinophilia-myalgia syndrome:[29]	Evidence level 2

The United States Food and Drug Administration (FDA) reported that an impurity know as 'Peak X' was identified in dietary supplements containing 5-HTP.[29] In 1991, one case of eosinophilia-myalgia syndrome (EMS) was associated with 5-HTP.[29] EMS is a serious systemic illness characterized by elevations of certain white blood cells and severe muscle pain.[29]

Increases fetal breathing movement:[30,31]	Evidence level 3

5-HTP was shown to prolong high-voltage electrocortical activity and increase the incidence of fetal breathing movements in animals.[30,31]

Unknown:	Evidence level 5

Although the safety of 5-HTP during pregnancy is unknown, it should be noted that there were no reports in the evidence-based medical literature of 5-HTP supplementation associated with abortion, teratogenicity, mutagenicity, uterine stimulation, menstrual stimulation (emmenagogue), or hormonal (estrogen, progesterone) activity.

Lactation

Increases serum levels of prolactin:[26]	Evidence level 1b

Oral administration of 5-HTP in 10 obese but otherwise healthy women was shown to increase serum levels of prolactin.[26] During pregnancy and lactation, prolactin levels normally increase.[27]

Unknown:	Evidence level 5

There are no reports in the evidence-based medical literature of 5-HTP supplementation being either safe or contraindicated during lactation.

COENZYME Q-10

Coenzyme Q-10 (Co Q-10) is fat soluble and a vitamin-like compound that is present in all cells and membranes and in addition to being a member of the mitochondrial respiratory chain.[32]

Main indications

Congestive heart failure:[33–35]	Evidence grade A
Hypertension:[36,37]	Evidence grade B2

Pregnancy

Unknown:	Evidence level 5

Although the safety of Co Q-10 during pregnancy is unknown, it should be noted that there were no reports in the evidence-based medical literature of Co Q-10 supplementation associated with abortion, teratogenicity, mutagenicity, uterine stimulation, menstrual stimulation (emmenagogue) or hormonal (estrogen, progesterone) activity.

Blood levels

Low serum levels associated with abortion:[38]	Evidence level 1b

A cohort study of 483 pregnancies found that low levels of Co Q-10 in maternal blood were observed in spontaneous abortions, in threatened late abortions, and in threatened preterm deliveries.[38] The authors concluded that Co Q-10 was a marker of pathological uterine contractile activity.[38]

Low serum levels associated with preeclampsia:[39,40]	Evidence level 1b

Two cohort study showed that during preeclampsia, there is a significant decrease in plasma levels of Co Q-10 compared with normal pregnant women.[39,40]

Lactation

Unknown:	Evidence level 5

There are no reports in the evidence-based medical literature of Co Q-10 supplementation being either safe or contraindicated during lactation.

BROMELAIN

Bromelain is a natural proteinase preparation derived from the stem of the pineapple.[41]

Main indications

Breast engorgement during lactation (with trypsin):[42]	Evidence grade A
Knee osteoarthritis:[43,44]	Evidence grade C
Ankylosing spondylitis:[45]	Evidence grade C

Pregnancy

Bromelain

Unknown:	Evidence level 5
Estrogenic[47]	Evidence level 4

Although the safety of bromelain during pregnancy is unknown, it should be noted that there were no reports in the evidence-based medical literature of bromelain supplementation associated with abortion, teratogenicity, mutagenicity, uterine stimulation, menstrual stimulation (emmenagogue), or hormonal (estrogen, progesterone) activity.

Pineapple

Emmenagogue:[46]	Evidence level 4
Potential abortifacient:[46]	Evidence level 4

With respect to pineapple, however, a review article on the potential value of plants as sources of anti-fertility agents reported that the leaf, fruit and juice of pineapple were emmenagogues and potential abortifacients, and that they had estrogenic acivity.[46,47]

Intravaginal use

May dilate cervical canal:[48]	Evidence level 1c
Avoid intravaginal use:[49,50]	Evidence level 1c

Through radiographic observation, intravaginal use of bromelain was shown to dilate and widen the cervical canal and to soften the cervix.[48] Two studies reported that the mucolytic activity of bromelain could be useful in cleaning the mucus plug in the cervical os to get better radiographs during cervicohysterograms.[49,50] Although not stated by the researchers, dilation of the cervix and dissolution of the cervical plug when bromelain is used intravaginally may adversely affect pregnancy outcome.

Lactation

Minimal risk:[42]	Evidence level 1a

A systematic review was conducted on the efficacy of various treatments to relieve symptoms of breast engorgement among breast-feeding women.[42] In combination with trypsin, bromelain was shown to significantly improve symptoms of breast engorgement.[42] No adverse effects were reported with respect to taking bromelain during lactation.[42]

FISH OILS

Eicosapentaenoic acid (EPA) and docosahexaenoic acid (DHA)

EPA and DHA are long-chain n-3 polyunsaturated fatty acids that are found in the tissues of marine mammals and oily fish.[4]

Main indications

Hyperlipidemia:[51,52]	Evidence grade A
Heart disease prevention:[53]	Evidence grade A
Hypertension:[54]	Evidence grade A

Pregnancy

Minimal risk:[55–58]	Evidence level 1a

A double-blind randomized controlled study of 590 pregnant women (19–35 years old) in weeks 17–19 of pregnancy showed no harmful effects of maternal supplementation with fish oils regarding pregnancy outcome, cognitive development, or growth.[58]

Longer gestational length:[58]	Evidence level 1a
Increased cerebral maturation:[58]	Evidence level 1a

Neonates with a high concentration of DHA in umbilical plasma had longer gestational length and mature EEG on the second day of life than neonates with a low concentration.[58]

Improves postnatal oxidative stress:[59]	Evidence level 1a
May reduce expression of allergic disease:[59]	Evidence level 1a

A randomized controlled trial of 83 pregnant atopic women showed that maternal supplementation with fish oil can attenuate neonatal lipid peroxidation, reduce postnatal oxidative stress, and reduce expression of allergic disease.[59]

Improves mental processing and IQ:[60]	Evidence level 1a

A randomized controlled trial of 341 mothers showed that children who were born to mothers who had taken cod liver oil during pregnancy and lactation scored higher on the Mental Processing Composite at 4 years of age as compared with children whose mothers had taken corn oil.[60] The children's mental processing scores at 4 years of age correlated significantly with maternal intake of DHA and EPA during pregnancy.[60]

Levels in the mother correlate to newborn levels:[55–57] **Evidence level 1b**

A cross-sectional study of 162 mothers found that omega-3 fatty acid intake by the mother was directly correlated to levels in the newborn.[55] An outcome study of 23 healthy pregnant women found that children born to mothers supplemented with fish oil in the last trimester of pregnancy start with a better DHA status at birth, which may be beneficial to neonatal neurodevelopment.[56]

Non-toxic:[61,62] **Evidence level 3**

Non-genotoxic:[61] **Evidence level 3**

Anti-mutagenic:[63] **Evidence level 3**

DHA produced negative results in genotoxicity assays and demonstrated a low acute oral toxicity in mice and rats.[61] EPA and DHA were shown to have anti-mutagenic activity in Chinese hamster cells.[63] EPA and DHA were shown to have low toxicity in human leukemic cell lines.[62]

Fish

Potential contamination:[64,65] **Evidence level 4**

Fish may contains contaminants such as methylmercury, dioxins and polychlorinated biphenyls (PCBs), that are harmful to pregnant and nursing mothers.[64] Although these safety concerns apply principally to fish meat, ensure that fish oil supplements do not contain methylmercury, dioxins, PCBs, and any other contaminants. Verify with manufacturer that there are laboratory reports indicating the absence of contaminants in their fish oil product.

Lactation

Minimal risk:[58] **Evidence level 1a**

A double-blind randomized controlled study of 590 pregnant women (19–35 years) in weeks 17–19 of pregnancy showed that supplementation with fish oil did not adversely affect lactation.[58]

Elevates milk DHA content:[58,66] **Evidence level 1a**

A double-blind randomized controlled study of 590 pregnant women (19–35 years) in weeks 17–19 of pregnancy showed that breast milk of mothers supplemented with cod liver oil contained more omega-3 fatty acids than breast milk of mothers supplemented with corn oil.[58] A study of eight lactating women showed that dietary intake of fish oil significantly elevated milk DHA content, which would elevate the newborns' DHA intake.[66] DHA is essential for brain, nervous tissue, and retinal development during the first year of life.[66]

Improves mental development:[67] **Evidence level 1a**

Improves mental processing and IQ:[60] **Evidence level 1a**

A randomized controlled trail of 56 newborns showed that early dietary supply of DHA was a major dietary determinant of improved performance on mental development indexes.[67] A randomized controlled trial of 341 mothers showed that children who were born to mothers who had taken cod liver oil during pregnancy and lactation scored higher on the Mental Processing Composite at 4 years of age as compared with children whose mothers had taken corn oil.[60]

Improves visual acuity development:[68] **Evidence level 1a**

A randomized controlled trail of 180 newborns showed that dietary DHA and arachidonic acid supplementation improved visual acuity development.[68]

Improves mucosal immunity:[69] **Evidence level 1a**

In a randomized controlled trial of 83 pregnant women, supplementation with fish oil during pregnancy significantly altered early post-partum breast milk fatty acid composition.[69] Omega-3 fatty acid levels were positively associated with IgA and sCD14 levels, suggesting a relation between fatty acid status and mucosal immune function.[69]

Use DHA in pre-term infants:[70] **Evidence level 1c**

Blood samples of pre-term infants showed that a too-high supply of EPA in addition to DHA might be harmful to mental development.[70]

Fish

Potential contamination:[64,65] **Evidence level 4**

Fish may contains contaminants such as methylmercury, dioxins and polychlorinated biphenyls (PCBs), that are harmful to pregnant and nursing mothers.[64] Although these safety concerns apply principally to fish meat, ensure that fish oil supplements do not contain methylmercury, dioxins, PCBs and any other contaminants. Verify with the manufacturer that there are laboratory reports indicating the absence of contaminants in their fish oil product.

SOY ISOFLAVONES

Soy isoflavones are heterocyclic phenols that are structurally similar to estradiol and to selective estrogen-receptor modulators (SERM). Soy isoflavones contain the isoflavone glucosides genistein and daidzein in their inactive conjugated forms.

Main indications

Hyperlipidemia:[71–73]	Evidence grade B1
Menopausal symptoms:[72,74]	Evidence grade B1
Breast cancer prevention:[75,76]	Evidence grade C

Pregnancy

Weak estrogenic activity:[77,78]	Evidence level 1a
Increases sex hormone binding globulin (SHBG):[79]	Evidence level 1b

A study on 18 post-menopausal women found that soy supplementation did not exert clinically important estrogenic effects on vaginal epithelium or endometrium.[77] Another study of 84 pre-menopausal women found short-term dietary soy has a weak estrogenic response on the breast.[78] A study on 20 post-menopausal women found that soy consumption significantly increased SHBG in subjects whose SHBG concentrations are in the low end of the concentration range.[79]

Potential allergen:[80]	Evidence level 1a

A randomized controlled trial of 288 pregnant women showed that a hypoallergenic diet, excluding allergens such as soy, during the third trimester of pregnancy and during lactation reduces food sensitization and allergy during the first year of life.[80]

Increased risk of hypospadias:[81]	Evidence level 1b

A prospective cohort study of 7928 boys born to mothers taking part in the Avon Longitudinal Study of Pregnancy and Childhood found that mothers who were vegetarian in pregnancy had higher odds of giving birth to a boy with hypospadias.[81] The researchers concluded that these results support the possibility that phytoestrogens, such as soy and soy milk, may have a deleterious effect on the developing male reproductive system.[81]

Conflicting evidence

May affect sexual development:[82–85]	Evidence level 3

Gestational and lactational exposure to genistein resulted in temporary, prepubertal urogenital abnormalities in male rats.[83] Males exposed to genistein had smaller anogenital distance and testis size, and delayed preputial separation.[83] Gestation and lactation exposure to genistein also caused long-term dysfunction in reproductive behavior, in which adult males exposed to genistein were less likely to mount, intromit, and ejaculate during mating tests.[83] Males exposed to genistein also had lower testosterone concentrations in adulthood.[83]

In two other studies, gestational and lactational exposure of mice to genistein at human exposure levels did not induce adverse effects on sperm quality, changes in testicular gene expression or any adverse effects on the reproductive organs in mice at the human intake dose level.[84,85]

Reduces body weight:[86] Evidence level 3

Does not affect endocrine function:[86] Evidence level 3

In rats, genistein supplementation was shown to reduced body weight at week 11, but not to affect endocrine parameters.[86]

Crosses the placenta:[87] Evidence level 3

In a study of human amniotic fluid following phytoestrogen ingestion, dietary phytoestrogens were quantified in 96.2% of second trimester amniotic fluid samples tested.[87] Second trimester amniotic fluid contained quantifiable levels of dietary phytoestrogens, including daidzein, genistein, formononetin, biochanin A, and coumestrol.[87]

May affect progesterone receptor:[88] Evidence level 3

Genistein was found to increase progesterone receptor (PR) in the uterine glandular epithelium, where PR is essential for regulating key female reproductive processes, such as uterine proliferation, implantation, and maintenance of pregnancy.[88] Increased PR expression suggests that genistein exposure during reproductive development may have long-term reproductive health consequences.[88]

Conflicting evidence

May increase or have a protective effect on mammary tumors:[89,90] Evidence level 3

Subcutaneous exposure to genistein, mimicking the effects of in utero estrogenic exposures, increased the incidence of mammary tumors in rats in a dose dependent manner, when compared with the controls.[89] However, another study showed that administration of genistein in the perinatal period had protective effects against induced mammary carcinoma in rats.[90]

Food amounts

Minimal risk:[91] — Evidence level 4

According to the United States Food and Drug Administration (FDA), soy consumption in foods amounts presents minimal risk during pregnancy.[91]

Lactation

Conflicting evidence

May affect sexual development:[82–85] — Evidence level 3

Gestational and lactational exposure to genistein resulted in temporary, prepubertal urogenital abnormalities in male rats.[83] Males exposed to genistein had smaller anogenital distance and testis size, and delayed preputial separation.[83] Gestation and lactation exposure to genistein also caused long-term dysfunction in reproductive behavior, in which adult males exposed to genistein were less likely to mount, intromit, and ejaculate during mating tests.[83] Males exposed to genistein also had lower testosterone concentrations in adulthood.[83]

In two other studies, gestational and lactational exposure of mice to genistein at human exposure levels did not induce adverse effects on sperm quality, changes in testicular gene expression or any adverse effects on the reproductive organs in mice at the human intake dose level.[84,85]

May or may not affect morphological changes in mammary glands:[82,92] — Evidence level 3

In one study, postnatal exposure to pharmacological levels of genistein induced profound morphological changes in the mammary glands of adult female rats, reflecting estrogenic activity.[92] In another study, in utero and lactational exposure to genistein at levels comparable to or greater than human exposures did not adversely affect mammary gland development in pubertal female mice.[82]

Food amounts

Minimal risk:[91] — Evidence level 4

According to the United States Food and Drug Administration (FDA), soy consumption in foods amounts presents minimal risk during lactation.[91]

LACTOBACILLUS SPP.

Lactobacillus refers to a group of lactic acid-producing, Gram-positive rods that are obligate and facultative anaerobes.[93] *Lactobacillus* species include *L. acidophilus*, *L. bulgaricus*, *L. casei rhamnosus*, *L. delbrueckii*, *L. fermentum*, *L. plantarum*, *L. reuteri*, *L. rhamnosus*, and *L. sporogenes*.[4]

Main indications

Diarrhea:[94,95]	Evidence grade A
Atopic disease:[96,97]	Evidence grade B1

Pregnancy

Minimal risk:[98]	Evidence level 1b

A total of 32 women with bacterial vaginosis in the first trimester of pregnancy were treated with intravaginal application of yoghurt, which contains *Lactobacillus* spp.[98] The yoghurt treatment restored the normal acidity and vaginal flora, without systemic effect to the mother or fetus.[98]

May reduce the risk of pre-term delivery:[99]	Evidence level 1b

A prospective study of the vaginal flora in the second trimester was undertaken in 1958 women with singleton pregnancies.[99] Absence of lactobacilli was identified as an independent risk factor and as a predictor for pre-term delivery at <33 weeks of gestation.[99] The study suggests that tests for determining the presence of vaginal lactobacilli may be clinically useful tools for identifying women at an increased risk of pre-term delivery at <33 weeks of gestation.[99]

Mother-to-newborn infant transmission:[100,101]	Evidence level 1c

A study of 86 pregnant women tested for vaginal lactobacilli showed that approximately one-fourth of infants acquire vaginal lactobacilli from their mothers at birth, and that the acquired lactobacilli do not last in the intestine of the infant long-term, but rather, are replaced by ones from milk or unknown sources after birth.[101] Six children whose mothers took supplementation with *Lactobacillus GG* during pregnancy showed temporary colonization of the gastrointestinal tract for as long as 6 months post delivery, and in some cases, as long as 24 months post delivery.[100]

Lactobacillus GG (L. rhamnosus)

Minimal risk:[96,97]	Evidence level 1a

A randomized controlled trial of 62 mother–infant pairs showed that administering probiotics to pregnant and lactating mothers increased the immunoprotective potential of breast milk.[96] The researchers observed that administering probiotics during pregnancy and lactation was safe and effective.[96] Another randomized controlled trial was conducted on 132 mother–infant pairs where *Lactobacillus GG* was used with apparent safety in lactating women for up to six months.[97]

Lactation

Lactobacillus GG (L. rhamnosus)

Minimal risk:[96,97]	Evidence level 1a

A randomized controlled trial of 62 mother–infant pairs showed that administering probiotics to pregnant and lactating mothers increased the immunoprotective potential of breast milk.[96] The researchers observed that administering probitoics during pregnancy and lactation was safe and effective.[96] Another randomized controlled trial was conducted on 132 mother–infant pairs where *Lactobacillus GG* was used with apparent safety in lactating women for up to 6 months.[97]

References

1. Barrager E, Veltmann JR, Jr, Schauss AG, Schiller RN. A multicentered, open-label trial on the safety and efficacy of methylsulfonylmethane in the treatment of seasonal allergic rhinitis. J Altern Complement Med 2002; 8:167–173.
2. Hucker HB, Ahmad PM, Miller E, Brobyn R. Metabolism of dimethyl sulphoxide to dimethyl sulphone in the rat and man. Nature 1966; 209:619–620.
3. Murav'ev IV, Venikova MS, PG, Riazantseva TA, Sigidin IaA. [Effect of dimethyl sulfoxide and dimethyl sulfone on a destructive process in the joints of mice with spontaneous arthritis]. Patol Fiziol Eksp Ter 1991:37–39.
4. Jellin JM, Batz F, Hitchens K. Natural Medicines Comprehensive Database, 3rd ed. Stockton, CA: Therapeutic Research Faculty, 2002:1530.
5. Richy F, Bruyere O, EO et al. Structural and symptomatic efficacy of glucosamine and chondroitin in knee osteoarthritis: a comprehensive meta-analysis. Arch Intern Med 2003; 163:1514–1522.
6. McAlindon TE, LaValley MP, Gulin J, Felson DT. Glucosamine and chondroitin for treatment of osteoarthritis: a systematic quality assessment and meta-analysis. JAMA 2000; 283:1469–1475.
7. www.naturalstandard.com. Glucosamine Natural Standard Monograph.
8. Scroggie DA, Albright A, Harris MD. The effect of glucosamine-chondroitin supplementation on glycosylated hemoglobin levels in patients with type 2 diabetes mellitus: a placebo-controlled, double-blinded, randomized clinical trial. Arch Intern Med 2003; 163:1587–1590.
9. Pouwels MJ, Jacobs JR, Span PN et al. Short-term glucosamine infusion does not affect insulin sensitivity in humans. J Clin Endocrinol Metab 2001; 86:2099–2103.
10. Hara Y, Suyama K. Biosynthesis of lactosamine in bovine mammary gland. Carbohydr Res 2001; 330:65–71.
11. Shoskes DA, Zeitlin SI, Shahed A, Rajfer J. Quercetin in men with category III chronic prostatitis: a preliminary prospective, double-blind, placebo-controlled trial. Urology 1999; 54:960–963.

12. Otsuka H, Inaba M, Fujikura T, Kunitomo M. Histochemical and functional characteristics of metachromatic cells in the nasal epithelium in allergic rhinitis: studies of nasal scrapings and their dispersed cells. J Allergy Clin Immunol 1995; 96:528–536.
13. Revuelta MP, Cantabrana B, Hidalgo A. Depolarization-dependent effect of flavonoids in rat uterine smooth muscle contraction elicited by $CaCl_2$. Gen Pharmacol 1997; 29:847–857.
14. Miodini P, Fioravanti L, Di Fronzo G, Cappelletti V. The two phyto-oestrogens genistein and quercetin exert different effects on oestrogen receptor function. Br J Cancer 1999; 80:1150–1155.
15. Huang Z, Fasco MJ, Kaminsky LS. Inhibition of estrone sulfatase in human liver microsomes by quercetin and other flavonoids. J Steroid Biochem Mol Biol 1997; 63:9–15.
16. Kellis JTJ, Vickery LE. Inhibition of human estrogen synthetase (aromatase) by flavones. Science 1984; 225:1032–1034.
17. Willhite CC. Teratogenic potential of quercetin in the rat. Food Chem Toxicol 1982; 20:75–79.
18. Ternaux JP, Portalier P. Effect of quercetine on survival and morphological properties of cultured embryonic rat spinal motoneurones. Neurosci Lett 2002; 332:33–36.
19. Tuan RS, Bigioni N. Ca(2+)-activated ATPase of the mouse chorioallantoic placenta: developmental expression, characterization and cytohistochemical localization. Development 1990; 110:505–513.
20. Aravindakshan M, Chauhan PS, Sundaram K. Studies on germinal effects of quercetin, a naturally occurring flavonoid. Mutat Res 1985; 144:99–106.
21. Sharoni Y, Teuerstein I, Shirman A, Feldman B, Levy J. Cyclic changes in rat uterine proliferation during the estrous cycle are preceded by changes in protein kinase activity. Endocrinology 1984; 115:2297–2302.
22. Bayat-Sarmadi M, Houdebine LM. Effect of various protein kinase inhibitors on the induction of milk protein gene expression by prolactin. Mol Cell Endocrinol 1993; 92:127–134.
23. Mitev VI, Sirakov LM. The difference between cytosol and membrane growth-related protein kinase activities in lactating mouse mammary gland. Int J Biochem 1989; 21:337–340.
24. Shaw K, Turner J Del Marc C. Tryptophan and 5-hydroxytryptophan for depression. Cochrane Database Syst Rev 2001:CD003198.
25. Caruso I, Sarzi Puttini P Cazzola M, Azzolini V. Double-blind study of 5-hydroxytryptophan versus placebo in the treatment of primary fibromyalgia syndrome. J Int Med Res 1990; 18:201–209.
26. Martinelli I, Mainini E, Mazzi C. [Effect of 5-hydroxytryptophan on the secretion of PRL, GH, TSH and cortisol in obesity]. Minerva Endocrinol 1992; 17:121–126.
27. Chen BL, Zhang ZH, Liu N, Huang KS. [Prolactin in normal pregnancy and severe pregnancy-induced hypertension]. Hunan Yi Ke Da Xue Xue Bao 2001; 26:67–69.
28. Hurtado Amador R, Ayala AR, Hernandez Marin I. [The impact of prolactinoma in human reproduction]. Ginecol Obstet Mex 2004; 72:3–9.
29. FDA. Center for Food Safety and Applied Nutrition, Office of Premarket Approval, EAFUS: A food additive database. vm.cfsan.fda.gov/~dms/eafus.html 2004.
30. Morrison JL, Chien C, Gruber N, Rurak D, Riggs W. Fetal behavioural state changes following maternal fluoxetine infusion in sheep. Brain Res Dev Brain Res 2001; 131:47–56.

31. Morrison JL, Carmichael L, Homan J, Richardson BS. The effects of 'sleep promoting agents' on behavioural state in the ovine fetus. Brain Res Dev Brain Res 1997; 103:1–8.
32. Turunen M, Olsson J, Dallner G. Metabolism and function of coenzyme Q. Biochim Biophys Acta 2004; 1660(1–2):171–199.
33. Morisco C, Trimarco B, Condorelli M. Effect of coenzyme Q10 therapy in patients with congestive heart failure: a long-term multicenter randomized study. Clin Investig 1993; 71(Suppl 8):S134–136.
34. Baggio E, Gandini R, Plancher A, Passeri M, Carmosino G. Italian multicenter study on the safety and efficacy of coenzyme Q10 as adjunctive therapy in heart failure. CoQ10 Drug Surveillance Investigators. Mol Aspects Med 1994; 1(Suppl 5):s287–294.
35. Soja AM, Mortensen SA. Treatment of congestive heart failure with coenzyme Q10 illuminated by meta-analyses of clinical trials. Mol Aspects Med 1997; 1(Suppl 8):S159–168.
36. Singh RB, Niaz MA, Rastogi S, Shukla PK, Thakur AS. Effect of hydrosoluble coenzyme Q10 on blood pressures and insulin resistance in hypertensive patients with coronary artery disease. J Hum Hypertens 1999; 13:203–208.
37. Hodgson JM, Watts GF, Playford D, Burke V, Croft KD. Coenzyme Q10 improves blood pressure and glycaemic control: a controlled trial in subjects with type 2 diabetes. Eur J Clin Nutr 2002; 56:1137–1142.
38. Noia G, Romano D, De Santis M et al. [The antioxidants (coenzyme Q10) in materno-fetal physiopathology]. Minerva Ginecol 1999; 51:385–391.
39. Teran E, Racines-Orbe M, Vivero S et al. Preeclampsia is associated with a decrease in plasma coenzyme Q10 levels. Free Radic Biol Med 2003; 35:1453–1456.
40. Palan PR, Shaban DW, Martino T, Mikhail MS. Lipid-soluble antioxidants and pregnancy: maternal serum levels of coenzyme Q10, alpha-tocopherol and gamma-tocopherol in preeclampsia and normal pregnancy. Gynecol Obstet Invest 2004; 58:8–13. Epub 2004 Feb 25.
41. Hale LP, Greer PK, Sempowski GD. Bromelain treatment alters leukocyte expression of cell surface molecules involved in cellular adhesion and activation. Clin Immunol 2002; 104:183–190.
42. Snowden HM, Renfrew MJ, Woolridge M. Treatments for breast engorgement during lactation (Cochrane Review). Cochrane Library, Issue 3, 2004. Oxford: Update Software.
43. Tilwe GH, Beria S, Turakhia NH, Daftary GV, Schiess W. Efficacy and tolerability of oral enzyme therapy as compared to diclofenac in active osteoarthrosis of knee joint: an open randomized controlled clinical trial. J Assoc Phys India 2001; 49:617–621.
44. Singer F, Singer C, Oberleitner H. Phlogenzym versus diclofenac in the treatment of activated osteoarthritis of the knee. A double-blind prospective randomized study. Int J Immunother 2001; 17:135–141.
45. Baerwald CH, Willeke A, Lies S, Goebel K-M, Engel HJ. Efficacy and tolerance of oral hydrolytic enzymes in ankylosing spondylitis as compared with indomethacin: a controlled double-blind prospective clinical trial. J Clin Res 1999; 2:17–34.
46. Farnsworth NR, Bingel AS, Cordell G, Crane FA, Fong HH. Potential value of plants as sources of new antifertility agents I. J Pharm Sci 1975; 64:535–598.
47. Farnsworth NR, Bingel AS, Cordell GA, Crane FA, Fong HH. Potential value of plants as sources of new antifertility agents II. J. Pharm Sci 1975; 64:717–753.
48. Youssef AF. The uterine isthmus and its sphincter mechanism: a clinical and radiographic study. Am J Obstet Gynecol 1960; 79:1161–1168.

49. Hunter RG, Henry GW, Heinicke RM. The action of Papain and Bromelain on the uterus. Am J Obstet Gynecol 1957; 73:867–881.
50. Hunter RG, Henry GW, Civin WH, Heincke RM. The action of papain and bromelain on the uterus. Am J Obstet Gynecol 1960; 79:428–431.
51. Grimsgaard S, Bonaa KH, Hansen J, Nordoy A. Highly purified eicosapentaenoic acid and docosahexaenoic acid in humans have similar triacylglycerol-lowering effects but divergent effects on serum fatty acids. Am J Clin Nutr 1997; 66:649–659.
52. Harris WS. n-3 fatty acids and serum lipoproteins: human studies. Am J Clin Nutr 1997; 65(Suppl 5):1645S–1654S.
53. Bucher HC, Hengstler P, Schindler C, Meier G. N-3 polyunsaturated fatty acids in coronary heart disease: a meta-analysis of randomized controlled trials. Am J Med 2002; 112:298–304.
54. Morris MC, Sacks F, Rosner B. Does fish oil lower blood pressure? A meta-analysis of controlled trials. Circulation 1993; 88:523–533.
55. Matorras R, Perteagudo L, Sanjurjo P, Ruiz JI. Intake of long chain w3 polyunsaturated fatty acids during pregnancy and the influence of levels in the mother on newborn levels. Eur J Obstet Gynecol Reprod Biol 1999; 83:179–184.
56. van Houwelingen AC, Sorensen JD, Hornstra G, Simonis MM et al. Essential fatty acid status in neonates after fish-oil supplementation during late pregnancy. Br J Nutr 1995; 74:723–731.
57. Connor WE, Lowensohn R, Hatcher L. Increased docosahexaenoic acid levels in human newborn infants by administration of sardines and fish oil during pregnancy. Lipids 1996; 31(Suppl):S183–187.
58. Helland IB, Saugstad OD, Smith L et al. Similar effects on infants of n-3 and n-6 fatty acids supplementation to pregnant and lactating women. Pediatrics 2001; 108:E82.
59. Barden AE, Mori TA, Dunstan J et al. Fish oil supplementation in pregnancy lowers F2–isoprostanes in neonates at high risk of atopy. Free Radic Res 2004; 38:233–239.
60. Helland IB, Smith L, Saarem K, Saugstad OD, Drevon CA. Maternal supplementation with very-long-chain n-3 fatty acids during pregnancy and lactation augments children's IQ at 4 years of age. Pediatrics 2003; 111:e39–e44.
61. Kroes R, Schaefer EJ, Squire R, Williams GM. A review of the safety of DHA45–oil. Food Chem Toxicol 2003; 41:1433–1446.
62. Lima TM, Kanunfre CC, Pompeia C, Verlengia R, Curi R. Ranking the toxicity of fatty acids on Jurkat and Raji cells by flow cytometric analysis. Toxicol In Vitro 2002; 16:741–747.
63. Kuroda Y, Shima N, Yazawa K, Kaji K. Desmutagenic and bio-antimutagenic activity of docosahexaenoic acid and eicosapentaenoic acid in cultured Chinese hamster V79 cells. Mutat Res 2001; 497:123–130.
64. www.naturalstandard.com. Omega-3 fatty acids, fish oil, alpha-linolenic acid–Natural Standard monograph.
65. Sakamoto M, Kubota M, Liu X et al. Maternal and fetal mercury and n-3 polyunsaturated fatty acids as a risk and benefit of fish consumption to fetus. Environ Sci Technol 2004; 38:3860–3863.
66. Harris WS, Connor WE, Lindsey S. Will dietary omega-3 fatty acids change the composition of human milk? Am J Clin Nutr 1984; 40:780–785.
67. Birch EE, Garfield S, Hoffman D, Uauy R, Birch DG. A randomized controlled trial of early dietary supply of long-chain polyunsaturated fatty acids and mental development in term infants. Dev Med Child Neurol 2000; 42:174–181.

68. Birch EE, Hoffman DR, Uauy R, Birch DG, Prestidge C. Visual acuity and the essentiality of docosahexaenoic acid and arachidonic acid in the diet of term infants. Pediatr Res 1998; 44:201–209.
69. Dunstan JA, Roper J, Mitoulas L, Hartmann PE, Simmer K, Prescott SL. The effect of supplementation with fish oil during pregnancy on breast milk immunoglobulin A, soluble CD14, cytokine levels and fatty acid composition. Clin Exp Allergy 2004; 34:1237–1242.
70. Bjerve KS, Brubakk AM, Fougner K, Johnsen H, Midthjell K, Vik T. Omega-3 fatty acids: essential fatty acids with important biological effects, and serum phospholipid fatty acids as markers of dietary omega 3–fatty acid intake. Am J Clin Nutr 1993; 57(Suppl 5):801S–805S; discussion 805S–806S.
71. Wong WW, Smith EO, Stuff J et al. Cholesterol-lowering effect of soy protein in normocholesterolemic and hypercholesterolemic men. Am J Clin Nutr 1998; 68(Suppl 6):1385S–1389S.
72. Washburn S, Burke GL, Morgan T, Anthony M. Effect of soy protein supplementation on serum lipoproteins, blood pressure, and menopausal symptoms in perimenopausal women. Menopause 1999; 6:7–13.
73. Crouse JR 3rd, Morgan T, Terry J et al. A randomized trial comparing the effect of casein with that of soy protein containing varying amounts of isoflavones on plasma concentrations of lipids and lipoproteins. Arch Intern Med 1999; 159:2070–2076.
74. Albertazzi P, Pansini F, Bonaccorsi G et al. The effect of dietary soy supplementation on hot flushes. Obstet Gynecol 1998; 91:6–11.
75. Murkies A, Dalais FS, Briganti E et al. Phytoestrogens and breast cancer in postmenopausal women: a case control study. Menopause 2000; 7:289–296.
76. Lee HP, Gourley L, Duffy S et al. Dietary effects on breast-cancer risk in Singapore. Lancet 1991; 337:1197–1200.
77. Duncan AM, Underhill KE, Xu X et al. Modest hormonal effects of soy isoflavones in postmenopausal women. J Clin Endocrinol Metab 1999; 84:3479–3484.
78. Hargreaves DF, Potten CS, Harding C, et al. Two-week dietary soy supplementation has an estrogenic effect on normal premenopausal breast. J Clin Endocrinol Metab 1999; 84:4017–4024.
79. Pino AM, Valladares LE, Palma M et al. Dietary isoflavones affect sex hormone-binding globulin levels in postmenopausal women. J Clin Endocrinol Metab 2000; 85:2797–2800.
80. Zeiger RS, Heller S, Mellon M et al. Effect of combined maternal and infant food-allergen avoidance on development of atopy in early infancy: a randomized study. J Allergy Clin Immunol 1989; 84:72–89.
81. North K, Golding J. A maternal vegetarian diet in pregnancy is associated with hypospadias. The ALSPAC Study Team. Avon Longitudinal Study of Pregnancy and Childhood. BJU Int 2000; 85:107–113.
82. Fielden MR, Fong CJ, Haslam S, Zacharewski TR. Normal mammary gland morphology in pubertal female mice following in utero and lactational exposure to genistein at levels comparable to human dietary exposure. Toxicol Lett 2002; 133:181–191.
83. Wisniewski AB, Klein SL, Lakshmann Y, Gearhart JP. Exposure to genistein during gestation and lactation demasculinizes the reproductive system in rats. J Urol 2003; 169:1582–1586.
84. Fielden MR, Samy SM, Chou K, Zacharewski TR. Effect of human dietary exposure levels of genistein during gestation and lactation on long-term reproductive development and sperm quality in mice. Food Chem Toxicol 2003; 41:447–454.

85. Kang KS, Che J, Lee YS. Lack of adverse effects in the F1 offspring maternally exposed to genistein at human intake dose level. Food Chem Toxicol 2002; 40:43–51.
86. Masutomi N, Shibutani M, Takagi H et al. Impact of dietary exposure to methoxychlor, genistein, or diisononyl phthalate during the perinatal period on the development of the rat endocrine/reproductive systems in later life. Toxicology 2003; 192:149–170.
87. Foster WG, Chan S, Platt L, Hughes CL, Jr. Detection of phytoestrogens in samples of second trimester human amniotic fluid. Toxicol Lett 2002; 129:199–205.
88. Hughes CL, Liu G, Beall S, Foster WG, Davis V. Effects of genistein or soy milk during late gestation and lactation on adult uterine organization in the rat. Exp Biol Med (Maywood) 2004; 229:108–117.
89. Hilakivi-Clarke L, Cho E, Onojafe I, Raygada M, Clarke R. Maternal exposure to genistein during pregnancy increases carcinogen-induced mammary tumorigenesis in female rat offspring. Oncol Rep 1999; 6:1089–1095.
90. Pei RJ, Sato M, Yuri T et al. Effect of prenatal and prepubertal genistein exposure on N-methyl-N-nitrosourea-induced mammary tumorigenesis in female Sprague-Dawley rats. In Vivo 2003; 17:349–357.
91. FDA. EAFUS: A food additive database. Center for Food Safety and Applied Nutrition, Office of Premarket Approva vm.cfsan.fda.gov/~dms/eafus.html 2004.
92. Foster WG, Younglai EV, Boutross-Tadross O, Hughes CL, Wade MG. Mammary gland morphology in Sprague-Dawley rats following treatment with an organochlorine mixture in utero and neonatal genistein. Toxicol Sci 2004; 77:91–100. Epub 2003 Sep 26.
93. Fujisawa T, Benno Y, Yaeshima T, Mitsuoka T. Taxonomic study of the *Lactobacillus acidophilus* group, with recognition of *Lactobacillus gallinarum* sp. nov. and *Lactobacillus johnsonii* sp. nov. and synonymy of *Lactobacillus acidophilus* group A3. Int J Syst Bacteriol 1992; 42:487–491.
94. Szajewska H, Kotowska M, Mrukowicz JZ, Armanska M, Mikolajczyk W. Efficacy of Lactobacillus GG in prevention of nosocomial diarrhea in infants. J Pediatr 2001; 138:361–365.
95. de Roos NM, Katan MB. Effects of probiotic bacteria on diarrhea, lipid metabolism, and carcinogenesis: a review of papers published between 1988 and 1998. Am J Clin Nutr 2000; 71:405–411.
96. Rautava S, Kalliomaki M, Isolauri E. Probiotics during pregnancy and breast-feeding might confer immunomodulatory protection against atopic disease in the infant. J Allergy Clin Immunol 2002; 109:119–121.
97. Kalliomaki M, Salminen S, Arvilommi H, Kero P, Koskinen P, Isolauri E. Probiotics in primary prevention of atopic disease: a randomised placebo-controlled trial. Lancet 2001; 357:1076–1079.
98. Neri A, Sabah G, Samra Z. Bacterial vaginosis in pregnancy treated with yoghurt. Acta Obstet Gynecol Scand 1993; 72:17–19.
99. Usui R, Ohkuchi A, Matsubara S et al. Vaginal lactobacilli and preterm birth. J Perinat Med 2002; 30:458–466.
100. Schultz M, Gottl C, Young R, Iwen P, Vanderhoof JA. Administration of oral probiotic bacteria to pregnant women causes temporary infantile colonization. J Pediatr Gastroenterol Nutr 2004; 38:293–297.
101. Matsumiya Y, Kato N, Watanabe K, Kato H. Molecular epidemiological study of vertical transmission of vaginal Lactobacillus species from mothers to newborn infants in Japanese, by arbitrarily primed polymerase chain reaction. J Infect Chemother 2002; 8:43–49.

INDEX